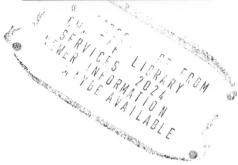

Sobotta
Atlas of Human Anatomy
Vol. 2

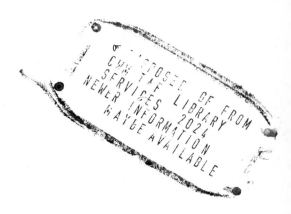

Sobotta
Atlas of
Human Anatomy

Edited by

HELMUT FERNER and JOCHEN STAUBESAND

Vol. 2: Thorax, Abdomen, Pelvis, Lower Extremities, Skin

10th English Edition with Nomenclature in English
Translated and Edited by WALTHER J. HILD
545 Illustrations, most in color

1983

Urban & Schwarzenberg · Baltimore–Munich

This book was founded by Johannes Sobotta, former Professor of Anatomy and Director of the Anatomical Institute of the University of Bonn,
followed by Hellmut Becher, former Professor of Anatomy and Director of the Anatomical Institute of the University of Münster.

Address of the English translator and editor:

Walther J. Hild, M.D., Professor and Chairman, Department of Anatomy, The University of Texas Medical Branch, Galveston, Texas 77550

Addresses of the German Editors:

Professor emerit. Dr. med. Helmut Ferner, I. Anatomische Lehrkanzel der Universität Wien
Währingerstraße 13, A-1090 Wien

Professor Dr. med. Jochen Staubesand, Direktor des Anatomischen Instituts (Lehrstuhl I) der Albert-Ludwigs-Universität, Freiburg
Albertstraße 17, 7800 Freiburg i. Br.

This atlas consists of two separate volumes:

Vol. 1: Head, Neck, Upper Extremities

Vol. 2: Thorax, Abdomen, Pelvis, Lower Extremities, Skin

Library of Congress Cataloging in Publication Data

Sobotta, Johannes, 1869–1945.
 Sobotta's Atlas of human anatomy.

 Translation of: Atlas der Anatomie des Menschen.
18th ed. 1982.
 Includes indexes.
 Contents: v. 1. Head, neck, upper extremities -- v. 2. Thorax, abdomen, pelvis, lower extremities, skin.
 1. Anatomy, Human--Atlases   I. Hild, Walther J.
II. Title. III. Title: Atlas of human anatomy.
[DNLM: 1. Anatomy--Regional--Atlases.   QS 17 S677a]
QM25.S676   1983   611'.0022'2   82-13604
  ISBN 0-8067-1710-6 (U.S. : v. 1)
  ISBN 0-8067-1720-3 (U.S. : v. 2)

German Editions:

1. Edition: J. F. Lehmanns Verlag, München 1904
2.–11. Edition: J. F. Lehmanns Verlag, München 1913–1944
    since 12. Edition: Urban & Schwarzenberg, 1948
13. Edition: 1953
14. Edition: 1956
15. Edition: 1957
16. Edition: 1967 (ISBN 3-541-02816-5)
17. Edition: 1972 (ISBN 3-541-02817-3)
18. Edition: 1982 (ISBN 3-541-02828-9)

Foreign Editions:

English Edition (with nomenclature in English)
Urban & Schwarzenberg

English Edition (with nomenclature in Latin)
Urban & Schwarzenberg

French Edition
Urban & Schwarzenberg

Turkish Edition
Urban & Schwarzenberg

Arabic Edition
Al Ahram, Cairo/Egypt

Italian Edition
USES, Florence, Italy

Greek Edition
Gregory Parisianos, Athens, Greece

Japanese Edition
Igaku-Shoin Ltd., Tokyo, Japan

Portuguese Edition
Editora Guanabara Koogan, Rio de Janeiro, Brazil

Spanish Edition
Ediciones Toray, Barcelona, Spain

Printed in Germany by Kastner & Callwey, München
© Urban & Schwarzenberg 1983

ISBN 0-8067-1720-3 Baltimore
ISBN 3-541-71720-3 Munich

Preface

The Sobotta Atlas of Human Anatomy has been a success by any standard.

For generations it has been indispensable to anatomists and artists, as well as an important reference for the practicing physician. Thoughts of changing such an integral part of the medical literature have not come easily. However, the teaching and learning of anatomy have changed dramatically, and the time has come for the Sobotta Atlas to do the same. This new edition reflects those changes, undertaken with the greatest care, and we are pleased to have had a part in the "remaking" of Sobotta.

The most important modification is that of organization. The Sobotta Atlas is now arranged in a regional format and follows the usual sequence of anatomic study. All information related to a specific area of the body – from the skin surface to the underlying organs to the skeleton – can now be found together in one volume. And, because this regional/topographical completeness is applied consistently throughout, it has been possible to reduce the three volumes of former editions to the two now available.

Another important change in this edition of Sobotta involves the illustrations. To make the leap into the modern era complete, many older illustrations have been repainted in more vivid color, a large number of the formerly black and white illustrations now appear in full color, and new radiographs have been added throughout both volumes. All of this has proved to be expensive, and we are especially grateful to the publishers for their enthusiastic support.

A new appendix (by Dr. F. Platz, Freiburg i. Br.) on the areas of arterial blood supply has been added.

The recommendations found in the 4th edition of Nomina Anatomica were followed whenever it was thought they were justified.

The editors would like to thank their many colleagues who supported them with help and advice. These include Prof. Dr. J. Altaras (Gießen), Prof. Dr. G. Kaufmann (Freiburg i. Br.) and Dr. S. Rau, lecturer (Freiburg i. Br.), who supplied us with radiographs and xeroradiographs; Prof. Dr. H. Roskamm (Bad Krozingen) who provided angiocardiographs of the ventricles; Prof. Dr. A. Kappert (Bern) who let us use originals from his "Leitfaden und Atlas der Angiologie" *(Textbook and Atlas of Angiology),* and Prof. Dr. R. May (Innsbruck) who made original illustrations of perforating veins in the foot and lower leg available to us. Dr. T. Grimm (Würzburg) supplied us with new material on the pattern of the dermal ridge of the finger and palm, as well as a revised text. We would also like to thank Dr. L. Wicke for a number of X-ray photographs from his "Atlas of Radiologic Anatomy" (Second Edition, Urban & Schwarzenberg, Baltimore–Munich, 1982) and Dr. R. Unsöld (Freiburg i. Br.) for computer tomograms with explanatory texts.

Our thanks are also due to our closest co-workers for their constant and reliable assistance and support. Dr. H. Schmiebusch and Frau M. Engler in particular helped in the great amount of editing required for the figures and texts. Dr. S. Zuleger took special interest in the chapter on the heart. Dr. H. Schmiebusch revised and extended the glossary.

The editors can look back at a long period of intensive and productive cooperation with Mr. Michael Urban, the managing partner of the Urban & Schwarzenberg publishing house, and his colleagues. Without their whole-hearted cooperation, the understanding they showed for our requests, and their technical expertise, the work for this new edition of the Sobotta Atlas could never have been completed on schedule.

Vienna and Freiburg i. Br.,
May 1982

H. FERNER
J. STAUBESAND

American Editor's Preface to the 10th English Edition

The new two-volume edition of the Sobotta Atlas of Human Anatomy has been rearranged in a regional format. This will enhance its usefulness as a reference work, and it can be consulted in the dissecting laboratory more efficiently in conjunction with various dissecting manuals. The anglicized nomenclature as used in North America has been consistently applied. A new and simplified index will facilitate rapid orientation.

I would like to thank various faculty members of the Department of Anatomy at UTMB for valuable advice. I am indebted to Mr. Braxton D. Mitchell and Ms. Nan Curtis Tyler of Urban & Schwarzenberg in Baltimore for their cooperation in every phase of translating and editing. Special thanks are due to my secretary, Ms. Phyllis Fletcher, whose superior typing and proofreading skills were essential for the completion on schedule of this English Edition.

Galveston, Texas, February 1983   WALTHER J. HILD

Table of Contents

Abbreviations

ant.	= anterior		int.	= interior		sup.	= superior
a. or aa.	= artery or arteries		inteross.	= interosseous		superf.	= superficial
art.	= articulation		lat.	= lateral		surf.	= surface
br.	= branch		lig. or ligg.	= ligament or ligaments		sut.	= suture
caud.	= caudal		m. or mm.	= muscle or muscles		transv.	= transverse
cran.	= cranial		med.	= medial		tuberc.	= tubercle
dist.	= distal		n. or nn.	= nerve or nerves		tuberos.	= tuberosity
dors.	= dorsal		obl.	= oblique		v. or vv.	= vein or veins
ext.	= external		post.	= posterior		vent.	= ventral
exten.	= extensor		prot.	= protuberance		vert.	= vertebra
flex.	= flexor		prox.	= proximal			
inf.	= inferior		r. or rr.	= ramus or rami			

General Terms of Direction and Position

The following terms designate the position of organs and parts of the body in their relationship to each other, sometimes irrespective of the position of the body in space. These designations are used not only in human anatomy, but also in medical practice and in comparative anatomy.

General designations

Anterior – posterior = in front – behind (e.g., anterior and posterior tibial arteries)

ventral – dorsal = toward the belly – toward the back

superior – inferior = above – below

cranial – caudal = toward the head – toward the tail

dexter – sinister = right – left (e.g., right and left common iliac arteries)

internal – external = located inside – located outside

superficial – deep = located superficially – located deeply (e.g., superficial and deep flexores digitorum muscles)

medius or *intermedius* = middle (in the middle between two other structures) (e.g., the middle nasal concha is located between the superior and inferior nasal concha)

medianus = located in the midline, median (e.g., median fissure of the spinal cord)
A "median sagittal section" divides the body into two mirror image-like portions.

medial – lateral = located toward the middle of the body – located toward the side of the body (e.g., medial and lateral inguinal fossae)

frontal = located in a frontal plane, also located toward the forehead (e.g., frontal process of maxilla)

longitudinal = parallel to the long axis (e.g., superior longitudinal muscle)

sagittal = in a plane perpendicular to the frontal plane (e.g., sagittal suture of the cranium)

transversal = in a transversal plane, at right angles to the long axis of the body or organ (e.g., transversus abdominis muscle)

transverse = running transversely (e.g., transverse process of a thoracic vertebra)

Designations for Directions and Positions of the Extremities

proximal – distal = located toward the root of the extremity – located toward the free end of the extremity (e.g., proximal and distal radioulnar joints)

For the upper extremity:

radial – ulnar = on the radial side – on the ulnar side (e.g., ulnar and radial arteries)

For the hand:

palmar – dorsal = toward the palm of the hand – toward the back of the hand (e.g., palmar aponeurosis)

For the lower extremity:

tibial – fibular (peroneal) = on the tibial side – on the fibular side

For the foot:

plantar – dorsal = toward the sole of the foot – toward the upper surface of the foot (e.g., lateral and medial plantar arteries, dorsal artery of the foot)

Short Explanation Concerning Derivation, Significance and Pronunciation of Anatomical Names

General

The Basle Anatomical Names (B.N.A.), adopted by the Anatomische Gesellschaft in 1895 and revised in 1955 as Paris Anatomical Names (P.N.A.), which are internationally used (Int. Anatomical Nomenclature Comm.: Nomina Anatomica; 4th ed. Excerpta Medica Amsterdam, Oxford 1977), have, for the most part, been used since antiquity. Only a relatively few names have been added over time. The large majority of the official names used today are derived from Latin, and many are derived from Greek and later Latinized to a greater or lesser degree. Occasionally, names are derived from oriental languages (Arabic, Aramaic). However, they have been Latinized in their grammatical form to such a degree that their original derivation can hardly be recognized.

Since the Greek alphabet differs markedly from the Latin, Greek names are written in Latin letters.

Spelling and Pronunciation of Names of Greek Derivation

The Greek Kappa (K) is changed to c, the Chi (ch) to ch, the Phi (ph) to ph, the Psi (ps) to ps, the Xi (X) to x, the Theta (th) to th, the so-called Spiritus asper to h. Gamma (g) before Gamma, Kappa (K), Chi (ch), and Xi (x) is pronounced as n (e.g. aggeion = angeion, agkos = ankos). Since Greek words that begin with Rho (r) carry the Spiritus asper over the Rho, they are spelled in Latin with rh, e.g. rhomboideus etc. Of the vowels and diphthongs of the Greek language the Omega (long O) and the Omikron (short O) are both spelled as O, the (short) Epsilon as well as the (long) Eta are both E; Ypsilon, Alpha, and Jota are spelled as in Greek. The diphthong Epsilon-Jota in its Latinized form (as in modern Greek) is pronounced i, e.g., Aristeides (gr.) Latinized = Aristides. Occasionally it is also pronounced as e as in tracheia (gr.) Latinized = trachea. The diphthong Omicron-Jota is spelled and pronounced as oe (oikos gr. = oecus lat., e.g. oeconomia), Alpha-Jota is changed to ae, Alpha-Ypsilon to au, Omikron-Ypsilon to u, Epsilon-Ypsilon to eu. The endings of nouns and adjectives are Latinized; e.g. sternon to sternum, isthmos to isthmus, and the adjective of thorax (thorakikos) to thoracicus. As a rule, the Latin declension is used (less frequently the Greek declension: e.g. hypophysis, gen. hypophyseos). Frequently, as was common in Roman times, Greek nouns are provided with Latin adjectival endings (e.g., centralis, derived from Latinized centrum, gr. kentron). Pronunciation and accentuation of Latinized names derived from Greek follow the Latin rule. The old rule of accentuation, vocalis ante vocalem brevis est (a vowel before a vowel is short), is generally valid and is neglected only if the vowel is derived from a Greek diphthong and therefore long. (Macron over the vowel = length; breve over the vowel = shortness; accent = accentuation; the Greek vowel Epsilon is given as e, Eta as ē).

A note regarding the color figures

The multicolor figures presented here are based on didactic considerations. Contrasts have been intensified to enhance the recognition of areas that are naturally difficult to discern. Hence, the colors used for various tissues (e.g., tendons, cartilage, bones, musculature) and pathways (arteries, veins, lymphatic vessels, nerves) are different from those found in living or dead bodies or in a preserved cadaver.

Any deviations in the tint or intensity of the colors found in this edition (e.g., in illustrations of muscles, blood vessels and nerves) exist primarily because the various illustrations were made over a long period of time. In addition to the artists who prepared the illustrations with Prof. Sobotta, later with Prof. Becher for the original collection (K. HAJEK, Prof. E. LEPIER, H. v. EICKSTEDT, W. WOHLSCHLEGEL), the following artists worked on the 18th edition: Elisabeth ALTHAUS: Figs. 51, 52, 53, 69, 70, 71, 72, 73, 74, 75, 76, 77, 78; Ulrike BRUGGER: Figs. 13, 62, 63, 100, 139, 156, 157, 158, 159, 166, 167, 179, 188, 232, 270, 271, 326, 327, 392, 459, 494, 495, 496, 497; Marie Anne ERHARD: Figs. 15, 16, 236, 238, 240; Luitgard KELLNER: Figs. 14, 177, 178, 224, 438; Li KÖRNER: Fig. 390 a; Christiane SCHAEFFER: Figs. 1, 230, 318, 391, 397; Lothar SCHNELLBÄCHER: Figs. 89, 90, 91, 136, 143, 154, 163, 208, 209, 212, 213, 221, 222, 223, 225, 226, 228, 229, 284, 294, 295, 298, 299, 307, 328, 332, 334; Fritz URICH: Figs. 68, 93, 383, 384, 385, 386 a, 386 b, 393, 395; Ingo WEGERL: Figs. 17, 19, 20, 45, 111, 112, 147, 148, 155, 180, 182, 185, 189, 257, 258, 267, 268, 273, 274, 275, 276, 277, 278, 280, 281, 282, 283, 288, 300, 301, 302, 303, 306, 308, 309, 320, 321, 394, 396, 401, 402, 403, 405, 407, 408, 409, 413, 418, 419, 435, 436, 437, 450, 451, 458, 460, 461, 462, 466, 467, 470, 471, 475, 476, 487, 488, 489, 490, 491, 498, 499, 504, 505; G. ZEH-KOSANKE: Figs. 130, 131, 132, 133, 134, 164, 165, 399, 400, 414, 415, 416, 417, 452, 453.

Trunk

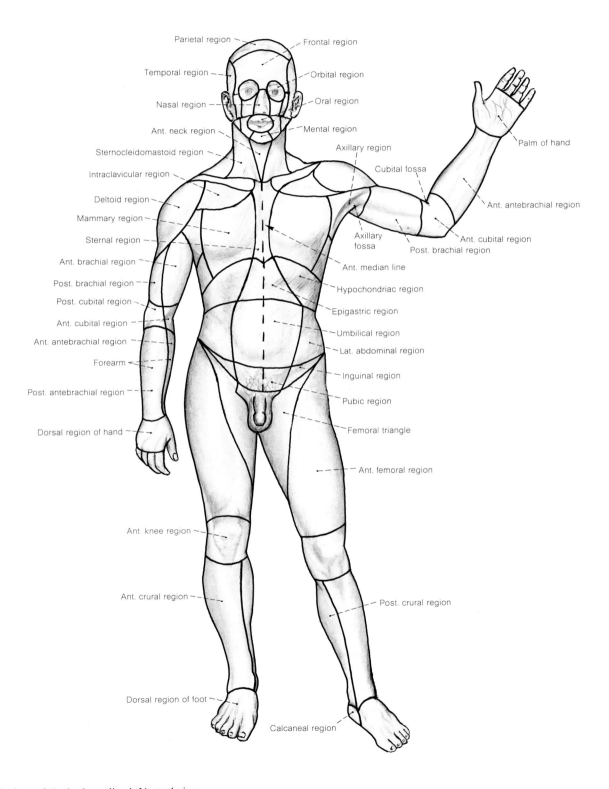

Parietal region

Frontal region

Temporal region

Orbital region

Nasal region

Oral region

Ant. neck region

Mental region

Sternocleidomastoid region

Axillary region

Intraclavicular region

Cubital fossa

Deltoid region

Mammary region

Sternal region

Ant. brachial region

Post. brachial region

Post. cubital region

Ant. cubital region

Ant. antebrachial region

Forearm

Post. antebrachial region

Dorsal region of hand

Ant. knee region

Ant. crural region

Dorsal region of foot

Calcaneal region

Palm of hand

Ant. antebrachial region

Axillary fossa

Ant. cubital region

Post. brachial region

Ant. median line

Hypochondriac region

Epigastric region

Umbilical region

Lat. abdominal region

Inguinal region

Pubic region

Femoral triangle

Ant. femoral region

Post. crural region

Fig. 1. Regions of the body outlined. Ventral view.

Chest Wall

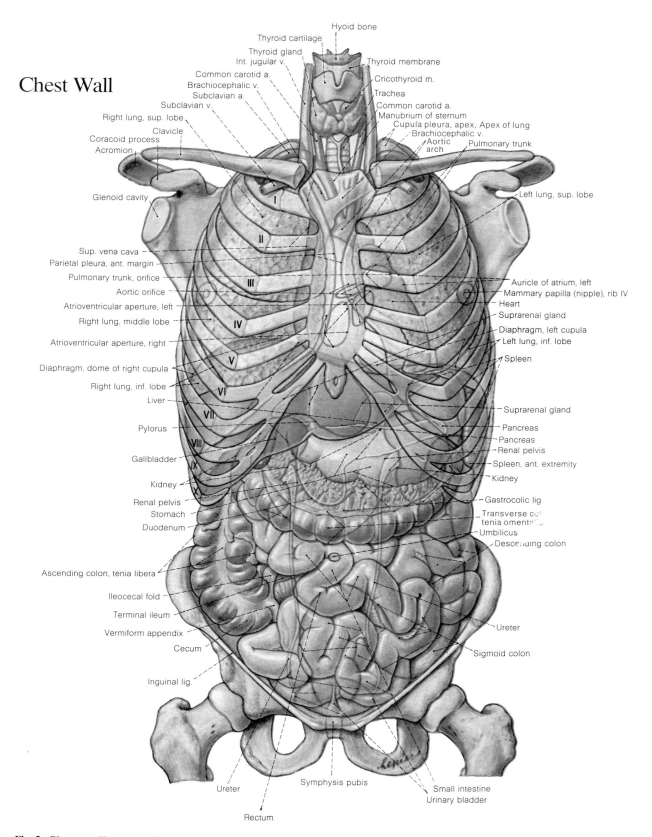

Fig. 2. Phantom silhouettes of the skeleton with the neck, chest, and abdominal viscera of an adult man. Ventral view. The greater omentum is removed from the transverse colon.

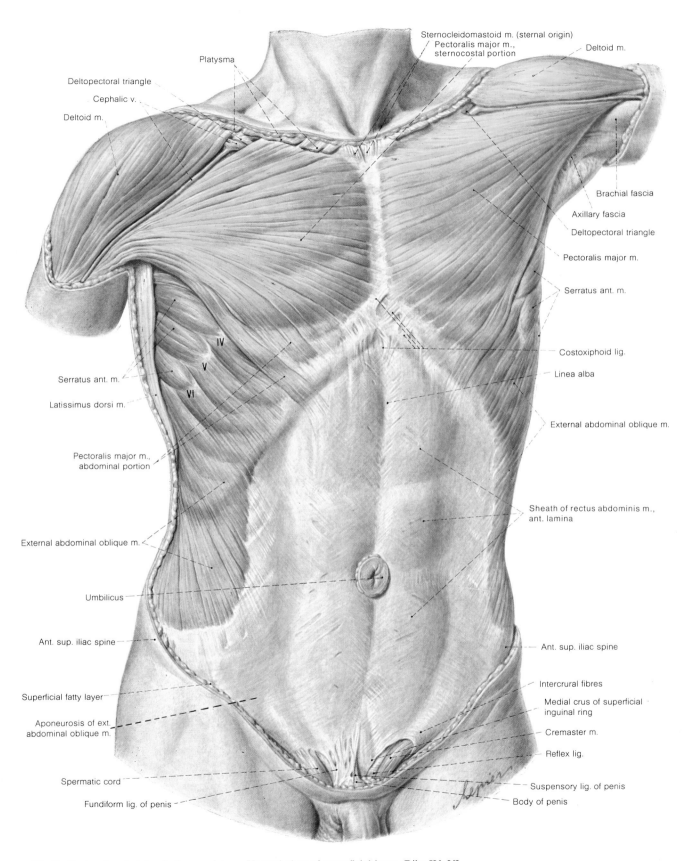

Sternocleidomastoid m. (sternal origin)
Pectoralis major m., sternocostal portion
Deltoid m.
Platysma
Deltopectoral triangle
Cephalic v.
Deltoid m.
Brachial fascia
Axillary fascia
Deltopectoral triangle
Pectoralis major m.
Serratus ant. m.
IV
V
VI
Costoxiphoid lig.
Linea alba
Serratus ant. m.
Latissimus dorsi m.
External abdominal oblique m.
Pectoralis major m., abdominal portion
Sheath of rectus abdominis m., ant. lamina
External abdominal oblique m.
Umbilicus
Ant. sup. iliac spine
Ant. sup. iliac spine
Intercrural fibres
Superficial fatty layer
Medial crus of superficial inguinal ring
Aponeurosis of ext. abdominal oblique m.
Cremaster m.
Reflex lig.
Spermatic cord
Suspensory lig. of penis
Fundiform lig. of penis
Body of penis

Fig. 3. Pectoral and abdominal musculature. Ventral view of superficial layer. Ribs IV–VI.

Thoracic Muscles (Figs. 3, 4, 5, 7)

Name	Origin	Insertion
1. Pectoralis major muscle Strong, predominantly fleshy; tendinous only at insertion	*Clavicular portion:* Sternal half of clavicle *Sternocostal portion:* Ventral surface of sternum and costal cartilages 2 to 6 *Abdominal portion:* A slip from the aponeurosis of the External abdominal oblique muscle	All fibers converge toward a flat tendon (5 cm broad) which is inserted into the crest of the greater tubercle of the humerus

Nerve: Lateral and medial pectoral nerves from the brachial plexus (C 5–T 1)

Function: Flexes, adducts, and rotates the arm medially. Powerful adduction (lowering the raised arm). In many cases, works with other muscles (Latissimus dorsi and Trapezius muscles)

Name	Origin	Insertion
2. Pectoralis minor muscle (Weak and moderately flat)	Ribs 2 to 5 near the junction	Coracoid process of scapula (medial border)

Nerve: Medial pectoral nerve (C 8–T 1)

Function: Depresses the shoulder, raises ribs in forced inspiration; seldom functions alone, but with the Serratus anterior and Trapezius muscles, etc.

Name	Origin	Insertion
3. Subclavius muscle	Short, thick tendon on 1st rib at junction of cartilage and bone	Acromial end of clavicle

Nerve: Subclavius nerve from the brachial plexus

Function: Adequate for such a small muscle; assists in drawing the shoulder forward and downward

Name	Origin	Insertion
4. Serratus anterior muscle	With fleshy digitations from first 9 ribs, consisting of 3 parts. The middle is the weakest; the caudal, the strongest	
(Superior part)	Ribs 1 and 2, somewhat converging	Superior angle of the scapula
(Middle part)	Ribs 2–4, diverging	Medial margin of scapula
(Inferior part)	Ribs 5–9, strongly converging	Inferior angle of scapula

Nerve: Long thoracic nerve from the brachial plexus (C 5, 6, 7)

Function: Holds scapula closely to the body, draws scapula forward as in a pushing action. Assists in flexion and abduction of the arm

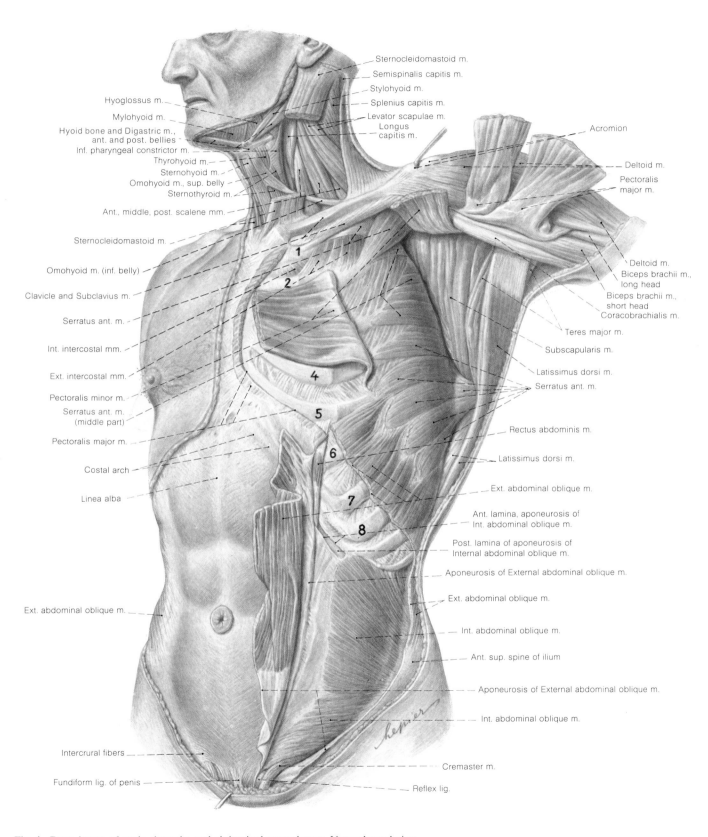

Sternocleidomastoid m.
Semispinalis capitis m.
Stylohyoid m.
Splenius capitis m.
Levator scapulae m.
Longus capitis m.

Hyoglossus m.
Mylohyoid m.
Hyoid bone and Digastric m., ant. and post. bellies
Inf. pharyngeal constrictor m.
Thyrohyoid m.
Sternohyoid m.
Omohyoid m., sup. belly
Sternothyroid m.
Ant., middle, post. scalene mm.
Sternocleidomastoid m.
Omohyoid m. (inf. belly)
Clavicle and Subclavius m.
Serratus ant. m.
Int. intercostal mm.
Ext. intercostal mm.
Pectoralis minor m.
Serratus ant. m. (middle part)
Pectoralis major m.
Costal arch
Linea alba
Ext. abdominal oblique m.
Intercrural fibers
Fundiform lig. of penis

Acromion
Deltoid m.
Pectoralis major m.
Deltoid m.
Biceps brachii m., long head
Biceps brachii m., short head
Coracobrachialis m.
Teres major m.
Subscapularis m.
Latissimus dorsi m.
Serratus ant. m.
Rectus abdominis m.
Latissimus dorsi m.
Ext. abdominal oblique m.
Ant. lamina, aponeurosis of Int. abdominal oblique m.
Post. lamina of aponeurosis of Internal abdominal oblique m.
Aponeurosis of External abdominal oblique m.
Ext. abdominal oblique m.
Int. abdominal oblique m.
Ant. sup. spine of ilium
Aponeurosis of External abdominal oblique m.
Int. abdominal oblique m.
Cremaster m.
Reflex lig.

Fig. 4. Deep layers of neck, thoracic, and abdominal musculature. Ventrolateral view.

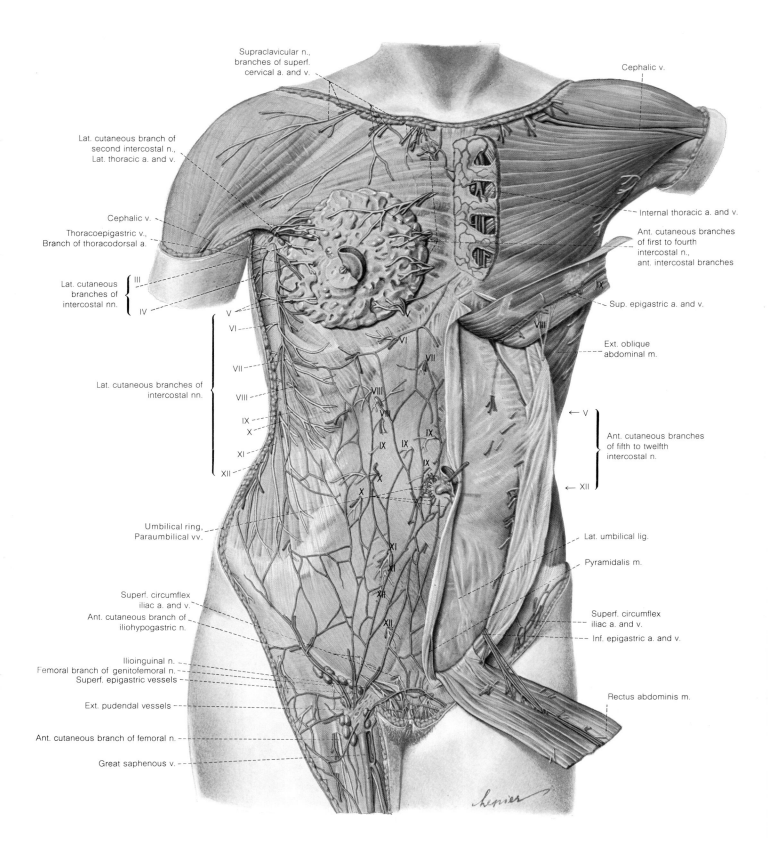

Supraclavicular n.,
branches of superf.
cervical a. and v.

Cephalic v.

Lat. cutaneous branch of
second intercostal n.,
Lat. thoracic a. and v.

Internal thoracic a. and v.

Cephalic v.

Ant. cutaneous branches
of first to fourth
intercostal n.,
ant. intercostal branches

Thoracoepigastric v.,
Branch of thoracodorsal a.

Lat. cutaneous
branches of
intercostal nn.

III

IV

Sup. epigastric a. and v.

V

VI

Ext. oblique
abdominal m.

Lat. cutaneous branches of
intercostal nn.

VII

VIII

IX
X

XI

XII

Ant. cutaneous branches
of fifth to twelfth
intercostal n.

Umbilical ring,
Paraumbilical vv.

Lat. umbilical lig.

Pyramidalis m.

Superf. circumflex
iliac a. and v.

Ant. cutaneous branch of
iliohypogastric n.

Superf. circumflex
iliac a. and v.

Inf. epigastric a. and v.

Ilioinguinal n.
Femoral branch of genitofemoral n.
Superf. epigastric vessels

Ext. pudendal vessels

Rectus abdominis m.

Ant. cutaneous branch of femoral n.

Great saphenous v.

Fig. 5. Nerves and vessels of the anterior thoracic and abdominal wall. Superficial layer on the left side of the picture.

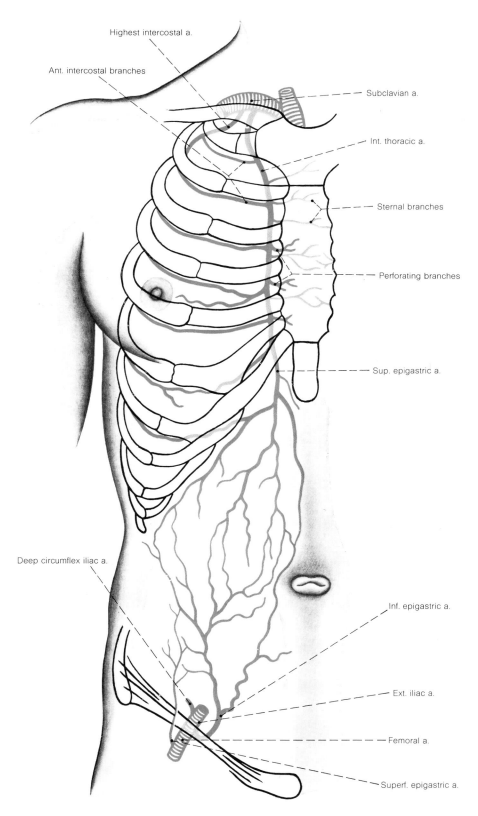

Highest intercostal a.

Ant. intercostal branches

Subclavian a.

Int. thoracic a.

Sternal branches

Perforating branches

Sup. epigastric a.

Deep circumflex iliac a.

Inf. epigastric a.

Ext. iliac a.

Femoral a.

Superf. epigastric a.

Fig. 6. Diagram showing the arterial anastomoses in the abdominal wall between subclavian artery ⤑ internal thoracic artery ⤑ superior epigastric artery coming from above, and external iliac artery ⤑ inferior epigastric artery coming from below. (After F. R. MERKEL: Handbuch der topographischen Anatomie. Vieweg, Braunschweig 1899.)

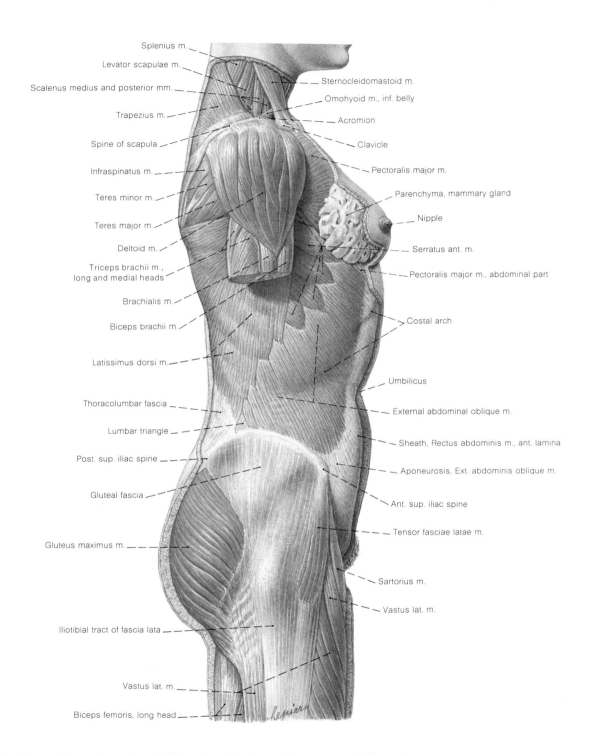

Splenius m.

Levator scapulae m.

Scalenus medius and posterior mm.

Trapezius m.

Spine of scapula

Infraspinatus m.

Teres minor m.

Teres major m.

Deltoid m.

Triceps brachii m., long and medial heads

Brachialis m.

Biceps brachii m.

Latissimus dorsi m.

Thoracolumbar fascia

Lumbar triangle

Post. sup. iliac spine

Gluteal fascia

Gluteus maximus m.

Iliotibial tract of fascia lata

Vastus lat. m.

Biceps femoris, long head

Sternocleidomastoid m.

Omohyoid m., inf. belly

Acromion

Clavicle

Pectoralis major m.

Parenchyma, mammary gland

Nipple

Serratus ant. m.

Pectoralis major m., abdominal part

Costal arch

Umbilicus

External abdominal oblique m.

Sheath, Rectus abdominis m., ant. lamina

Aponeurosis, Ext. abdominis oblique m.

Ant. sup. iliac spine

Tensor fasciae latae m.

Sartorius m.

Vastus lat. m.

Fig. 7. Musculature of the neck, trunk, and thigh of an adult female. Mammary gland dissected.

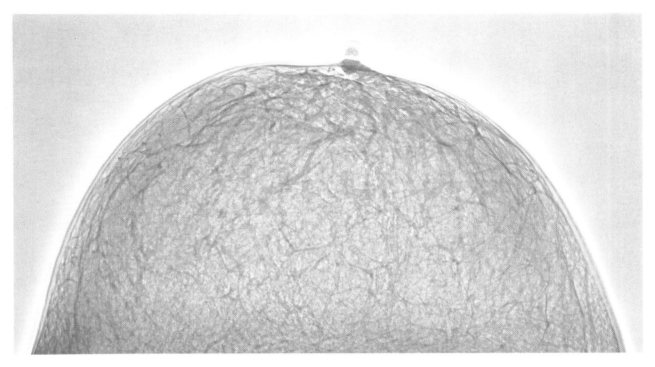

Fig. 8. Craniocaudal xeroradiograph of the female mammary gland: density differences between fat (light), supporting tissue and vessels (dark) are recognizable as structural images. (Courtesy Prof. Dr. G. KAUFFMANN, Zentrum Radiologie des Klinikums der Universität Freiburg i. Brsg.)

Developmental stages of the mammary gland (from O. HÖVELS [Ed.]: Wartmann, Wiesbaden 1977)

B 1	Prepubertal: no palpable glandular substance, only the nipple is prominent.	
B 2	Budding stage: slight enlargement of the gland in the area of the areola. Enlargement of the areolar diameter as compared to B 1.	
B 3	Further enlargement of gland and areola. Gland now larger than areola. The latter, however, without its own contours.	
B 4	Bud breast: Areola and nipple are elevated above the gland.	
B 5	Fully developed breast: Areola does not protrude above the general contour of the breast.	

Stage B 4 can be absent (in 25% of all girls). Development may be arrested at Stage B 4 or may continue to Stage B much later.

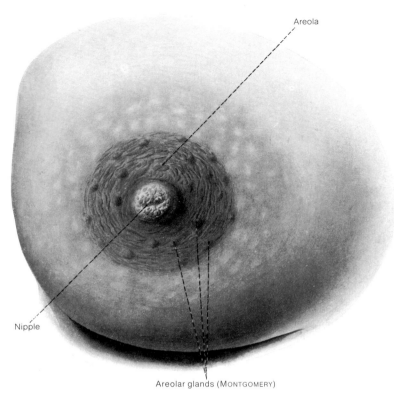

Areola

Nipple

Areolar glands (MONTGOMERY)

Fig. 9. Right breast of a pregnant woman.

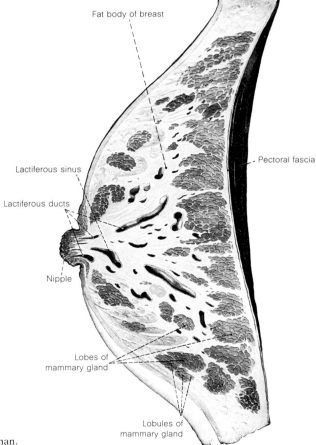

Fat body of breast

Pectoral fascia

Lactiferous sinus

Lactiferous ducts

Nipple

Lobes of
mammary gland

Lobules of
mammary gland

Fig. 10. Sagittal section through the right breast of a pregnant woman.

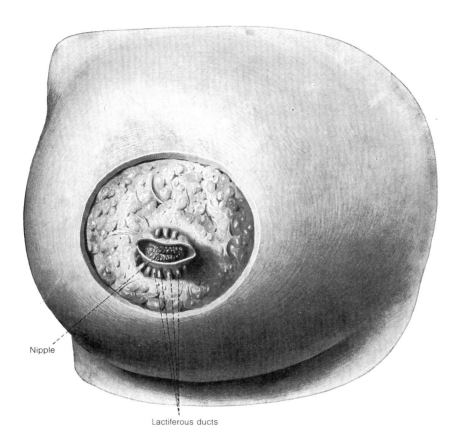

Nipple

Lactiferous ducts

Fig. 11. Right breast of a pregnant woman. A ring-shaped piece of skin surrounding the nipple has been removed. The margin of the skin near the nipple has been reflected in order to display the lactiferous ducts.

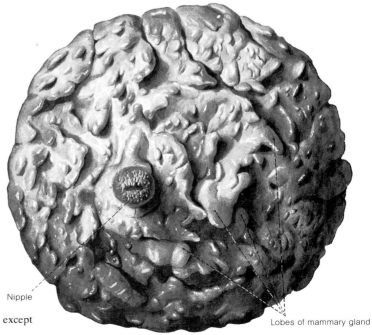

Nipple

Lobes of mammary gland

Fig. 12. Right mammary gland of a pregnant woman. Skin, except for nipple, and most of the fat have been removed.

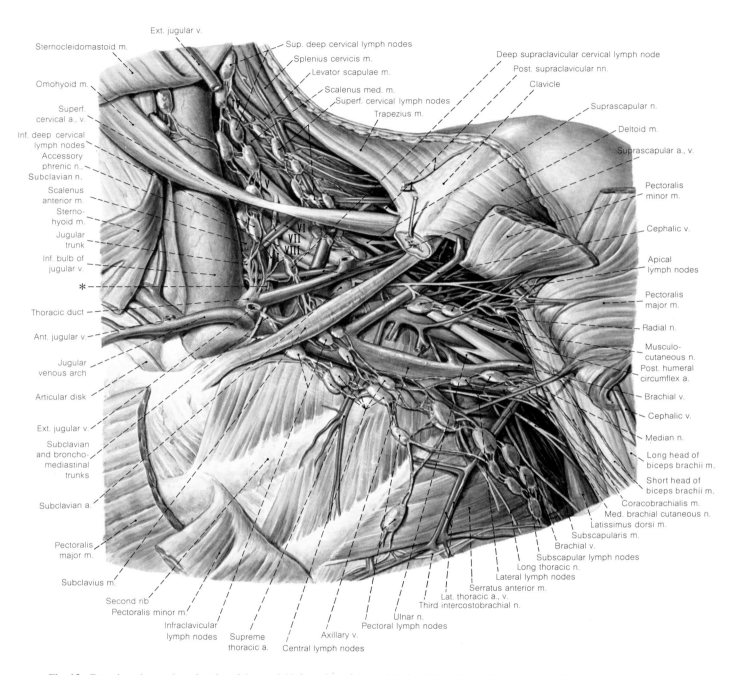

Ext. jugular v.

Sternocleidomastoid m.

Omohyoid m.

Superf. cervical a., v.

Inf. deep cervical lymph nodes

Accessory phrenic n., Subclavian n.

Scalenus anterior m.

Sterno-hyoid m.

Jugular trunk

Inf. bulb of jugular v.

*

Thoracic duct

Ant. jugular v.

Jugular venous arch

Articular disk

Ext. jugular v.

Subclavian and broncho-mediastinal trunks

Subclavian a.

Pectoralis major m.

Subclavius m.

Second rib
Pectoralis minor m.

Infraclavicular lymph nodes

Supreme thoracic a.

Central lymph nodes

Axillary v.

Ulnar n.

Pectoral lymph nodes

Third intercostobrachial n.

Lat. thoracic a., v.

Serratus anterior m.

Lateral lymph nodes

Long thoracic n.

Subscapular lymph nodes

Brachial v.

Subscapularis m.

Latissimus dorsi m.

Med. brachial cutaneous n.

Coracobrachialis m.

Short head of biceps brachii m.

Long head of biceps brachii m.

Median n.

Cephalic v.

Brachial v.

Post. humeral circumflex a.

Musculo-cutaneous n.

Radial n.

Pectoralis major m.

Apical lymph nodes

Cephalic v.

Pectoralis minor m.

Suprascapular a., v.

Deltoid m.

Suprascapular n.

Clavicle

Post. supraclavicular nn.

Deep supraclavicular cervical lymph node

Sup. deep cervical lymph nodes

Splenius cervicis m.

Levator scapulae m.

Scalenus med. m.

Superf. cervical lymph nodes

Trapezius m.

Fig. 13. Deep lymph vessels and nodes of the caudal left section of the neck, left axilla and part of the thoracic wall. In the neck, the Sterno-cleidomastoid muscle and a large part of the clavicle was resected. In the thorax, the Pectoralis major and minor muscles were divided. The label for the articular disk indicates where the clavicle had been attached. "Virchow's node or gland" belongs to the group of deep cervical lymph nodes. It lies near the opening of the thoracic duct in the angle between the internal jugular vein and subclavian artery, just dorsal to the clavicle and deep to the origin of the Sternocleidomastoid muscle. This lymph node has special clinical significance because of the tendency of liver and stomach cancer to metastasize to it. * = Virchow's gland; I = first thoracic nerve; IV–VIII = fourth to eighth cervical nerves.

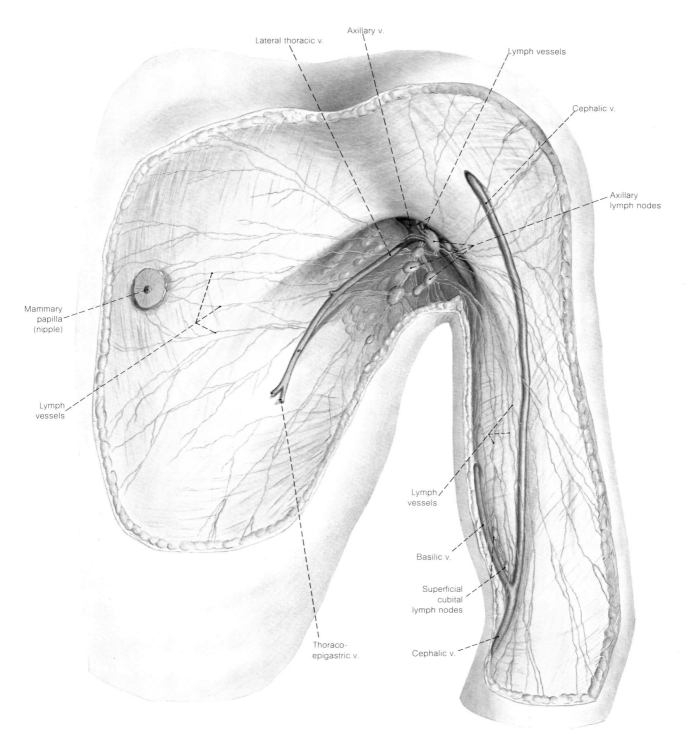

Axillary v.

Lateral thoracic v.

Lymph vessels

Cephalic v.

Axillary
lymph nodes

Mammary
papilla
(nipple)

Lymph
vessels

Lymph
vessels

Basilic v.

Superficial
cubital
lymph nodes

Thoraco-
epigastric v.

Cephalic v.

Fig. 14. Superficial lymph vessels and nodes of the arm, thoracic wall, and axilla. The lymph vessels were injected with India ink. The skin of the thorax, shoulder, flexor surface of the arm, and part of the forearm was removed.

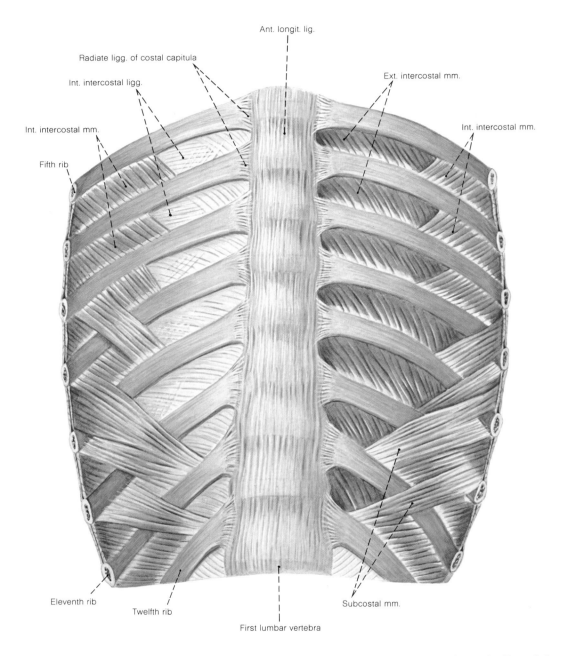

Fig. 15. The fifth to the twelfth thoracic vertebrae and the vertebral ends of the corresponding ribs, with their muscles. Frontal view. On the left, the internal intercostal ligaments were removed.

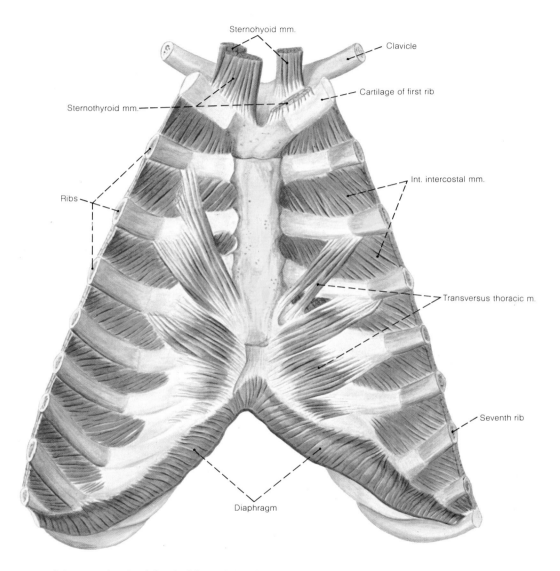

Fig. 16. The sternum and the sternal ends of the clavicles and the ribs, with the associated muscles from behind.

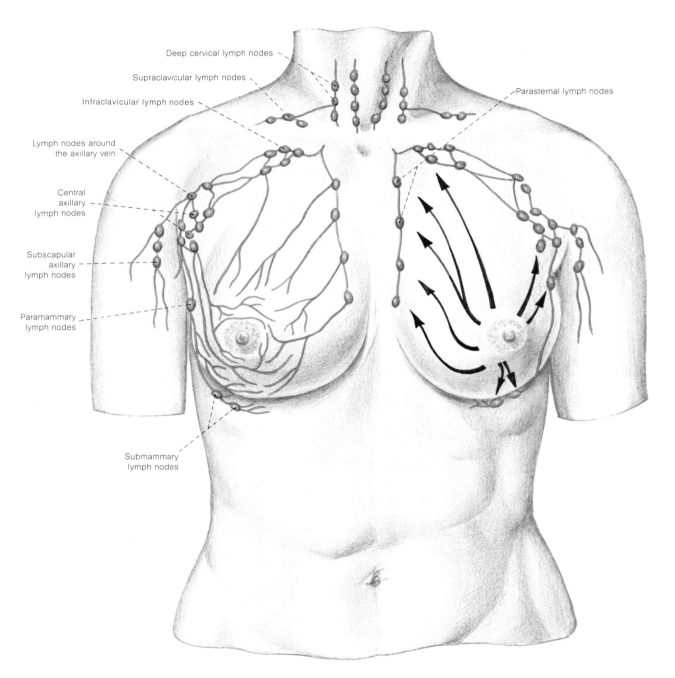

Deep cervical lymph nodes

Supraclavicular lymph nodes

Infraclavicular lymph nodes

Lymph nodes around
the axillary vein

Central
axillary
lymph nodes

Subscapular
axillary
lymph nodes

Paramammary
lymph nodes

Submammary
lymph nodes

Parasternal lymph nodes

Fig. 17. Lymphatic drainage of the female breast and the site of the regional lymph nodes and their connections (after Bäsler 1978). (From Benninghoff/Goerttler: Lehrbuch der Anatomie des Menschen, Vol. 2, 12th ed. [Eds. H. Ferner and J. Staubesand]. Urban & Schwarzenberg, Munich–Vienna–Baltimore 1979.)

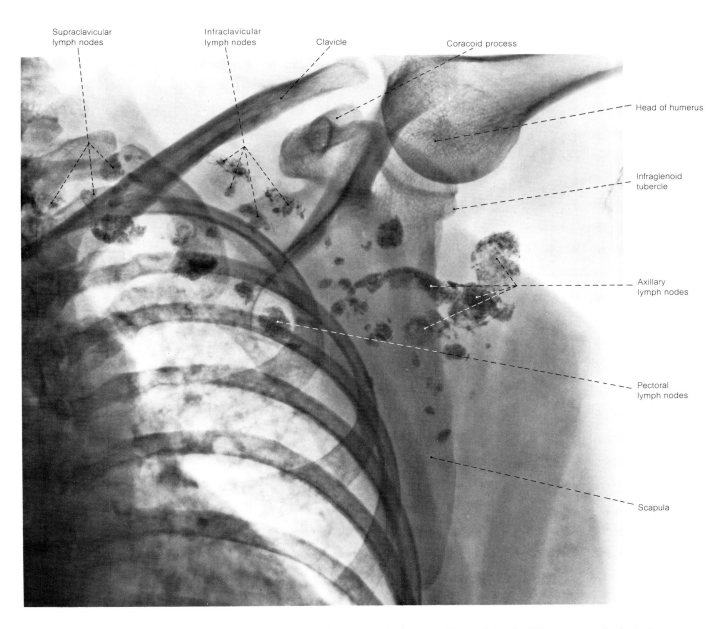

Fig. 18. Lymphadenogram of pectoral and axillary lymph nodes (Nodal phase). (From L. WICKE, Atlas der Röntgenanatomie, 2nd ed. Urban & Schwarzenberg, Munich–Vienna–Baltimore 1980.)

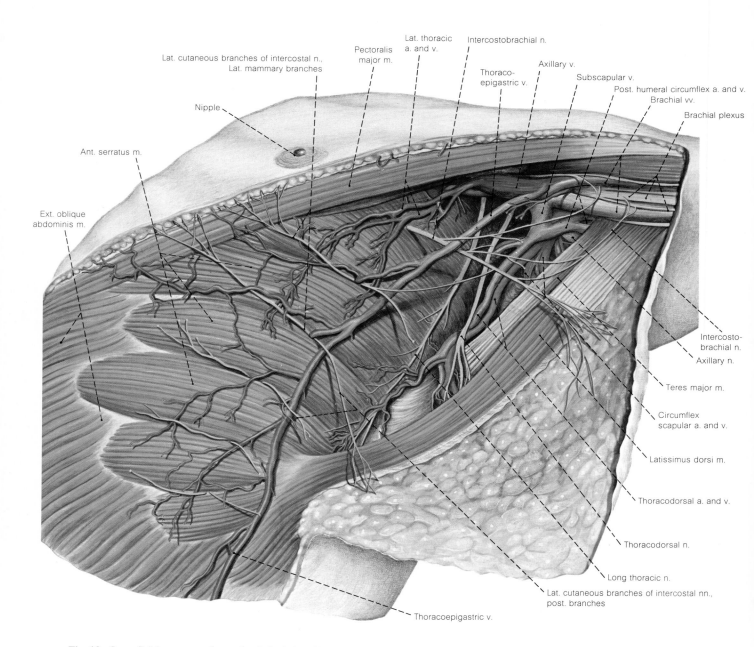

Lat. cutaneous branches of intercostal n.,
Lat. mammary branches

Pectoralis
major m.

Lat. thoracic
a. and v.

Intercostobrachial n.

Thoraco-
epigastric v.

Axillary v.

Subscapular v.

Post. humeral circumflex a. and v.
Brachial vv.

Brachial plexus

Nipple

Ant. serratus m.

Ext. oblique
abdominis m.

Intercosto-
brachial n.

Axillary n.

Teres major m.

Circumflex
scapular a. and v.

Latissimus dorsi m.

Thoracodorsal a. and v.

Thoracodorsal n.

Long thoracic n.

Lat. cutaneous branches of intercostal nn.,
post. branches

Thoracoepigastric v.

Fig. 19. Superficial nerves and vessels of the left axilla. Skin and subcutaneous fat have been reflected, the muscle fascia removed.

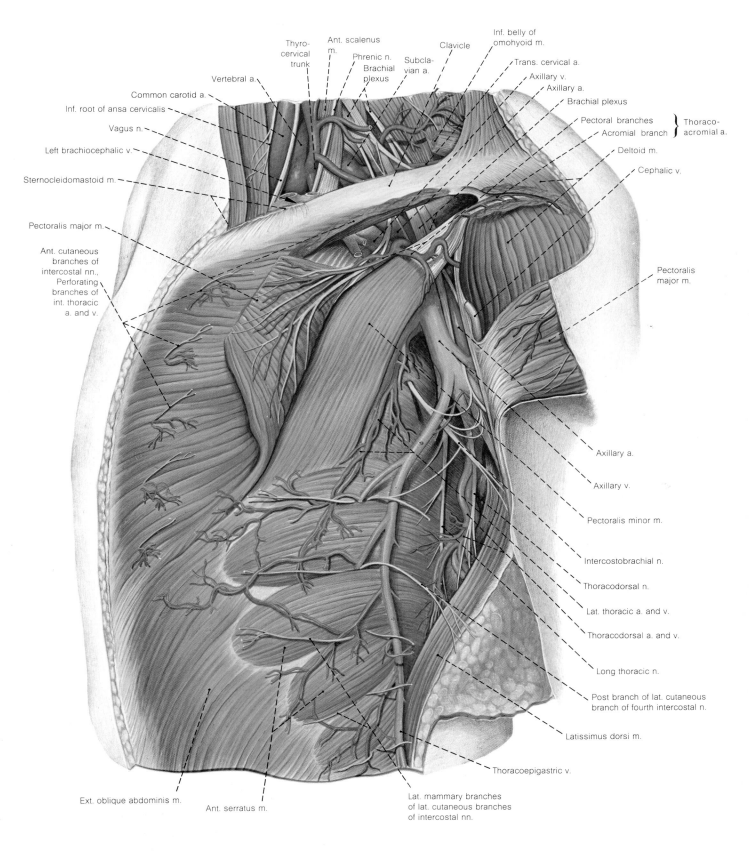

Thyro-cervical trunk

Ant. scalenus m.

Phrenic n.
Brachial plexus

Subclavian a.

Clavicle

Inf. belly of omohyoid m.

Trans. cervical a.

Axillary v.

Axillary a.

Brachial plexus

Pectoral branches
Acromial branch } Thoraco-acromial a.

Deltoid m.

Cephalic v.

Vertebral a.

Common carotid a.

Inf. root of ansa cervicalis

Vagus n.

Left brachiocephalic v.

Sternocleidomastoid m.

Pectoralis major m.

Ant. cutaneous branches of intercostal nn., Perforating branches of int. thoracic a. and v.

Pectoralis major m.

Axillary a.

Axillary v.

Pectoralis minor m.

Intercostobrachial n.

Thoracodorsal n.

Lat. thoracic a. and v.

Thoracodorsal a. and v.

Long thoracic n.

Post branch of lat. cutaneous branch of fourth intercostal n.

Latissimus dorsi m.

Thoracoepigastric v.

Ext. oblique abdominis m.

Ant. serratus m.

Lat. mammary branches of lat. cutaneous branches of intercostal nn.

Fig. 20. Deeper and vessels of the left axilla. Pectoralis major muscle cut and reflected.

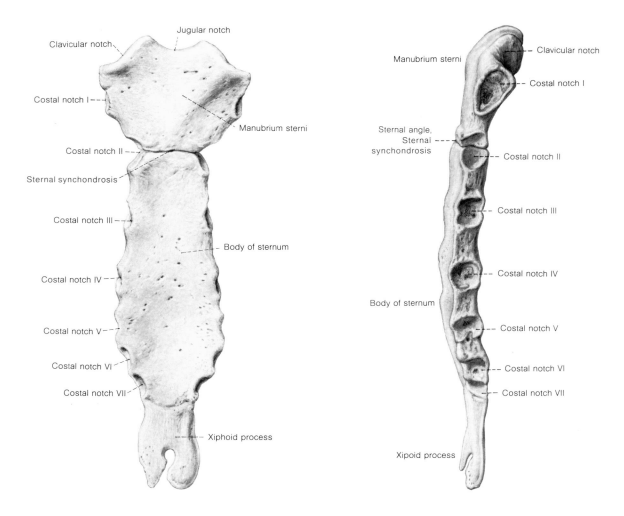

Clavicular notch

Jugular notch

Costal notch I

Manubrium sterni

Costal notch II

Sternal synchondrosis

Costal notch III

Body of sternum

Costal notch IV

Costal notch V

Costal notch VI

Costal notch VII

Xiphoid process

Manubrium sterni

Sternal angle, Sternal synchondrosis

Body of sternum

Xipoid process

Clavicular notch

Costal notch I

Costal notch II

Costal notch III

Costal notch IV

Costal notch V

Costal notch VI

Costal notch VII

Fig. 21. Sternum of an adult. Ventral view.

Fig. 22. Sternum of an adult. Lateral view.

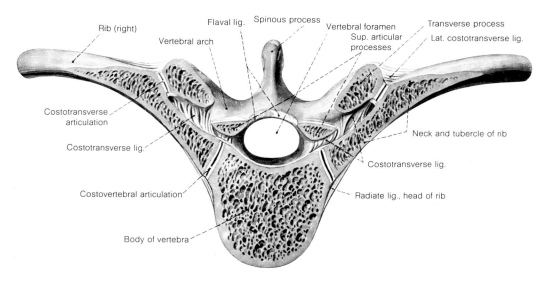

Rib (right)

Flaval lig.

Spinous process

Vertebral arch

Vertebral foramen

Sup. articular processes

Transverse process

Lat. costotransverse lig.

Costotransverse articulation

Costotransverse lig.

Costovertebral articulation

Body of vertebra

Neck and tubercle of rib

Costotransverse lig.

Radiate lig., head of rib

Fig. 23. Horizontal section through a thoracic vertebra, with the costovertebral articulations.

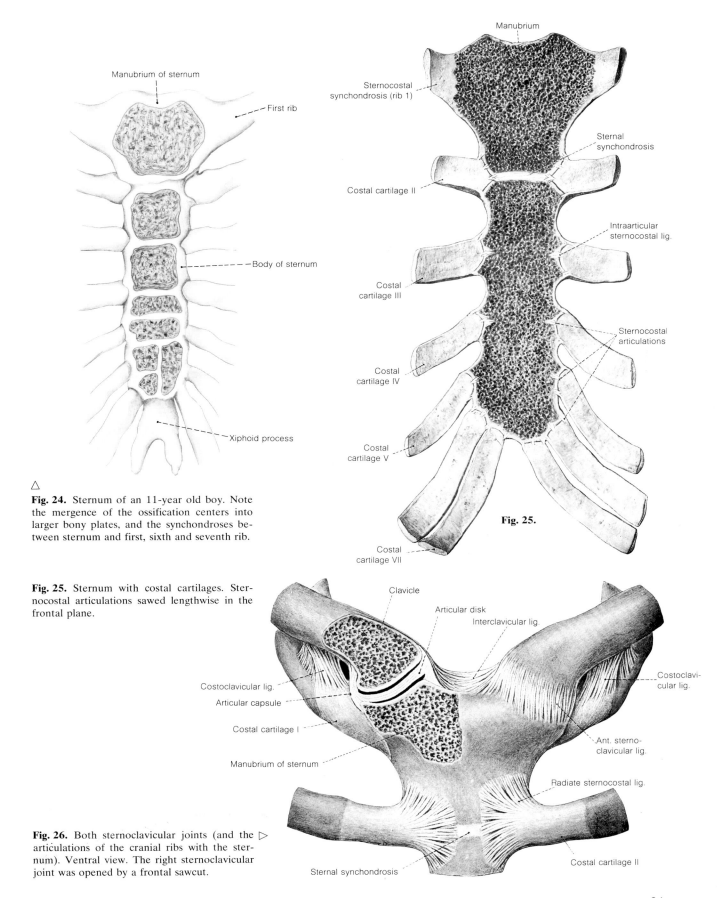

Manubrium of sternum

First rib

Body of sternum

Xiphoid process

Manubrium

Sternocostal synchondrosis (rib 1)

Sternal synchondrosis

Costal cartilage II

Intraarticular sternocostal lig.

Costal cartilage III

Sternocostal articulations

Costal cartilage IV

Costal cartilage V

Fig. 25.

Costal cartilage VII

Clavicle

Articular disk

Interclavicular lig.

Costoclavicular lig.

Articular capsule

Costoclavicular lig.

Costal cartilage I

Ant. sternoclavicular lig.

Manubrium of sternum

Radiate sternocostal lig.

Sternal synchondrosis

Costal cartilage II

Fig. 24. Sternum of an 11-year old boy. Note the mergence of the ossification centers into larger bony plates, and the synchondroses between sternum and first, sixth and seventh rib.

Fig. 25. Sternum with costal cartilages. Sternocostal articulations sawed lengthwise in the frontal plane.

Fig. 26. Both sternoclavicular joints (and the ▷ articulations of the cranial ribs with the sternum). Ventral view. The right sternoclavicular joint was opened by a frontal sawcut.

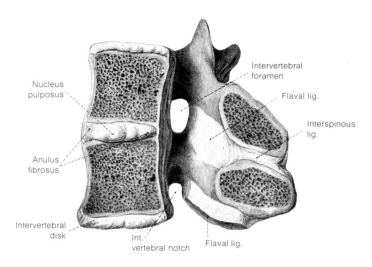

Nucleus
pulposus

Intervertebral
foramen

Flaval lig.

Interspinous
lig.

Anulus
fibrosus

Intervertebral
disk

Int.
vertebral notch

Flaval lig.

Fig. 27. Two thoracic vertebrae with their ligaments (ligamenta flava). Cut through the median sagittal plane.

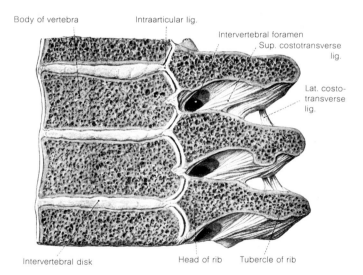

Body of vertebra

Intraarticular lig.

Intervertebral foramen

Sup. costotransverse lig.

Lat. costo-
transverse
lig.

Intervertebral disk

Head of rib

Tubercle of rib

Fig. 28. Sawcut through the vertebral bodies, the costovertebral articulations and the vertebral ends of the ribs. The cut is at a 45° angle to the median plane. The interarticular crest is closely bound up with the intervertebral disk through the intraarticular ligament. The rib belongs to the body of the vertebra below.

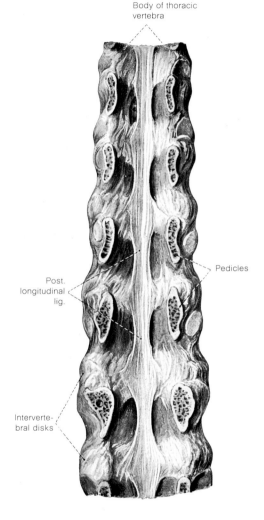

Body of thoracic
vertebra

Pedicles

Post.
longitudinal
lig.

Interverte-
bral disks

Fig. 29. Posterior longitudinal ligament and intervertebral disk of the caudal region of the thoracic vertebral column. Vertebral canal opened by removing the vertebral arches from the dorsal side.

NOTE: The costal heads articulate with their corresponding vertebrae at the upper margin of the vertebral body in the superior costal facet, with the intervertebral disk by means of the intraarticular ligament from the intraarticular crest, and with the next higher vertebral body at its lower margin in the inferior costal facet. Only the eleventh and the twelfth thoracic vertebrae have a whole costal facet at the upper lateral aspect of the vertebral body. The first thoracic vertebra is peculiar in that it possesses, besides a whole costal facet for the first rib, an inferior costal facet for the second rib.

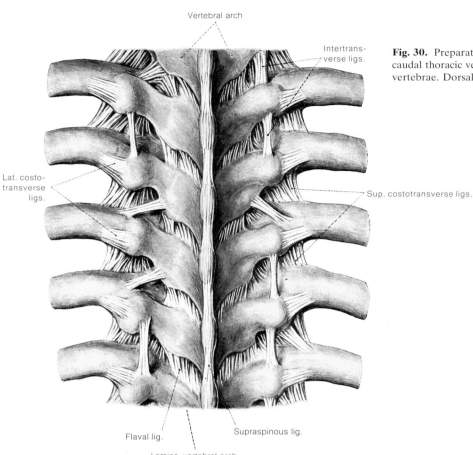

Vertebral arch

Intertransverse ligs.

Lat. costotransverse ligs.

Sup. costotransverse ligs.

Flaval lig.

Supraspinous lig.

Lamina, vertebral arch

Fig. 30. Preparation of the ligaments of the middle and caudal thoracic vertebrae and ribs. Articulations of the vertebrae. Dorsal view.

NOTE: The second to ninth thoracic vertebrae possess, on each side, three articular facets for ribs: each an upper demifacet on the vertebra body for the corresponding rib, each a lower demifacet on the vertebral body for the following rib, and each one facet on the transverse process for the corresponding side.

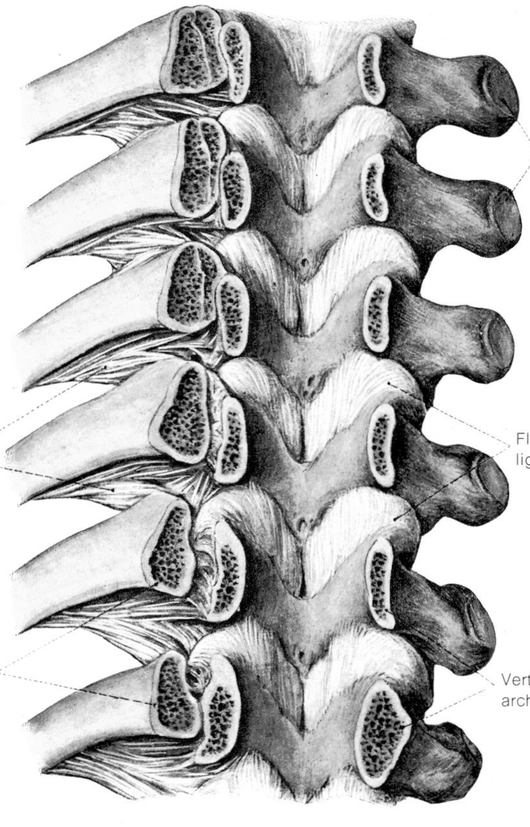

Costotransverse facet

Costotransverse ligs.

Flaval ligs.

Ribs

Vertebral arch

Fig. 31. Ligamenta flava of the thoracic vertebrae. (Seen from inside the vertebral canal.) The vertebral bodies are sawed off to display the lamina. The ribs on the left are disarticulated and removed; on the right, they are in their natural position.

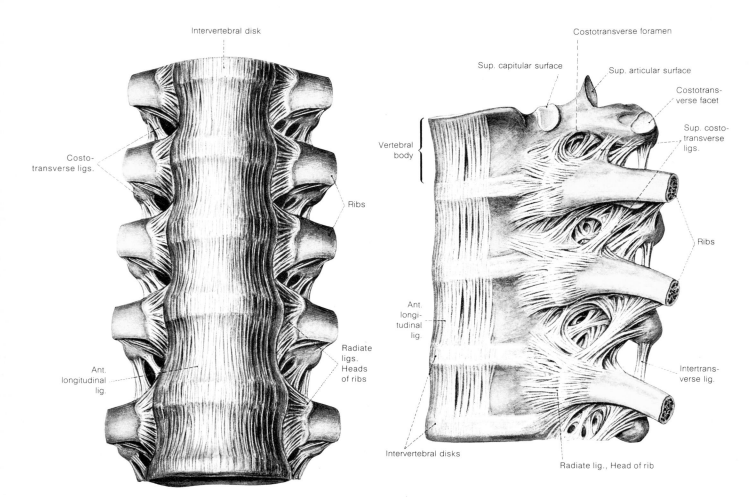

Fig. 32. Preparation of the anterior longitudinal ligament of the caudal section of the thoracic vertebral column with the costovertebral articulations. Ventral view.

Fig. 33. Preparation of the middle and caudal thoracic vertebrae and ribs. The most cranial rib was disarticulated and removed. Left lateral view.

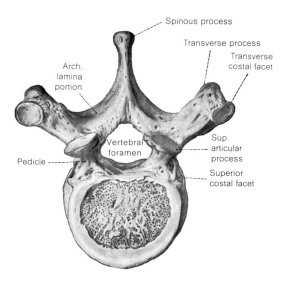

Fig. 34. Sixth thoracic vertebra seen from above.

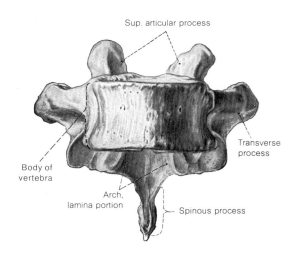

Fig. 35. Tenth thoracic vertebra in ventral view.

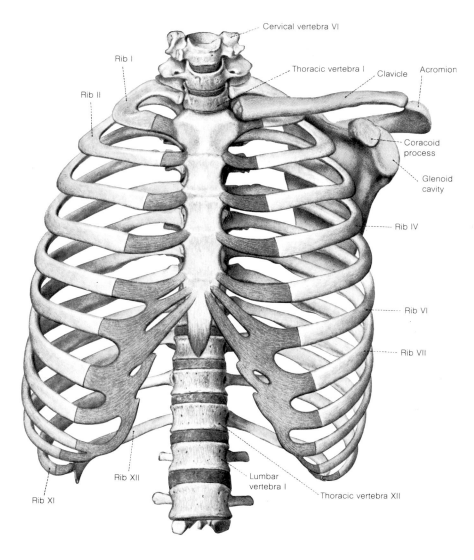

Fig. 36. Thorax, moderate inspiration. Ventral view. Left shoulder girdle blue.

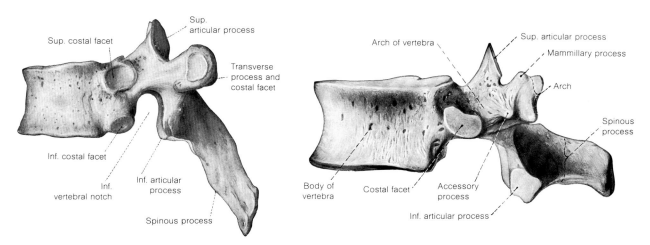

Fig. 37. Sixth thoracicvertebra in left lateral view.

Fig. 38. Twelfth thoracic vertebra in left lateral view.

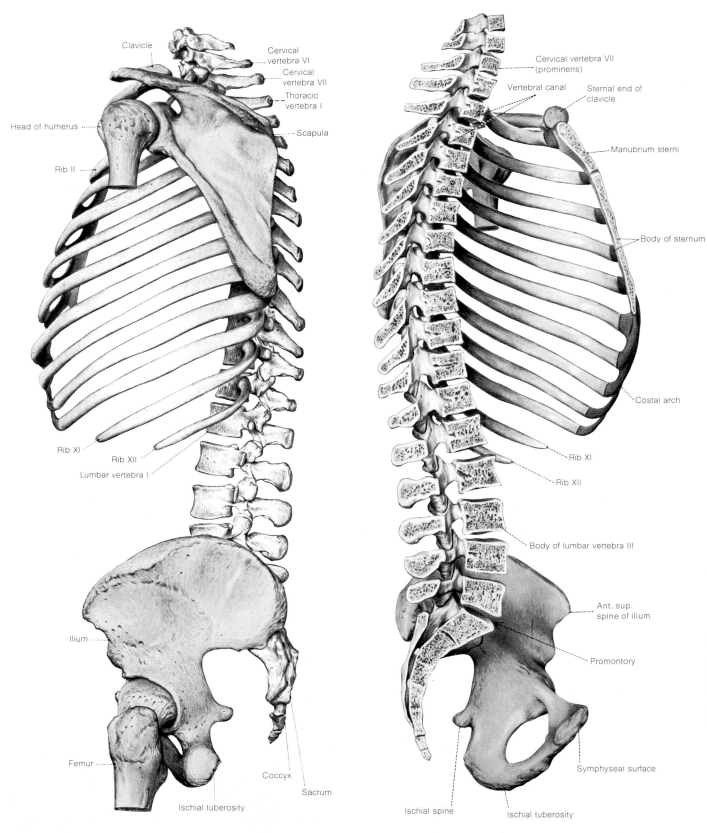

Clavicle

Cervical
vertebra VI

Cervical
vertebra VII

Thoracic
vertebra I

Head of humerus

Scapula

Rib II

Rib XI

Rib XII

Lumbar vertebra I

Ilium

Femur

Coccyx

Sacrum

Ischial tuberosity

Cervical vertebra VII
(prominens)

Vertebral canal

Sternal end of
clavicle

Manubrium sterni

Body of sternum

Costal arch

Rib XI

Rib XII

Body of lumbar vertebra III

Ant. sup.
spine of ilium

Promontory

Symphyseal surface

Ischial spine

Ischial tuberosity

Fig. 39. Skeleton of the trunk with shoulder and pelvic girdles and proximal part of the femur in blue. Left median half viewed from the left side.

Fig. 40. Skeleton of the trunk with shoulder and pelvic girdles in blue. Left median half viewed from the right.

26

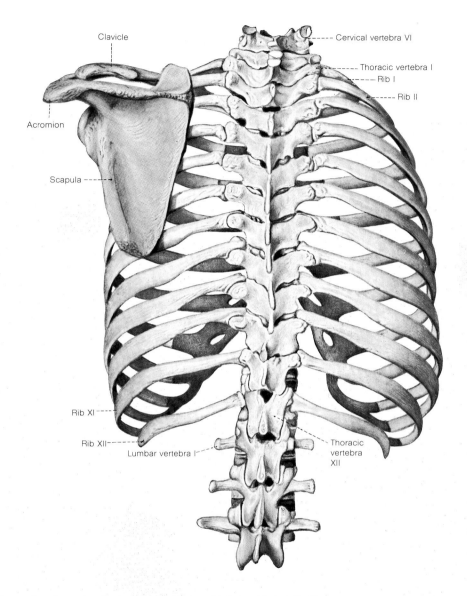

Clavicle

Cervical vertebra VI

Thoracic vertebra I
Rib I
Rib II

Acromion

Scapula

Rib XI

Rib XII

Lumbar vertebra I

Thoracic
vertebra
XII

Fig. 41. Thorax (moderate inspiration) in dorsal view. Left shoulder girdle blue.

NOTE: The insertion of the second rib meets the sternal angle, i.e., where the manubrium meets the body of the sternum (synchondrosis). This bulge across the sternum is always palpable under the skin as an indication of the ending of the second rib.

NOTE: The superior thoracic aperture is bounded by the first thoracic vertebra, the first rib, the manubrium sterni with its jugular notch. The inferior thoracic aperture is bounded by the 12th thoracic vertebra, the 12th rib, and the cartilaginous costal arch. The upper seven ribs are called true ribs because they are attached by cartilage to the sternum. The remaining 5 are called false ribs because they do not directly attach to the sternum. Three of them form the costal arch; and the 11th and 12th are referred to as floating ribs.

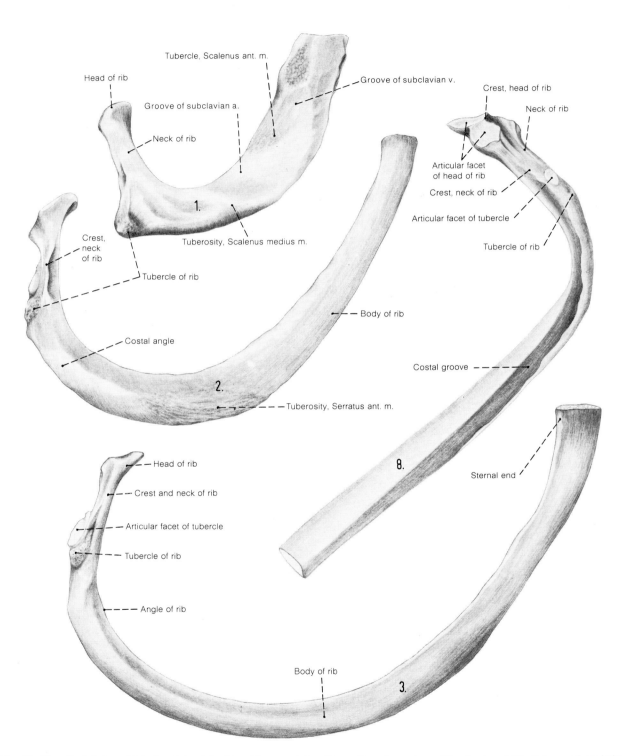

Fig. 42. First, 2nd, 3rd, and 8th ribs of the right side without costal cartilages. Seen from above. The shortened 8th rib is seen from below.

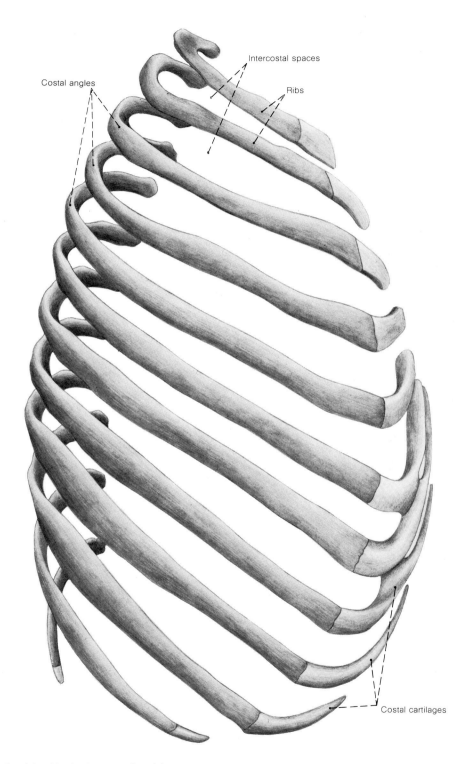

Costal angles

Intercostal spaces

Ribs

Costal cartilages

Fig. 43. The ribs of the right side, in the natural position.

Trunk

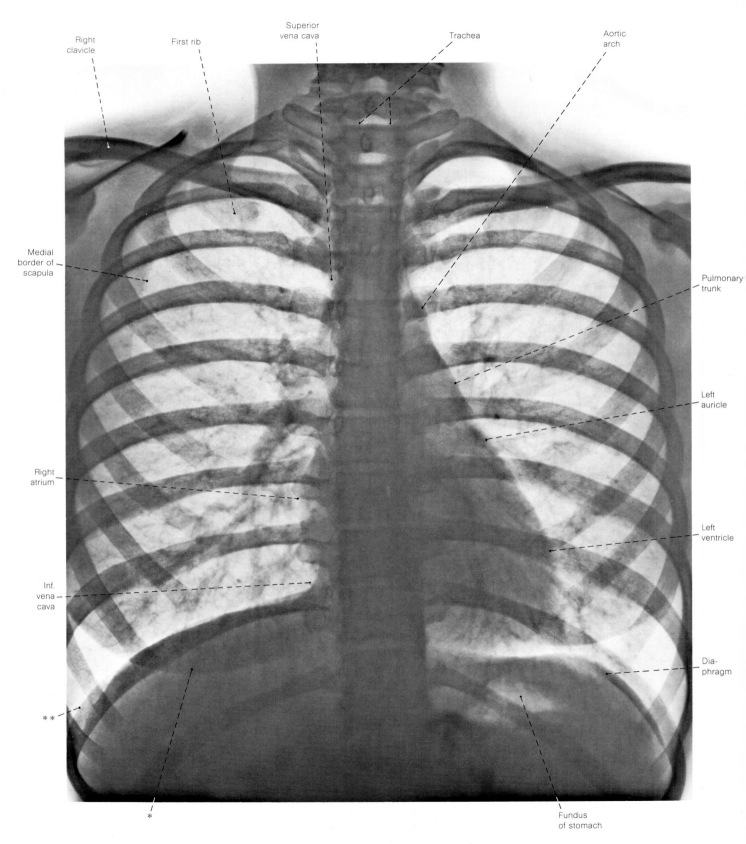

Right clavicle

First rib

Superior vena cava

Trachea

Aortic arch

Medial border of scapula

Pulmonary trunk

Left auricle

Right atrium

Left ventricle

Inf. vena cava

Dia-phragm

**

*

Fundus of stomach

Fig. 44. P.-a. roentgenogram of the thorax. (From L. WICKE: Atlas der Röntgenanatomie, 2nd ed. Urban & Schwarzenberg, Munich–Vienna–Baltimore 1980.) * Breast contour. ** Costodiaphragmatic recess.

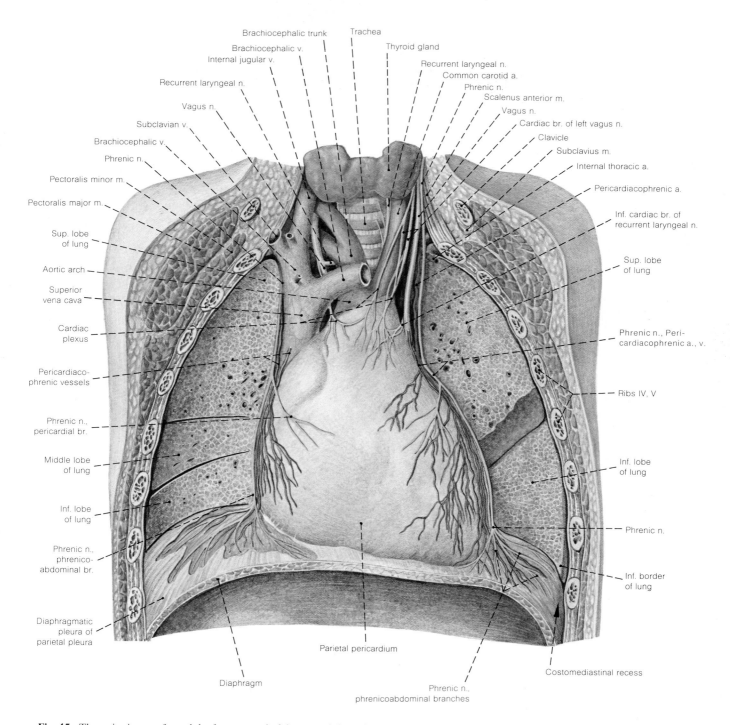

Brachiocephalic trunk
Brachiocephalic v.
Internal jugular v.
Recurrent laryngeal n.
Vagus n.
Subclavian v.
Brachiocephalic v.
Phrenic n.
Pectoralis minor m.
Pectoralis major m.
Sup. lobe of lung
Aortic arch
Superior vena cava
Cardiac plexus
Pericardiaco-phrenic vessels
Phrenic n., pericardial br.
Middle lobe of lung
Inf. lobe of lung
Phrenic n., phrenico-abdominal br.
Diaphragmatic pleura of parietal pleura

Trachea
Thyroid gland
Recurrent laryngeal n.
Common carotid a.
Phrenic n.
Scalenus anterior m.
Vagus n.
Cardiac br. of left vagus n.
Clavicle
Subclavius m.
Internal thoracic a.
Pericardiacophrenic a.
Inf. cardiac br. of recurrent laryngeal n.
Sup. lobe of lung
Phrenic n., Peri-cardiacophrenic a., v.
Ribs IV, V
Inf. lobe of lung
Phrenic n.
Inf. border of lung
Costomediastinal recess

Diaphragm
Parietal pericardium
Phrenic n., phrenicoabdominal branches

Fig. 45. Thoracic viscera of an adult after removal of the ventral thoracic wall and a ventral plane section of both lungs except for a portion of the left, which was partly removed. Ventral view. The mediastinal pleura is dissected off the pericardium in order to expose the phrenic nerves as well as the pericardiophrenic vessels. The thymus was entirely removed.

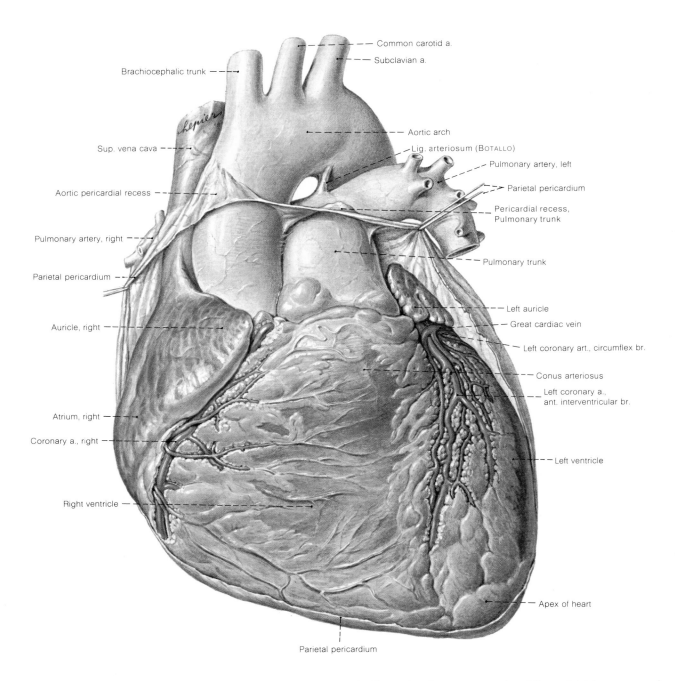

Common carotid a.

Subclavian a.

Brachiocephalic trunk

Aortic arch

Lig. arteriosum (BOTALLO)

Sup. vena cava

Pulmonary artery, left

Parietal pericardium

Aortic pericardial recess

Pericardial recess, Pulmonary trunk

Pulmonary artery, right

Pulmonary trunk

Parietal pericardium

Left auricle

Great cardiac vein

Auricle, right

Left coronary art., circumflex br.

Conus arteriosus

Left coronary a., ant. interventricular br.

Atrium, right

Coronary a., right

Left ventricle

Right ventricle

Apex of heart

Parietal pericardium

Fig. 46. Ventral view of the heart and the trunks of the great vessels. The pericardium was opened and the parietal layer removed. The larger branches of the coronary arteries were dissected. Note the pockets in the folds of the pericardium where it reflects upon the pulmonary trunk and aorta.

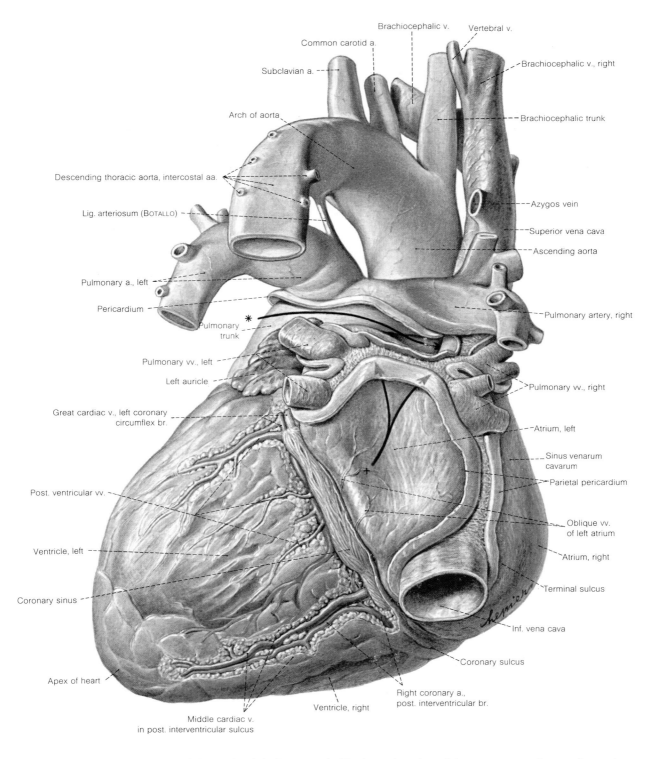

Brachiocephalic v.

Vertebral v.

Common carotid a.

Brachiocephalic v., right

Subclavian a.

Brachiocephalic trunk

Arch of aorta

Azygos vein

Descending thoracic aorta, intercostal aa.

Superior vena cava

Lig. arteriosum (BOTALLO)

Ascending aorta

Pulmonary a., left

Pericardium

Pulmonary artery, right

Pulmonary trunk

*

Pulmonary vv., left

Left auricle

Pulmonary vv., right

Great cardiac v., left coronary circumflex br.

Atrium, left

Sinus venarum cavarum

Post. ventricular vv.

Parietal pericardium

Ventricle, left

Oblique vv. of left atrium

Coronary sinus

Atrium, right

Terminal sulcus

Inf. vena cava

Apex of heart

Coronary sulcus

Middle cardiac v. in post. interventricular sulcus

Ventricle, right

Right coronary a., post. interventricular br.

Fig. 47. Dorsal view of the heart and the trunks of the large vessels. The larger branches of the coronary vessels were dissected.
* Arrow in the transverse pericardial sinus.
+ Split arrow in the oblique pericardial sinus.

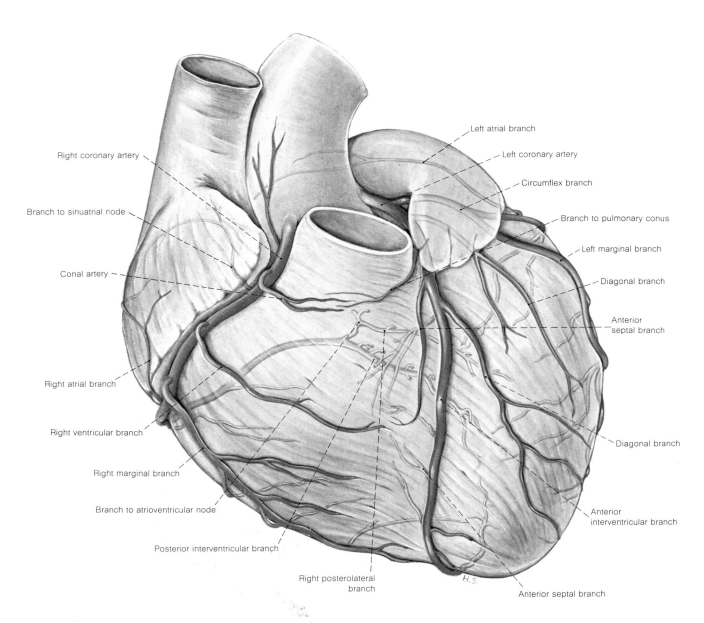

Right coronary artery

Branch to sinuatrial node

Conal artery

Right atrial branch

Right ventricular branch

Right marginal branch

Branch to atrioventricular node

Posterior interventricular branch

Right posterolateral
branch

Left atrial branch

Left coronary artery

Circumflex branch

Branch to pulmonary conus

Left marginal branch

Diagonal branch

Anterior
septal branch

Diagonal branch

Anterior
interventricular branch

Anterior septal branch

H.S.

Fig. 48. The coronary arteries; injection preparation.

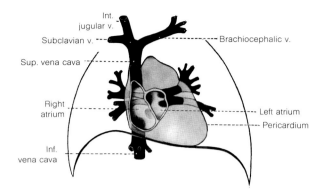

Fig. 49. The venous cross formed by veins entering the heart; the long arm of the cross is formed by the superior vena cava, the venous sinus of the right atrium, and the inferior vena cava. The cross arm consists of the two right and two left pulmonary veins converging to open into the left atrium (after BENNINGHOFF).

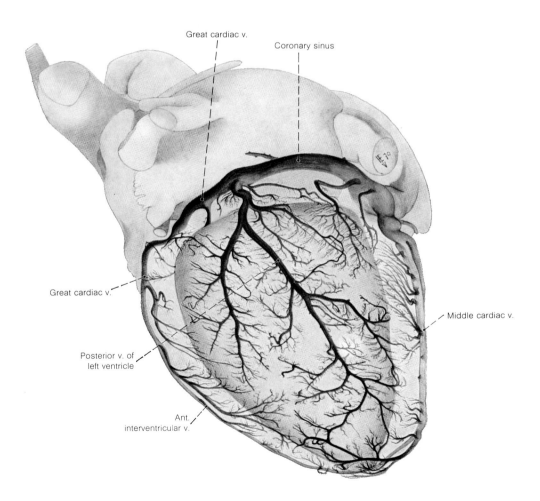

Fig. 50. The left side of the heart. Demonstration of the entry of veins into the coronary sinus. Observe the venous anastomosis in the region of the apex of the heart.

Coronary angiography has gained increasing importance in the diagnosis and therapy of coronary artery diseases. With this technique, individual coronary distribution types ("balanced type": Fig. 51, "left dominance": Fig. 52, "right dominance": Fig. 33) can be recognized as well as stenoses and obliterations the knowledge of which is of decisive significance for possible surgical intervention. The schemata of M. KALTENBACH and F. SPAHN (1975) indicate the principal coronary distribution patterns. (M. KALTENBACH and F. SPAHN: Koronarographische Nomenklatur und Typologie der Koronararterien des Menschen. Z. Kardiol. 64 [1975].)

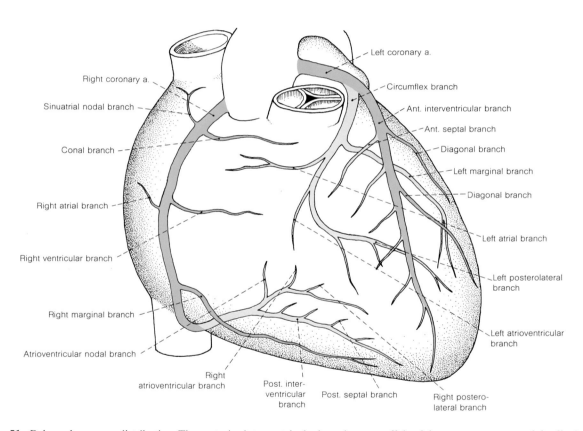

Fig. 51. Balanced coronary distribution. The posterior intraventricular branch comes off the right coronary artery, and the diaphragmatic wall of the left ventricle is supplied by the right posterolateral branch.

Fig. 52. Left dominance of coronary distribution. The left coronary artery alone supplies the left ventricle and the interventricular septum. ▷ The posterior interventricular branch here is a branch of the left coronary artery.

Fig. 53. Right dominance of coronary distribution. The right posterolateral branch is large, the circumflex branch small. The posterior wall of the left ventricle is supplied predominantly from the right coronary artery.

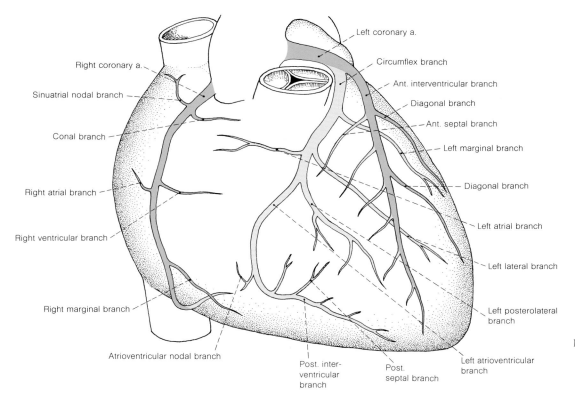

Right coronary a.

Sinuatrial nodal branch

Conal branch

Right atrial branch

Right ventricular branch

Right marginal branch

Atrioventricular nodal branch

Left coronary a.

Circumflex branch

Ant. interventricular branch

Diagonal branch

Ant. septal branch

Left marginal branch

Diagonal branch

Left atrial branch

Left lateral branch

Left posterolateral branch

Post. interventricular branch

Post. septal branch

Left atrioventricular branch

Fig. 52.

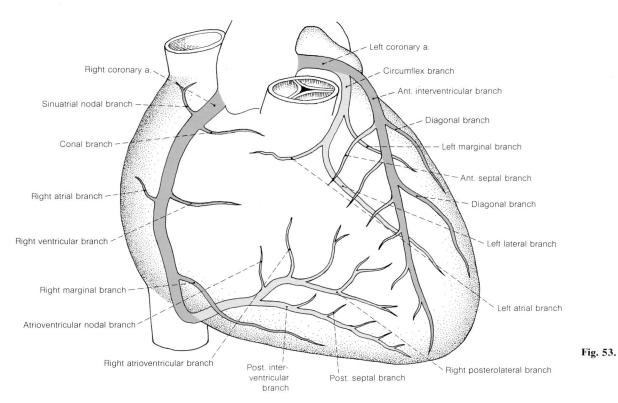

Right coronary a.

Sinuatrial nodal branch

Conal branch

Right atrial branch

Right ventricular branch

Right marginal branch

Atrioventricular nodal branch

Right atrioventricular branch

Left coronary a.

Circumflex branch

Ant. interventricular branch

Diagonal branch

Left marginal branch

Ant. septal branch

Diagonal branch

Left lateral branch

Left atrial branch

Right posterolateral branch

Post. interventricular branch

Post. septal branch

Fig. 53.

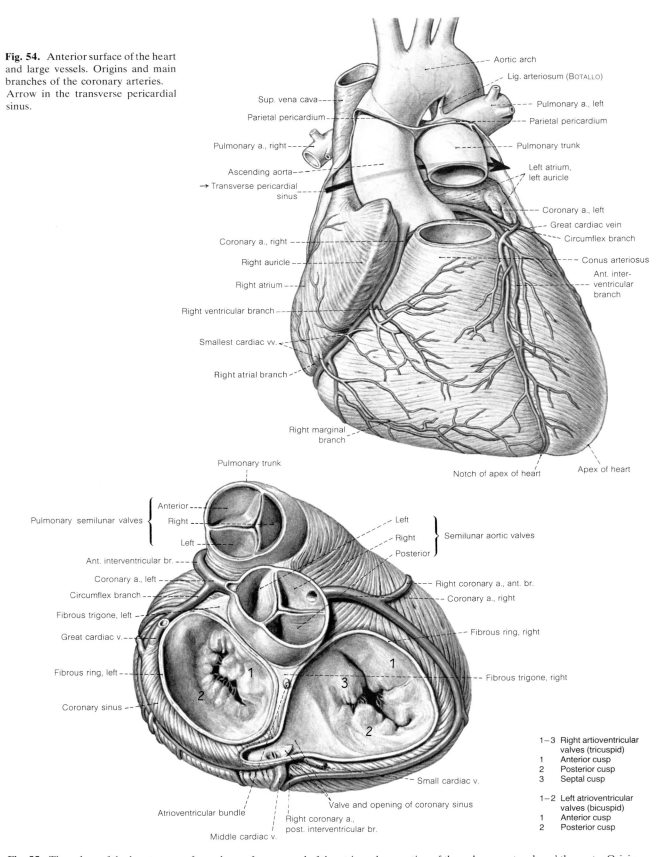

Fig. 54. Anterior surface of the heart and large vessels. Origins and main branches of the coronary arteries. Arrow in the transverse pericardial sinus.

Aortic arch

Lig. arteriosum (BOTALLO)

Sup. vena cava

Parietal pericardium

Pulmonary a., left

Parietal pericardium

Pulmonary a., right

Pulmonary trunk

Ascending aorta

Left atrium, left auricle

→ Transverse pericardial sinus

Coronary a., left

Great cardiac vein

Circumflex branch

Coronary a., right

Conus arteriosus

Right auricle

Ant. inter-ventricular branch

Right atrium

Right ventricular branch

Smallest cardiac vv.

Right atrial branch

Right marginal branch

Notch of apex of heart

Apex of heart

Pulmonary trunk

Anterior

Pulmonary semilunar valves

Right

Left

Left

Right

Posterior

Semilunar aortic valves

Ant. interventricular br.

Coronary a., left

Right coronary a., ant. br.

Circumflex branch

Coronary a., right

Fibrous trigone, left

Great cardiac v.

Fibrous ring, right

Fibrous ring, left

Fibrous trigone, right

Coronary sinus

Small cardiac v.

Atrioventricular bundle

Valve and opening of coronary sinus

Right coronary a., post. interventricular br.

Middle cardiac v.

1–3 Right artioventricular valves (tricuspid)
1   Anterior cusp
2   Posterior cusp
3   Septal cusp

1–2 Left atrioventricular valves (bicuspid)
1   Anterior cusp
2   Posterior cusp

Fig. 55. The valves of the heart as seen from above after removal of the atria and separation of the pulmonary trunk and the aorta. Origin, course, and main branches of the heart vessels. Orifice of the coronary sinus.

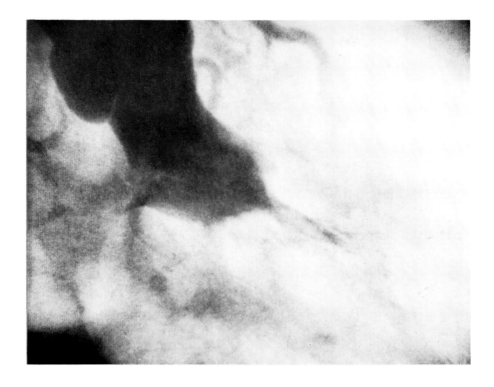

Fig. 56. Levocardiogram in systole. Original: Prof. Dr. H. ROSKAMM, Bad Krozingen.

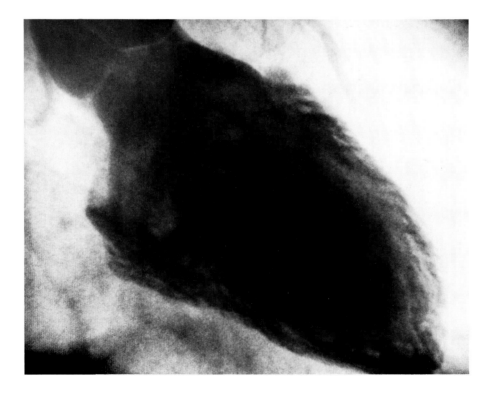

Fig. 57. Levocardiogram in diastole. Original: Prof. Dr. H. ROSKAMM, Bad Krozingen.

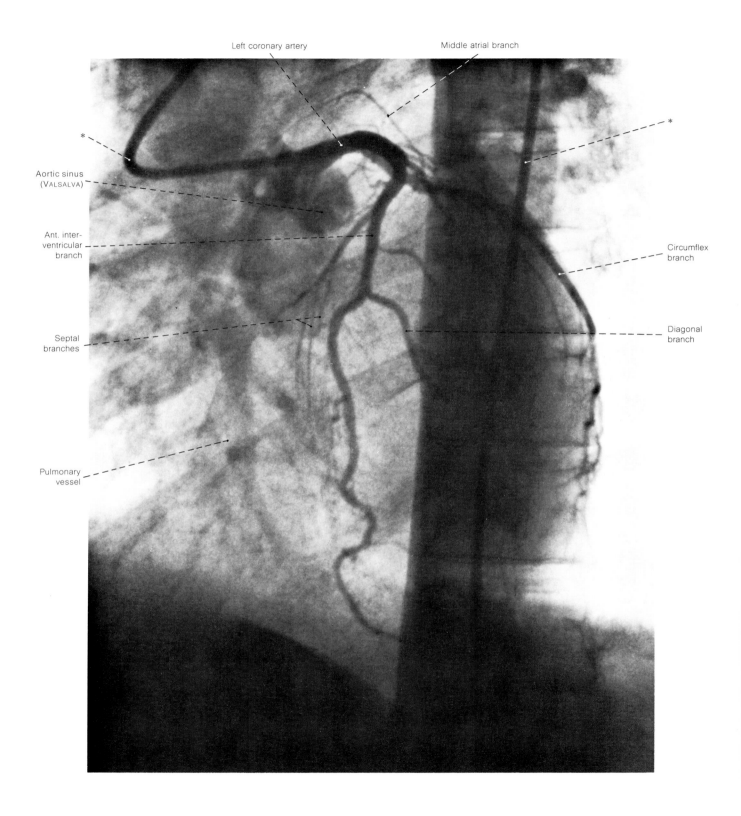

Left coronary artery

Middle atrial branch

*

*

Aortic sinus
(VALSALVA)

Circumflex
branch

Ant. inter-
ventricular
branch

Septal
branches

Diagonal
branch

Pulmonary
vessel

Fig. 58. Left coronary arteriogram (left antero-oblique projection). (From L. WICKE: Atlas der Röntgenanatomie, 2nd ed. Urban & Schwarzenberg, Munich–Vienna–Baltimore 1980.) * Catheter.

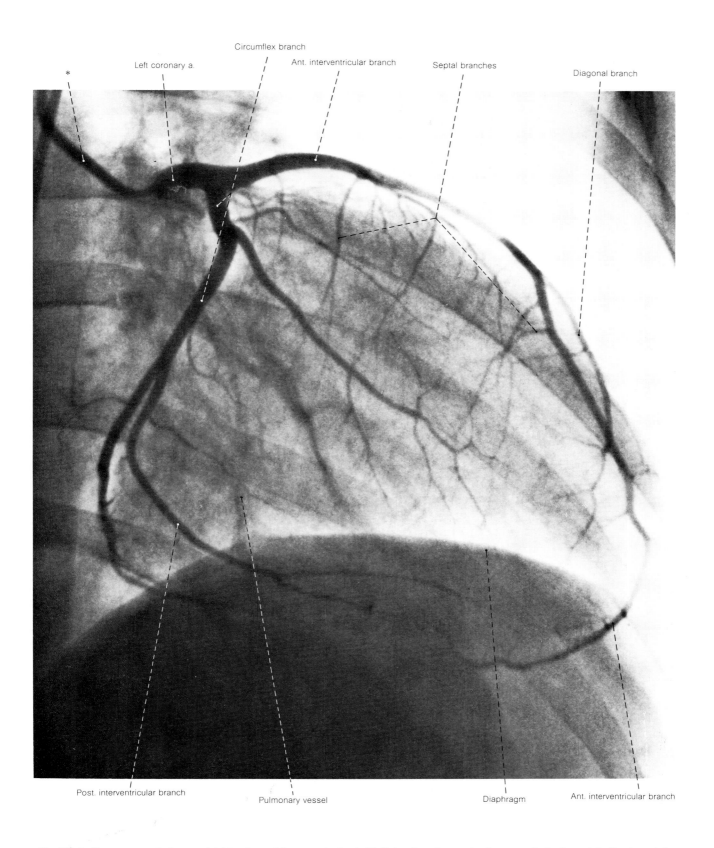

Fig. 59. Left coronary arteriogram (right antero-oblique projection). Well developed posterior interventricular branch indicating a left coronary artery dominance. (From L. WICKE, 1977.) * Catheter.

White numerals:

1 Pectoralis major m.	7 Latissimus dorsi m.
2 Pectoralis minor m.	8 Infraspinatus m.
3 Intercostales mm.	9 Rhomboideus m.
4 Serratus anterior m.	10 Trapezius m.
5 Subscapularis m.	11 Erector spinae m.
6 Teres major m.	12 Scapula

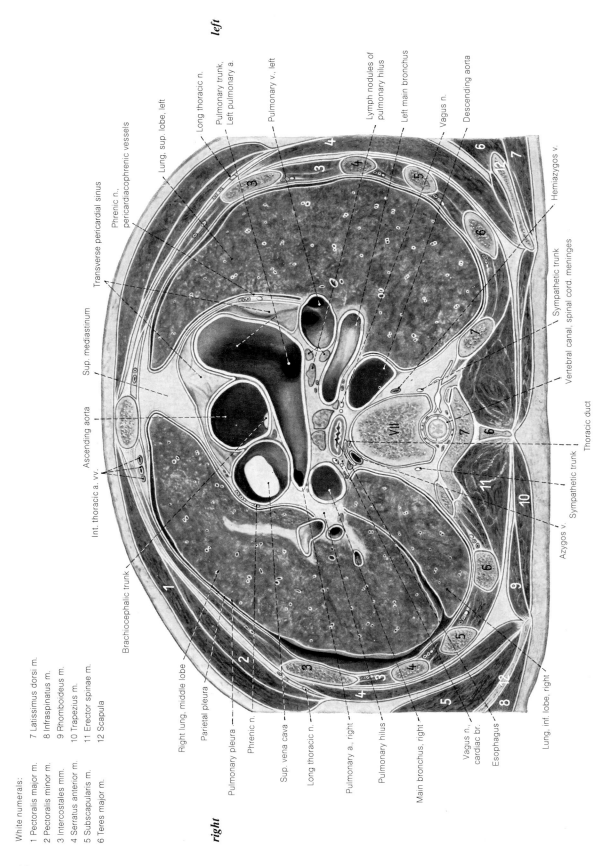

right

left

Transverse pericardial sinus

Sup. mediastinum

Ascending aorta

Int. thoracic a. vv.

Brachiocephalic trunk

Right lung, middle lobe

Parietal pleura

Pulmonary pleura

Phrenic n.

Sup. vena cava

Long thoracic n.

Pulmonary a., right

Pulmonary hilus

Main bronchus, right

Vagus n.,
cardiac br.

Esophagus

Lung. inf. lobe, right

Phrenic n.,
pericardiacophrenic vessels

Lung. sup. lobe, left

Long thoracic n.

Pulmonary trunk,
Left pulmonary a.

Pulmonary v., left

Lymph nodules of
pulmonary hilus

Left main bronchus

Vagus n.

Descending aorta

Hemiazygos v.

Sympathetic trunk

Vertebral canal, spinal cord, meninges

Thoracic duct

Sympathetic trunk

Azygos v.

VII

Fig. 60. Transverse section through the thorax at the level of the thoracic vertebra VII. The arabic numbers in black (3–7) on both sides refer to the ribs. In the dorsal midline, 7 refers to the vertebral arch of that segment (VII). Below it, 6 is the spinous process of vertebra VI. Section viewed from the caudal aspect.

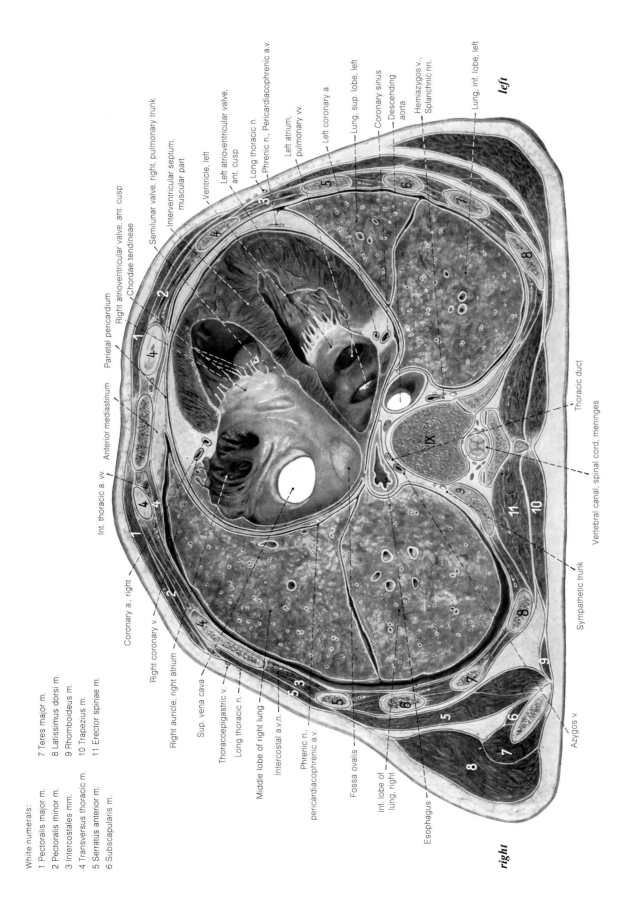

White numerals:

1 Pectoralis major m.
2 Pectoralis minor m.
3 Intercostales mm.
4 Transversus thoracic m.
5 Serratus anterior m.
6 Subscapularis m.

7 Teres major m.
8 Latissimus dorsi m.
9 Rhomboideus m.
10 Trapezius m.
11 Erector spinae m.

Fig. 61. Transverse section of the thorax at the level of the body of thoracic vertebra IX. The arabic numbers in black (4–9) indicate the cut ribs. Section viewed from the caudal aspect.

right

left

Semilunar valve, right, pulmonary trunk
Interventricular septum, muscular part
Ventricle, left
Left atrioventricular valve, ant. cusp
Long thoracic n.
Phrenic n., Pericardiacophrenic a.v.
Left atrium, pulmonary vv.
Left coronary a.
Lung, sup. lobe, left
Coronary sinus
Descending aorta
Hemiazygos v., Splanchnic nn.
Lung, inf. lobe, left

Right atrioventricular valve, ant. cusp
Chordae tendineae
Parietal pericardium
Anterior mediastinum
Int. thoracic a. vv.

Coronary a., right
Right coronary v.
Right auricle, right atrium
Sup. vena cava
Thoracoepigastric v.
Long thoracic n.
Middle lobe of right lung
Intercostal a.v.n.
Phrenic n., pericardiacophrenic a.v.
Fossa ovalis
Inf. lobe of lung, right
Esophagus
Azygos v.

Thoracic duct
Vertebral canal, spinal cord, meninges
Sympathetic trunk

43

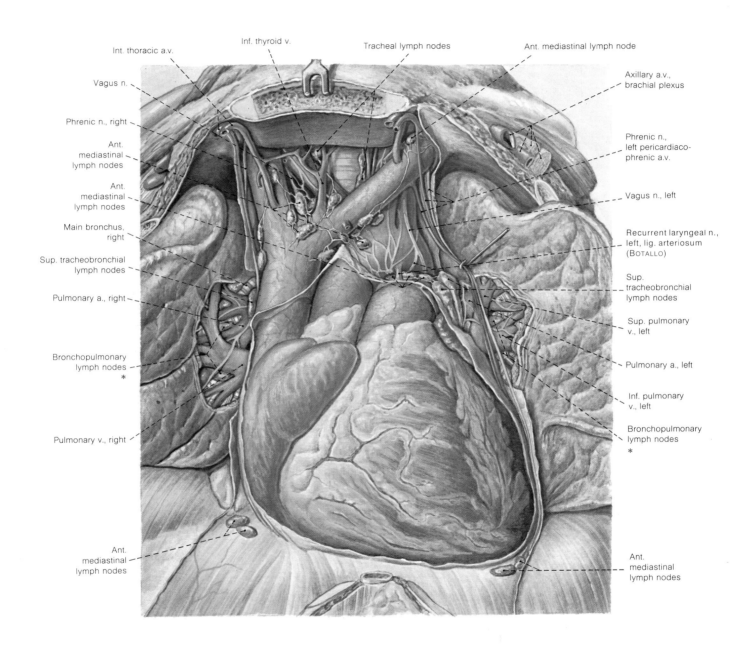

Int. thoracic a.v.

Inf. thyroid v.

Tracheal lymph nodes

Ant. mediastinal lymph node

Vagus n.

Phrenic n., right

Ant. mediastinal lymph nodes

Ant. mediastinal lymph nodes

Main bronchus, right

Sup. tracheobronchial lymph nodes

Pulmonary a., right

Bronchopulmonary lymph nodes *

Pulmonary v., right

Ant. mediastinal lymph nodes

Axillary a.v., brachial plexus

Phrenic n., left pericardiaco-phrenic a.

Vagus n., left

Recurrent laryngeal n., left, lig. arteriosum (BOTALLO)

Sup. tracheobronchial lymph nodes

Sup. pulmonary v., left

Pulmonary a., left

Inf. pulmonary v., left

Bronchopulmonary lymph nodes *

Ant. mediastinal lymph nodes

Fig. 62. Lymph nodes of the thoracic viscera. Ventral view. The thorax was opened from the front, the manubrium sterni was sawed through and pulled cranially. The thymus and sternocostal surface of the pericardium was removed. The ventral parts of the roots of the lungs were dissected free. * "Hilus glands"

Fig. 63. Lymph nodes of the thoracic organs. Dorsal view. The thoracic viscera have been removed from the thoracic cavity. The lungs were ▷ cut off at the pulmonary roots. Part of the diaphragm is attached to the pericardium. The passage of the inferior vena cava and the esophagus through the diaphragm is depicted. The thoracic aorta and azygos vein were cut off. The lymph nodes are named according to the structures they are near.

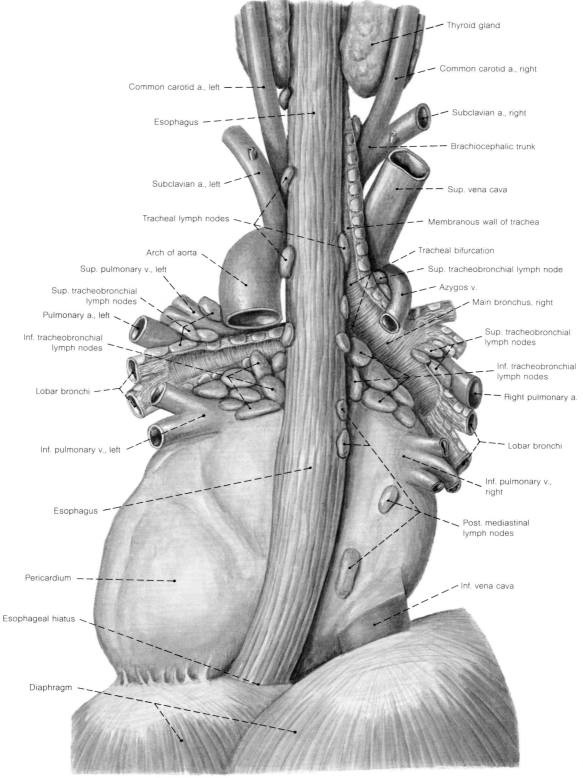

Thyroid gland

Common carotid a., right

Common carotid a., left

Subclavian a., right

Esophagus

Brachiocephalic trunk

Sup. vena cava

Subclavian a., left

Tracheal lymph nodes

Membranous wall of trachea

Arch of aorta

Tracheal bifurcation

Sup. pulmonary v., left

Sup. tracheobronchial lymph node

Sup. tracheobronchial lymph nodes

Azygos v.

Pulmonary a., left

Main bronchus, right

Inf. tracheobronchial lymph nodes

Sup. tracheobronchial lymph nodes

Inf. tracheobronchial lymph nodes

Lobar bronchi

Right pulmonary a.

Inf. pulmonary v., left

Lobar bronchi

Inf. pulmonary v., right

Esophagus

Post. mediastinal lymph nodes

Pericardium

Inf. vena cava

Esophageal hiatus

Diaphragm

Fig. 63.

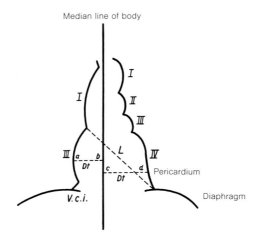

Fig. 64. Diagram of x-rayed heart shadow, saggital plane (after SCHULTZE-LUBOSCH). Right: I = superior vena cava and ascending aorta; III = right atrium. – Left: I = descending aorta; II = pulmonary arch; III = left atrium; IV = left ventricle. – Vci = inferior vena cava; Dt = average transverse diameter (ab + cd = 13–14 cm); L = longitudinal axis of heart (15–16 cm) from upper end of right atrium to the apex.

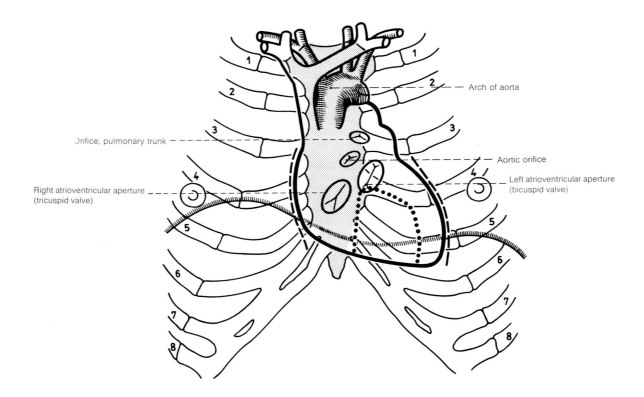

Fig. 65. Sternocostal projection of the heart and its valves on the thoracic wall. Broken lines: Lateral boundary of the relatively large area of cardiac dullness. Dotted lines: Boundary of the maximum cardiac dullness. In percussion, the determination of relative and absolute cardiac dullness plays an important role.

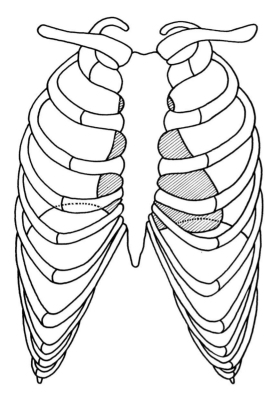

Fig. 66. Heart in expiration position.

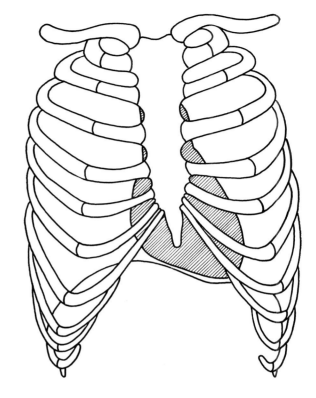

Fig. 67. Heart in inspiration position.

Standard points for the auscultation of the heart[1].

For the auscultation of the heart, customarily 7 points for the position of the stethoscope are recommended whose topographical positions are listed as follows. They are designated by the abbreviations S1–S7:

S1: Area of the maximal cardiac dullness parasternal in the left IVth intercostal space (mitral valve).

S2: Over the apex of the heart in the medioclavicular area of the left Vth intercostal space (mitral valve).

S3: Over the sternal end of the right IInd intercostal space (aortic valve).

S4: Over the sternal end of the left IInd intercostal space (aortic or pulmonary valve).

S5: Additional auscultation point (5th point of ERB) over the sternal end of the left IIIrd intercostal space (aortic valve).

S6: Over the sternal end of the right Vth intercostal space (tricuspid valve).

S7: Anterior axillary line left (mitral valve).

[1] From J. SCHMIDT-VOIGT: Herzauskultation audiovisuell. J. F. LEHMANN, Munich 1973.

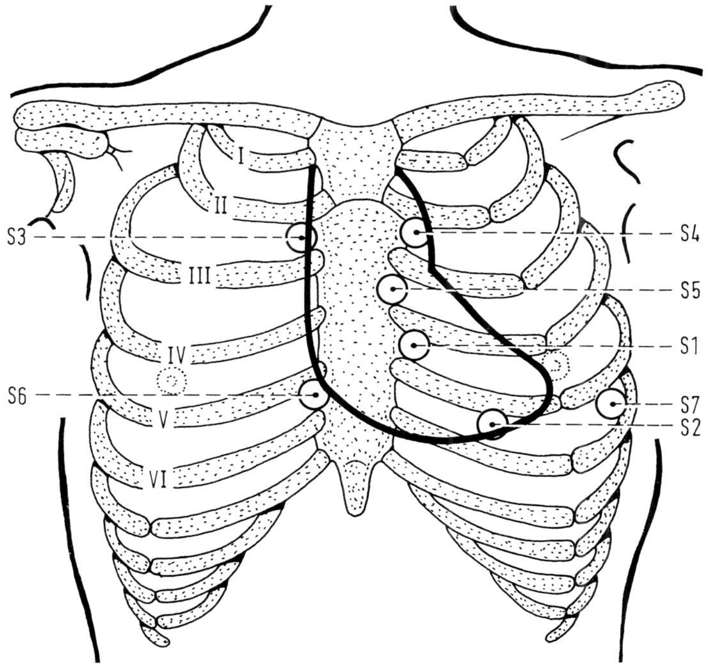

Fig. 68. Standard points for the auscultation of the heart.

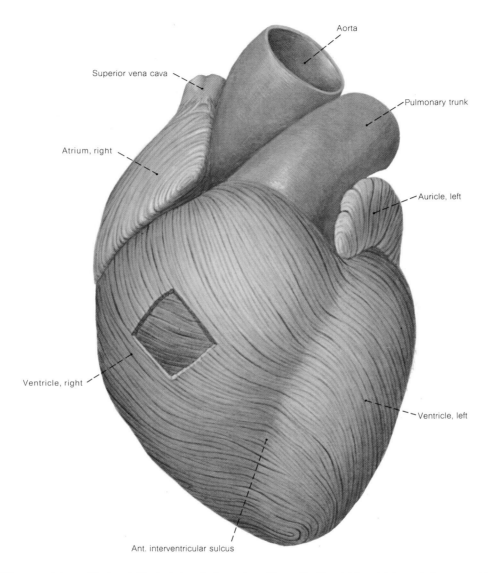

Aorta

Superior vena cava

Pulmonary trunk

Atrium, right

Auricle, left

Ventricle, right

Ventricle, left

Ant. interventricular sulcus

Fig. 69. The musculature of the heart. Ventral view. In the region of the wall of the right ventricle, a window was cut in the superficial muscle layer in order to see the difference in the direction of the muscle fiber bundles in the deeper layer.

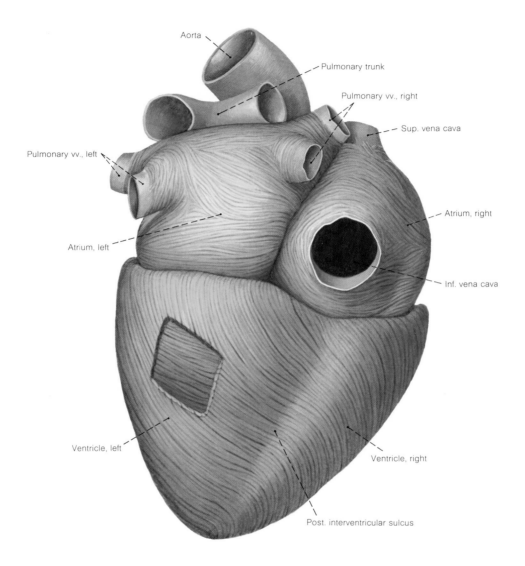

Aorta

Pulmonary trunk

Pulmonary vv., right

Sup. vena cava

Pulmonary vv., left

Atrium, right

Atrium, left

Inf. vena cava

Ventricle, left

Ventricle, right

Post. interventricular sulcus

Fig. 70. The musculature of the heart. Dorsal view. In the region of the wall of the left ventricle, a square piece is cut in the superficial layer in order to see the difference in the direction of the muscle fiber bundles in the deeper layer.

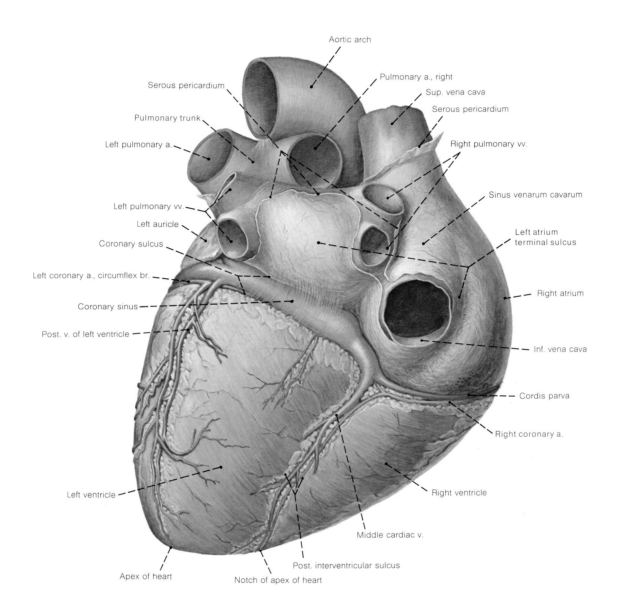

Aortic arch

Serous pericardium

Pulmonary a., right

Sup. vena cava

Serous pericardium

Pulmonary trunk

Left pulmonary a.

Right pulmonary vv.

Left pulmonary vv.

Sinus venarum cavarum

Left auricle

Coronary sulcus

Left atrium
terminal sulcus

Left coronary a., circumflex br.

Coronary sinus

Right atrium

Post. v. of left ventricle

Inf. vena cava

Cordis parva

Right coronary a.

Left ventricle

Right ventricle

Middle cardiac v.

Apex of heart

Post. interventricular sulcus

Notch of apex of heart

Fig. 71. The diaphragmatic surface of the heart. The pericardium was removed, with the exception of the place of attachment of the large vessels.

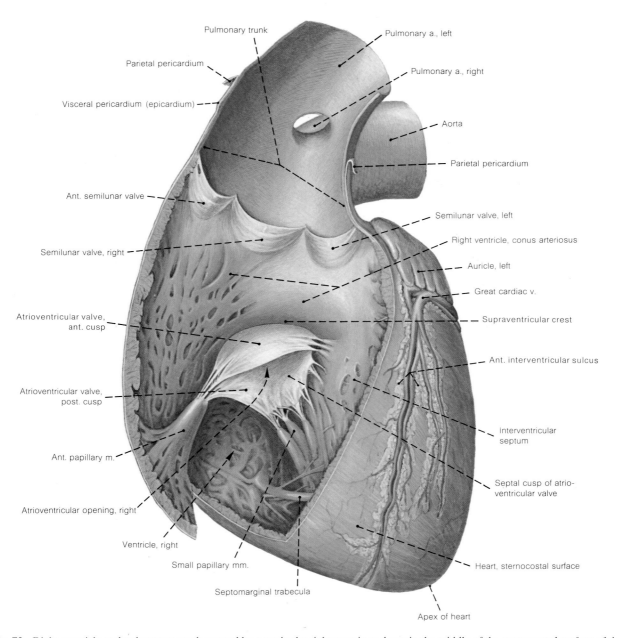

Pulmonary trunk

Pulmonary a., left

Parietal pericardium

Pulmonary a., right

Visceral pericardium (epicardium)

Aorta

Parietal pericardium

Ant. semilunar valve

Semilunar valve, left

Right ventricle, conus arteriosus

Semilunar valve, right

Auricle, left

Great cardiac v.

Atrioventricular valve, ant. cusp

Supraventricular crest

Ant. interventricular sulcus

Atrioventricular valve, post. cusp

Interventricular septum

Ant. papillary m.

Septal cusp of atrio-ventricular valve

Atrioventricular opening, right

Ventricle, right

Heart, sternocostal surface

Small papillary mm.

Septomarginal trabecula

Apex of heart

Fig. 72. Right ventricle and pulmonary trunk opened by a cut in the right margin and one in the middle of the sternocostal surface of the heart. Note: The flap with the Papillary muscle pulled laterally so the right ventricle at the right atrioventricular opening was visible and shows the atrioventricular (tricuspid) valve. Also the pulmonary trunk was opened to display three pulmonary semilunar valve cusps.

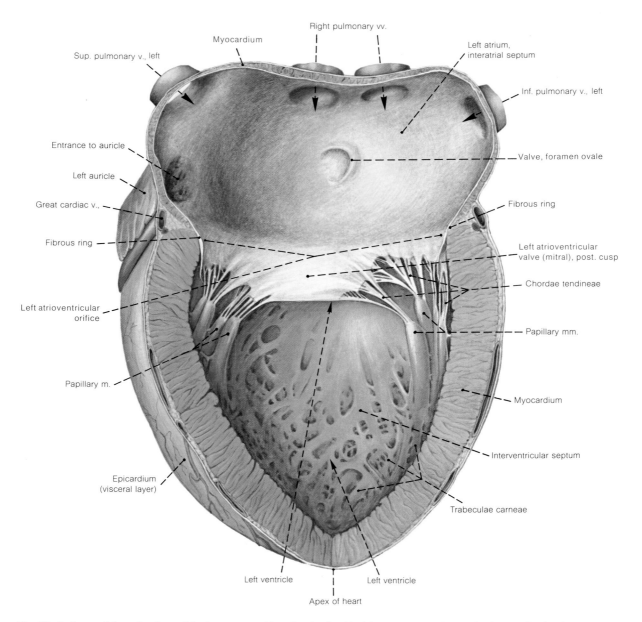

Sup. pulmonary v., left

Myocardium

Right pulmonary vv.

Left atrium,
interatrial septum

Inf. pulmonary v., left

Entrance to auricle

Left auricle

Great cardiac v.,

Fibrous ring

Valve, foramen ovale

Fibrous ring

Left atrioventricular
valve (mitral), post. cusp

Chordae tendineae

Left atrioventricular
orifice

Papillary mm.

Papillary m.

Myocardium

Interventricular septum

Epicardium
(visceral layer)

Trabeculae carneae

Left ventricle

Left ventricle

Apex of heart

Fig. 73. Left ventricle and atrium of the heart opened by a longitudinal incision. The left atrioventricular opening is slit and pulled out so that the dorsal flap of the left atrioventricular valve is seen from above.

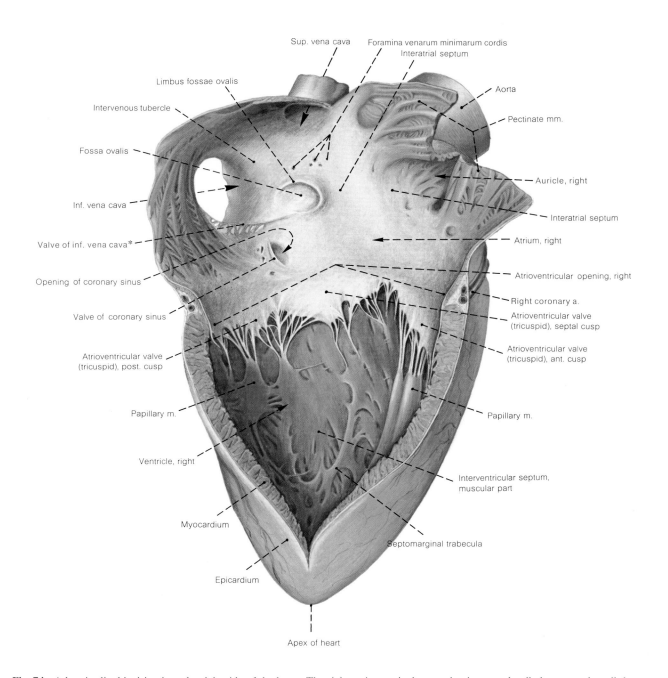

Sup. vena cava

Foramina venarum minimarum cordis
Interatrial septum

Limbus fossae ovalis

Aorta

Intervenous tubercle

Pectinate mm.

Fossa ovalis

Auricle, right

Inf. vena cava

Interatrial septum

Valve of inf. vena cava*

Atrium, right

Opening of coronary sinus

Atrioventricular opening, right

Valve of coronary sinus

Right coronary a.

Atrioventricular valve
(tricuspid), septal cusp

Atrioventricular valve
(tricuspid), ant. cusp

Atrioventricular valve
(tricuspid), post. cusp

Papillary m.

Papillary m.

Ventricle, right

Interventricular septum,
muscular part

Myocardium

Epicardium

Septomarginal trabecula

Apex of heart

Fig. 74. A longitudinal incision into the right side of the heart. The right atrioventricular opening is cut and pulled open so that all three valves of the right atrioventricular valve may be seen. * EUSTACHI valvula.

53

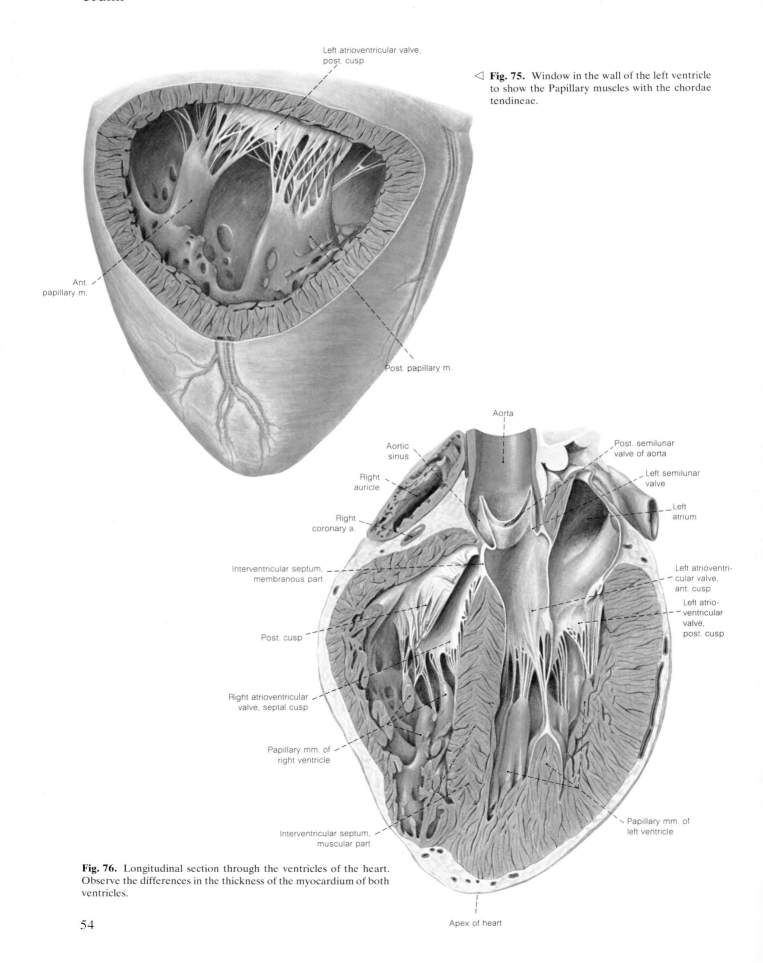

Left atrioventricular valve, post. cusp

◁ **Fig. 75.** Window in the wall of the left ventricle to show the Papillary muscles with the chordae tendineae.

Ant. papillary m.

Post. papillary m.

Aorta

Aortic sinus

Post. semilunar valve of aorta

Right auricle

Left semilunar valve

Right coronary a.

Left atrium

Interventricular septum, membranous part

Left atrioventricular valve, ant. cusp

Left atrioventricular valve, post. cusp

Post. cusp

Right atrioventricular valve, septal cusp

Papillary mm. of right ventricle

Papillary mm. of left ventricle

Interventricular septum, muscular part

Fig. 76. Longitudinal section through the ventricles of the heart. Observe the differences in the thickness of the myocardium of both ventricles.

Apex of heart

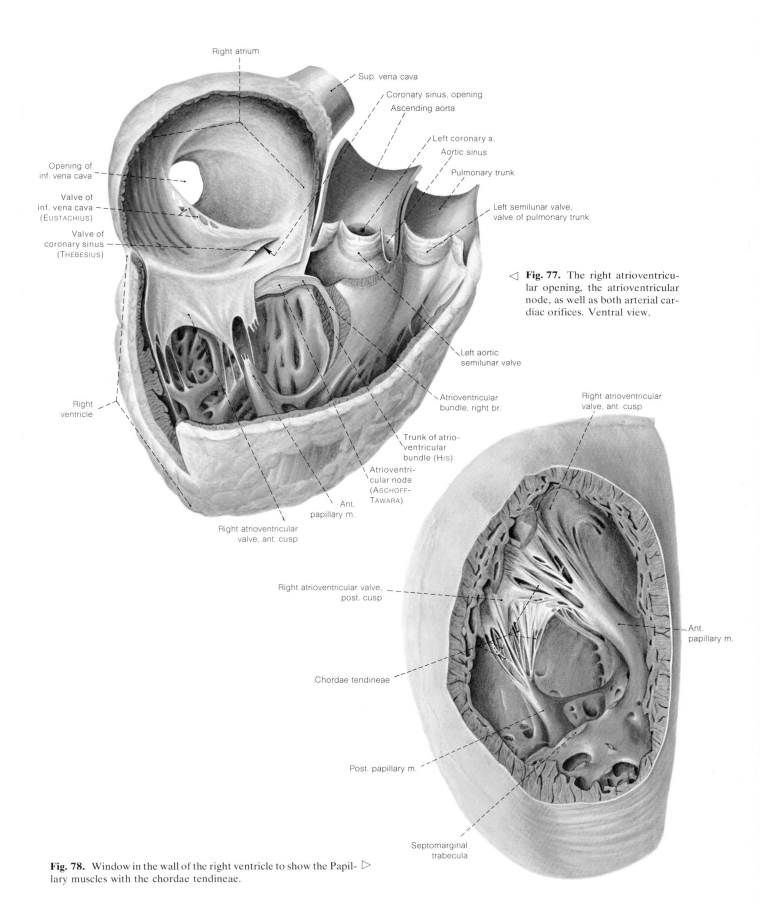

Right atrium

Sup. vena cava

Coronary sinus, opening

Ascending aorta

Left coronary a.

Aortic sinus

Pulmonary trunk

Opening of inf. vena cava

Valve of inf. vena cava (EUSTACHIUS)

Valve of coronary sinus (THEBESIUS)

Left semilunar valve, valve of pulmonary trunk

Left aortic semilunar valve

Right ventricle

Atrioventricular bundle, right br.

Trunk of atrioventricular bundle (HIS)

Atrioventricular node (ASCHOFF-TAWARA)

Ant. papillary m.

Right atrioventricular valve, ant. cusp

◁ **Fig. 77.** The right atrioventricular opening, the atrioventricular node, as well as both arterial cardiac orifices. Ventral view.

Right atrioventricular valve, ant. cusp

Right atrioventricular valve, post. cusp

Ant. papillary m.

Chordae tendineae

Post. papillary m.

Septomarginal trabecula

Fig. 78. Window in the wall of the right ventricle to show the Papil- ▷ lary muscles with the chordae tendineae.

55

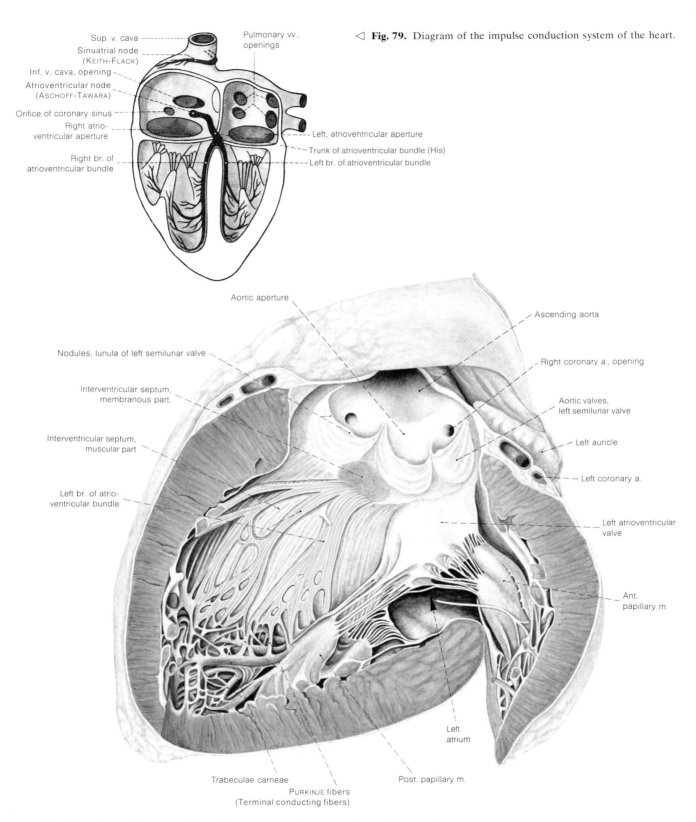

Sup. v. cava

Sinuatrial node
(KEITH-FLACK)

Inf. v. cava, opening

Atrioventricular node
(ASCHOFF-TAWARA)

Orifice of coronary sinus

Right atrio-
ventricular aperture

Right br. of
atrioventricular bundle

Pulmonary vv.,
openings

◁ **Fig. 79.** Diagram of the impulse conduction system of the heart.

Left, atrioventricular aperture

Trunk of atrioventricular bundle (His)

Left br. of atrioventricular bundle

Aortic aperture

Ascending aorta

Nodules, lunula of left semilunar valve

Right coronary a., opening

Interventricular septum,
membranous part.

Aortic valves,
left semilunar valve

Interventricular septum,
muscular part

Left auricle

Left coronary a.

Left br. of atrio-
ventricular bundle

Left atrioventricular
valve

Ant.
papillary m.

Left
atrium

Trabeculae carneae

PURKINJE fibers
(Terminal conducting fibers)

Post. papillary m.

Fig. 80. Left ventricle opened. Note: The interventricular septum with the left crus of the atrioventricular fasciculus, and the opening of the aorta. (From PERNKOPF: Atlas der topographischen und angewandten Anatomie des Menschen, Vol. 2, 2nd ed. [Ed. H. FERNER]. Urban & Schwarzenberg, Munich–Vienna–Baltimore 1980.)

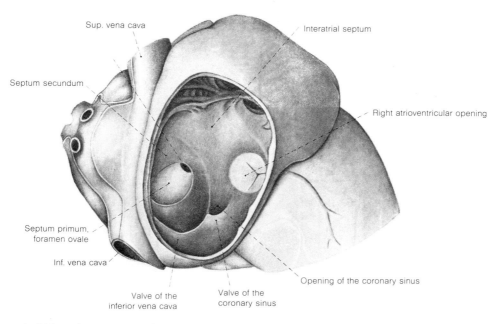

Fig. 81. Right atrium of a 310 mm human embryo (after BORN and TANDLER) opened to display the foramen ovale. * = open connection between right and left atrium.

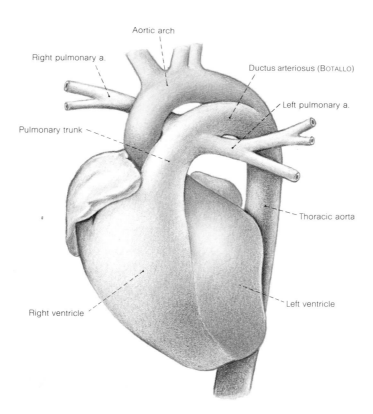

Fig. 82. Heart of a neonate. Intermixing of blood in the descending aorta due to the shunt through the ductus arteriosus (BOTALLO).

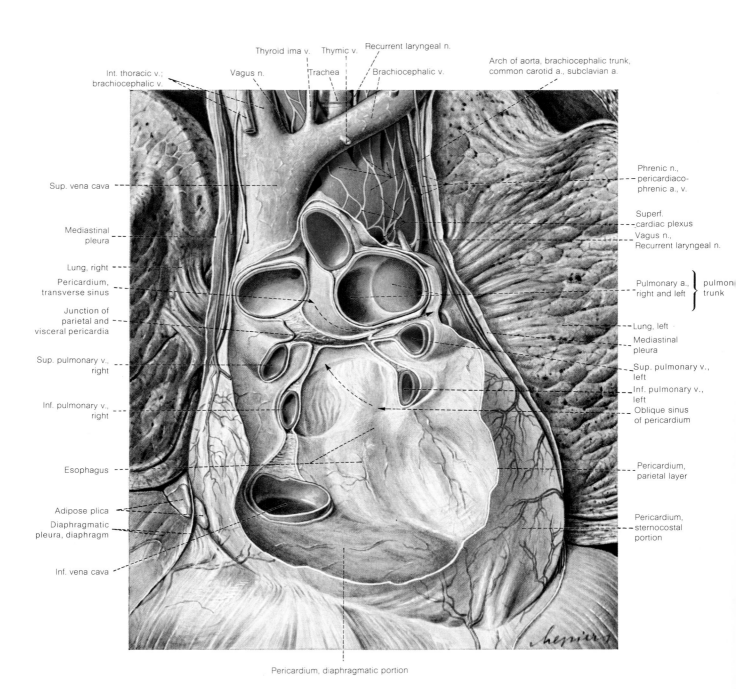

Thyroid ima v. Thymic v. Recurrent laryngeal n.

Int. thoracic v.;
brachiocephalic v.

Vagus n.

Trachea

Brachiocephalic v.

Arch of aorta, brachiocephalic trunk,
common carotid a., subclavian a.

Sup. vena cava

Mediastinal
pleura

Lung, right

Pericardium,
transverse sinus

Junction of
parietal and
visceral pericardia

Sup. pulmonary v.,
right

Inf. pulmonary v.,
right

Esophagus

Adipose plica

Diaphragmatic
pleura, diaphragm

Inf. vena cava

Phrenic n.,
pericardiaco-
phrenic a., v.

Superf.
cardiac plexus

Vagus n.,
Recurrent laryngeal n.

Pulmonary a., right and left } pulmon. trunk

Lung, left

Mediastinal
pleura

Sup. pulmonary v.,
left

Inf. pulmonary v.,
left

Oblique sinus
of pericardium

Pericardium,
parietal layer

Pericardium,
sternocostal
portion

Pericardium, diaphragmatic portion

Fig. 83. Ventral view of the dorsal wall of the pericardium, after removal of the heart. The ventral wall of the pericardium was opened in the craniocaudal direction and partially removed. The eight vessels that leave or enter the heart were cut close to the pericardium (compare with Fig. 45).

Vascular Trunks

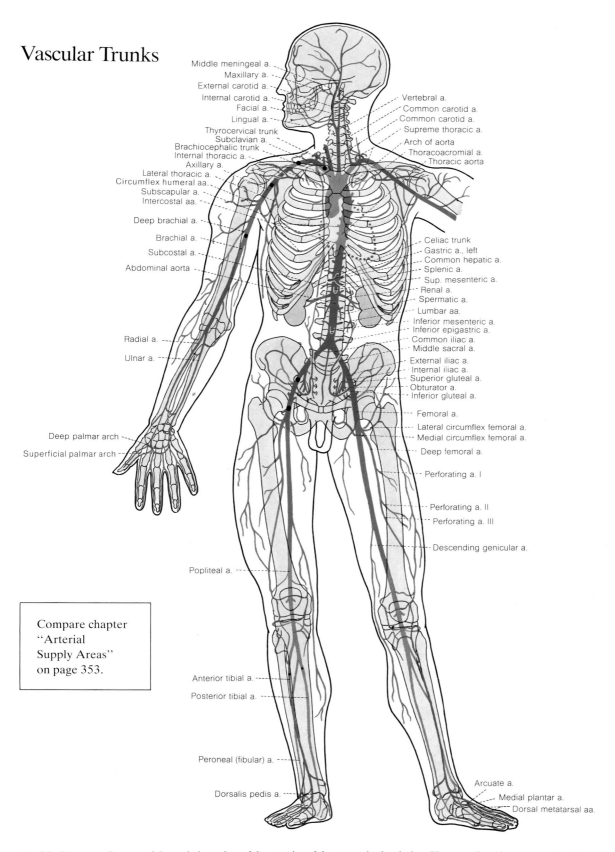

Middle meningeal a.
Maxillary a.
External carotid a.
Internal carotid a.
Facial a.
Lingual a.
Thyrocervical trunk
Subclavian a.
Brachiocephalic trunk
Internal thoracic a.
Axillary a.
Lateral thoracic a.
Circumflex humeral aa.
Subscapular a.
Intercostal aa.
Deep brachial a.
Brachial a.
Subcostal a.
Abdominal aorta
Radial a.
Ulnar a.
Deep palmar arch
Superficial palmar arch

Vertebral a.
Common carotid a.
Common carotid a.
Supreme thoracic a.
Arch of aorta
Thoracoacromial a.
Thoracic aorta
Celiac trunk
Gastric a., left
Common hepatic a.
Splenic a.
Sup. mesenteric a.
Renal a.
Spermatic a.
Lumbar aa.
Inferior mesenteric a.
Inferior epigastric a.
Common iliac a.
Middle sacral a.
External iliac a.
Internal iliac a.
Superior gluteal a.
Obturator a.
Inferior gluteal a.
Femoral a.
Lateral circumflex femoral a.
Medial circumflex femoral a.
Deep femoral a.
Perforating a. I
Perforating a. II
Perforating a. III
Descending genicular a.

Popliteal a.

Anterior tibial a.
Posterior tibial a.

Peroneal (fibular) a.

Dorsalis pedis a.

Arcuate a.
Medial plantar a.
Dorsal metatarsal aa.

Compare chapter
"Arterial
Supply Areas"
on page 353.

Fig. 84. Phantom diagram of the main branches of the arteries of the systemic circulation. Heart outlined in red dots. The black dots on the arteries are surgically useful pressure points for the interruption of bloodflow to the extremities.

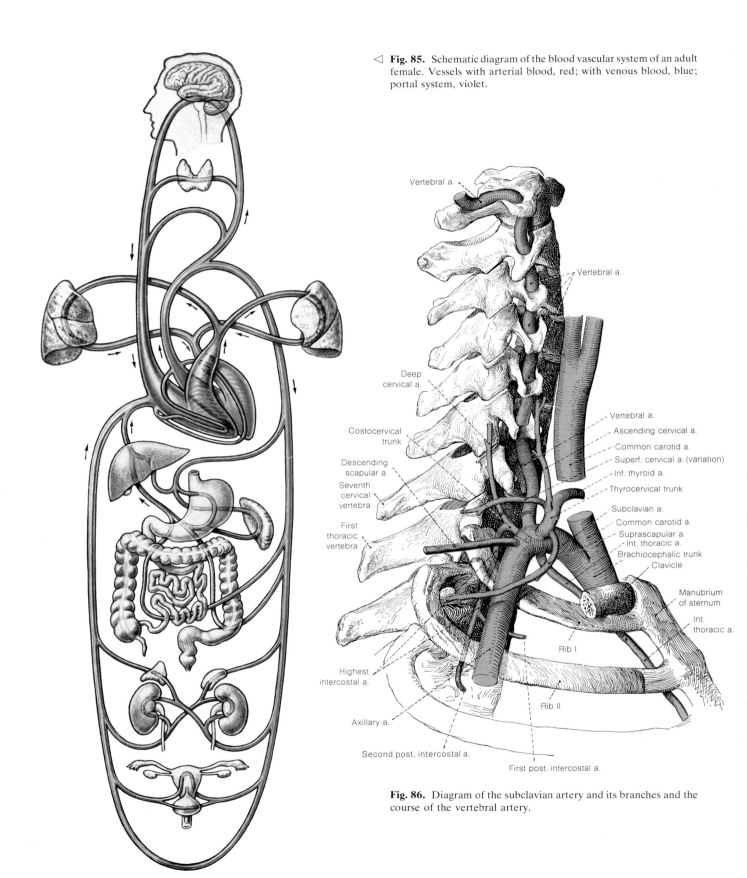

◁ **Fig. 85.** Schematic diagram of the blood vascular system of an adult female. Vessels with arterial blood, red; with venous blood, blue; portal system, violet.

Vertebral a.

Vertebral a.

Deep cervical a.

Vertebral a.

Ascending cervical a.

Costocervical trunk

Common carotid a.

Superf. cervical a. (variation)

Descending scapular a.

Inf. thyroid a.

Thyrocervical trunk

Seventh cervical vertebra

Subclavian a.

Common carotid a.

First thoracic vertebra

Suprascapular a.

Int. thoracic a.

Brachiocephalic trunk

Clavicle

Manubrium of sternum

Int. thoracic a.

Rib I

Highest intercostal a.

Rib II

Axillary a.

Second post. intercostal a.

First post. intercostal a.

Fig. 86. Diagram of the subclavian artery and its branches and the course of the vertebral artery.

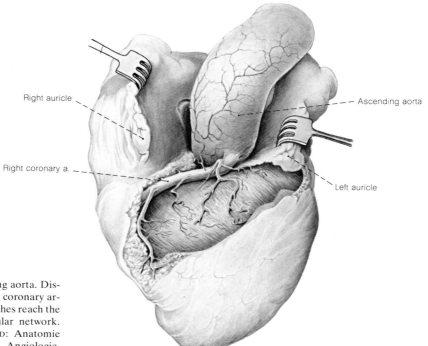

Right auricle

Right coronary a.

Ascending aorta

Left auricle

Fig. 87. Vasa vasorum of the ascending aorta. Dissection of the initial section of the right coronary artery from which small retrograde branches reach the aortic wall where they form a vascular network. Latex injection. (From J. STAUBESAND: Anatomie der Blutgefässe. In: M. RATSCHOW: Angiologie. Thieme, Stuttgart 1959.)

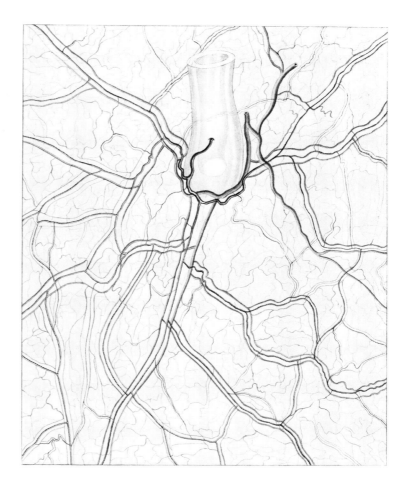

Fig. 88. Thoracic aorta in a transparent total preparation after India ink injection of the vasa vasis and ablation of the tunica adventitia. From the stem of an intercostal artery orginates a recurrent branch which enters into the network of the vascular artery. Below this, one recognizes a capillary spongework in the outer layers of the tunica media. (From J. STAUBESAND, Anat. Anz. 107, 332−339, 1959.)

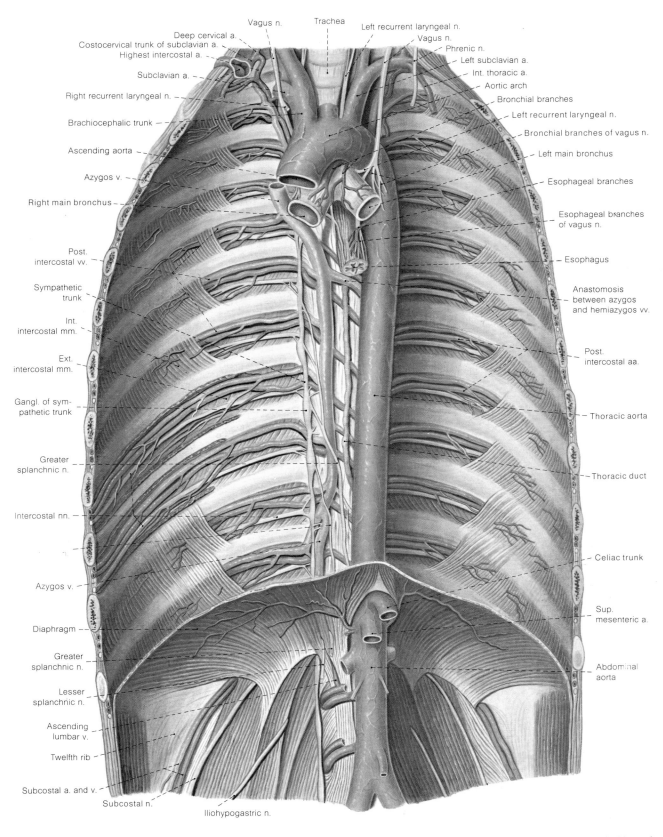

Fig. 89. Nerves and vessels of intercostal spaces and posterior mediastinum. Thoracic and abnormal aorta. Sympathetic trunk. Ventral view.

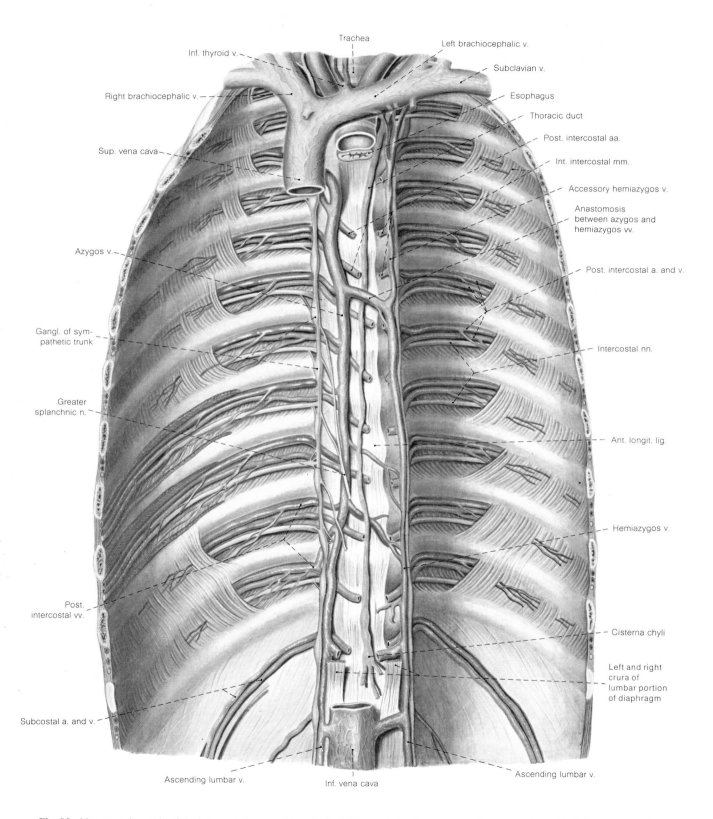

Trachea

Inf. thyroid v.

Left brachiocephalic v.

Subclavian v.

Right brachiocephalic v.

Esophagus

Thoracic duct

Post. intercostal aa.

Sup. vena cava

Int. intercostal mm.

Accessory hemiazygos v.

Anastomosis between azygos and hemiazygos vv.

Azygos v.

Post. intercostal a. and v.

Gangl. of sympathetic trunk

Intercostal nn.

Greater splanchnic n.

Ant. longit. lig.

Hemiazygos v.

Post. intercostal vv.

Cisterna chyli

Left and right crura of lumbar portion of diaphragm

Subcostal a. and v.

Ascending lumbar v.

Inf. vena cava

Ascending lumbar v.

Fig. 90. Nerves and vessels of the intercostal spaces; thoracic duct. The aorta has been removed, the superior and inferior vena cava have been cut off at the entry into the pericardial sac and caudal to the diaphragm, respectively.

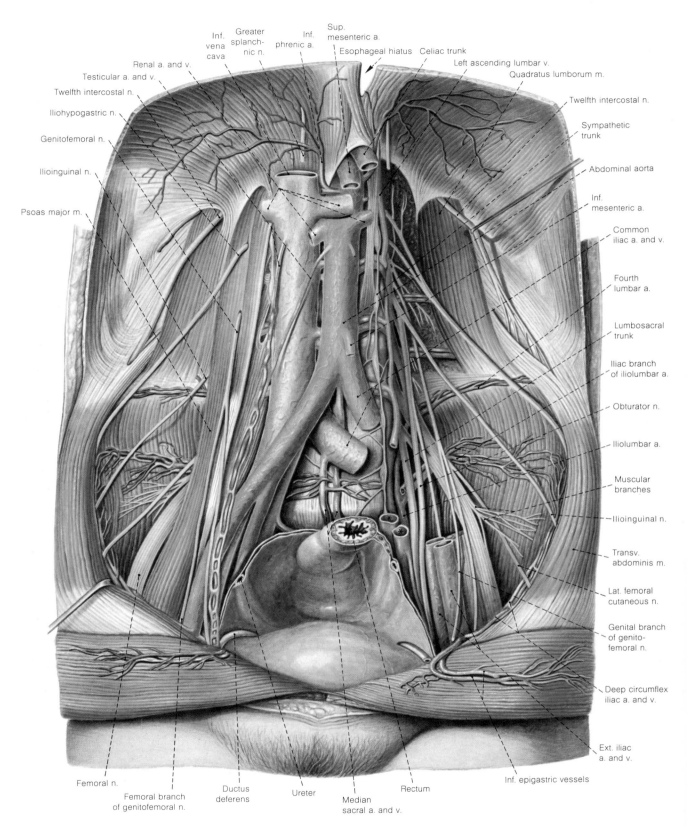

Fig. 91. Nerves and blood vessels of the posterior abdominal wall, lumbar plexus. The right psoas major muscle and portions of the common iliac vessels have been removed. ** = internal iliac vessels.

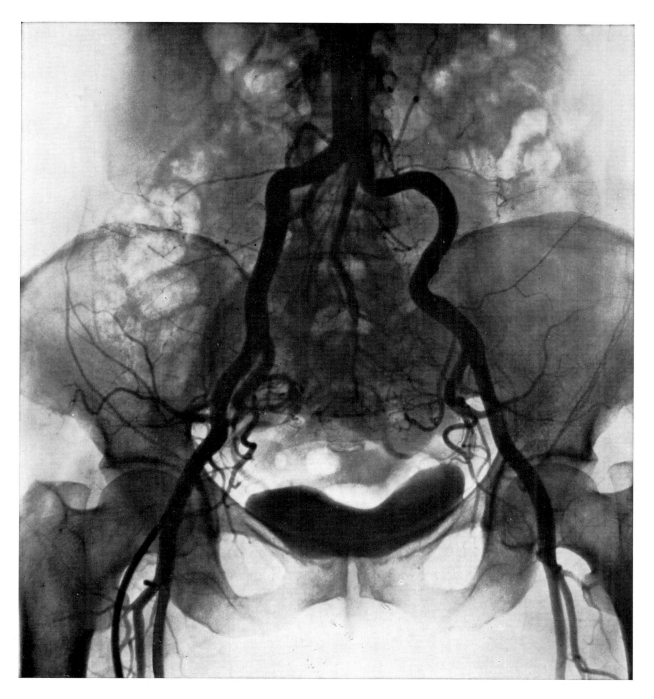

Fig. 92. Arteriogram of the lower abdominal aorta, iliac arteries and their branches. Observe the course of the median sacral artery and its branches. Contrast medium that has been eliminated by the kidneys can be seen in the urinary bladder. (Sagittal film by Dr. H. SCHMIDT, Pforzheim.)

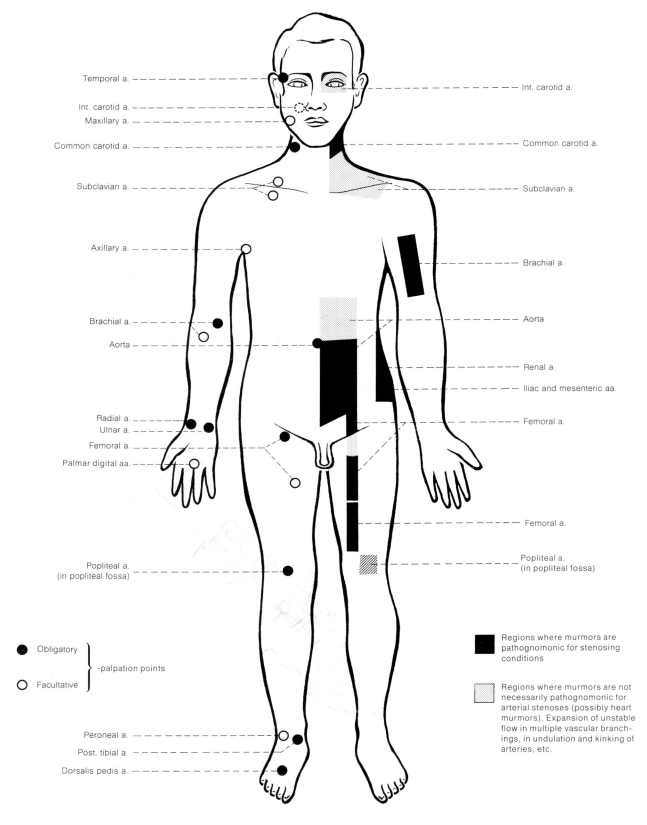

Temporal a.

Int. carotid a.

Int. carotid a.

Maxillary a.

Common carotid a.

Common carotid a.

Subclavian a.

Subclavian a.

Axillary a.

Brachial a.

Brachial a.

Aorta

Aorta

Renal a.

Iliac and mesenteric aa.

Radial a.

Ulnar a.

Femoral a.

Femoral a.

Palmar digital aa.

Femoral a.

Popliteal a.
(in popliteal fossa)

Popliteal a.
(in popliteal fossa)

● Obligatory

○ Facultative

} -palpation points

Peroneal a.

Post. tibial a.

Dorsalis pedis a.

■ Regions where murmors are pathognomonic for stenosing conditions

▨ Regions where murmors are not necessarily pathognomonic for arterial stenoses (possibly heart murmors). Expansion of unstable flow in multiple vascular branchings, in undulation and kinking of arteries, etc.

Fig. 93. Typical palpation and auscultation point of major arteries. (From A. Kappert: Lehrbuch und Atlas der Angiologie. 10th ed. Huber, Bern–Stuttgart–Vienna 1981.)

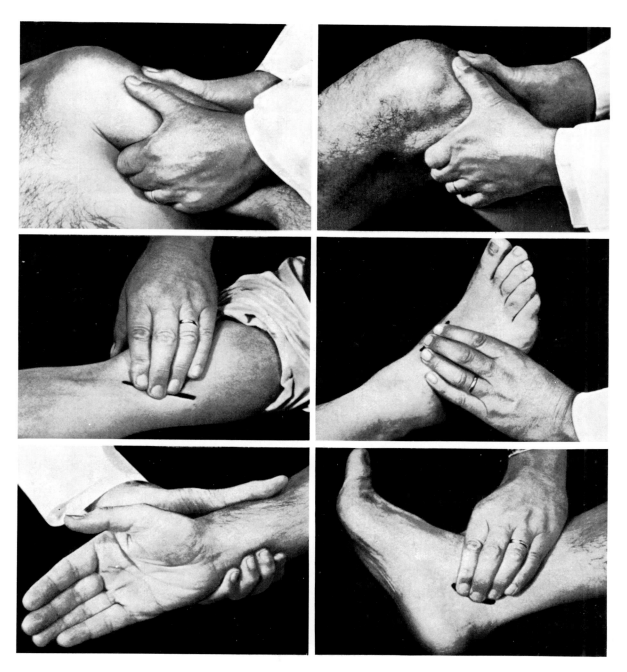

Fig. 94. Palpation of arterial pulses. From top to bottom left axillary a., brachial a., ulnar a.; right popliteal a., dorsalis pedis a., post. tibial a. (From A. KAPPERT: Lehrbuch und Atlas der Angiologie. 10th ed. Huber, Bern–Stuttgart–Vienna 1981.)

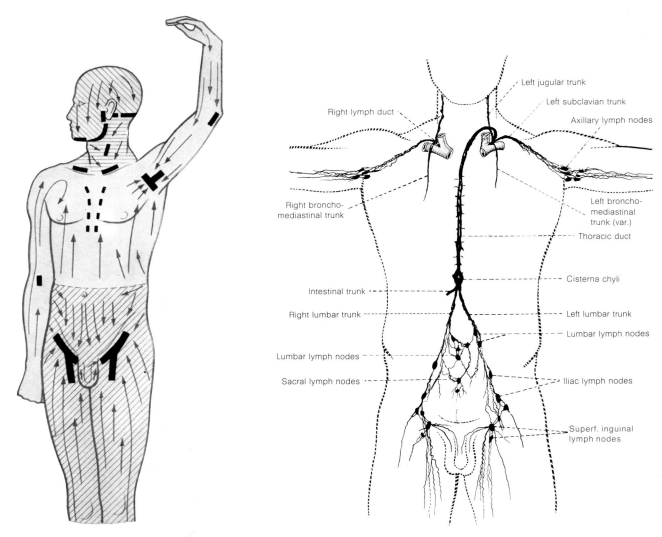

Fig. 95. Schematic descriptions of the most important regional lymph nodes (▬) and the four (I–IV) main areas of their sources (→). (From B. LEIBER: Der menschliche Lymphknoten. Urban & Schwarzenberg, Munich–Berlin 1961.)

Fig. 96. Schematic representation of the large lymph vessels of the human body. (From BENNINGHOFF/GOERTTLER: Lehrbuch der Anatomie des Menschen, Vol. 2, 12th ed. [Eds. H. FERNER und J. STAUBESAND]: Urban & Schwarzenberg, Munich–Vienna–Baltimore 1979.)

Region	Name of lymph nodes	Site
Head (I)	Submental Submandibular Superficial and deep parotid Retroauricular Occipital	under the chin on submandibular gland in front of ear and in parotid gland behind the ear on the insertion of the Trapezius m.
Neck (II)	Sup. superficial cervical Inf. superficial cervical	on the Sternocleidomastoid m. near the angle of the jaw in the side of the cervical triangle over the clavicle
Thorax and upper limb (III)	Superficial axillary	axilla
Lower half of the body (IV)	Superficial inguinal	groin

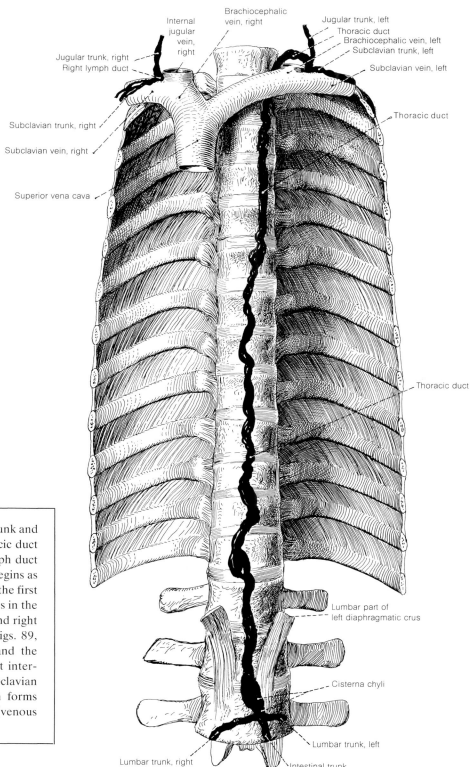

Internal
jugular
vein,
right

Brachiocephalic
vein, right

Jugular trunk, left
Thoracic duct
Brachiocephalic vein, left
Subclavian trunk, left

Subclavian vein, left

Jugular trunk, right
Right lymph duct

Thoracic duct

Subclavian trunk, right

Subclavian vein, right

Superior vena cava

Thoracic duct

The right bronchomediastinal trunk and the thoracic inflow of the thoracic duct are not shown. The largest lymph duct of the body, the thoracic duct, begins as the cysterna chyli at the level of the first or second lumbar vertebra. It lies in the thoracic cavity close to dorsal and right of the descending aorta. (See Figs. 89, 97.) It is between the aorta and the azygos vein, ventral to the right intercostal arteries, and joins the subclavian near the angle which this vein forms with the internal jugular vein (venous angle).

Lumbar part of
left diaphragmatic crus

Cisterna chyli

Lumbar trunk, left

Lumbar trunk, right

Intestinal trunk

Fig. 97. Schematic view of the principal lymphatic trunks. The right bronchomediastinal trunk and the thoracic inflow to the thoracic duct are not represented (compare Figs. 89 and 90).

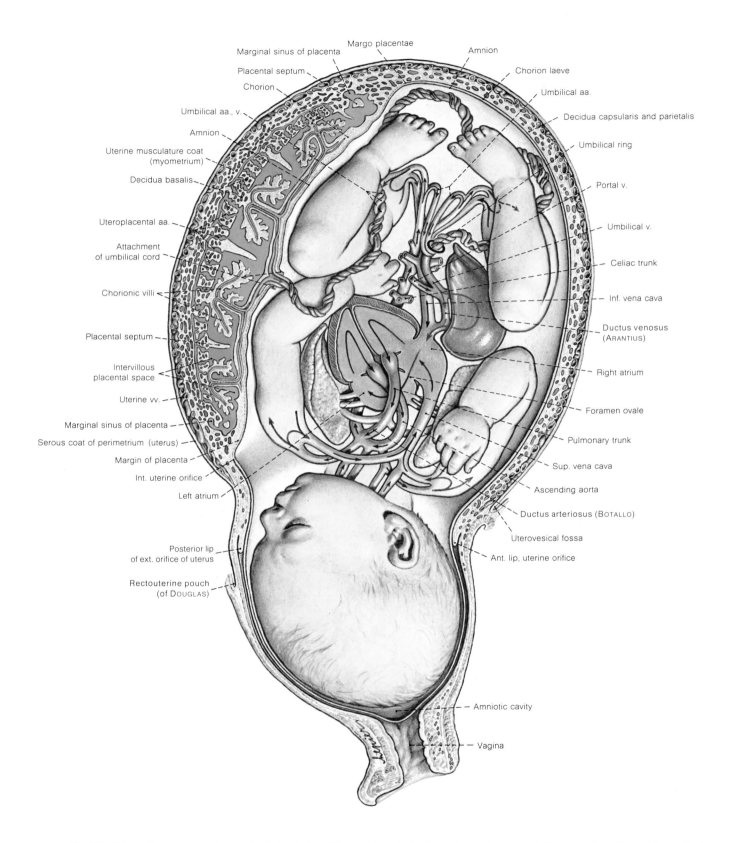

Marginal sinus of placenta

Margo placentae

Amnion

Placental septum

Chorion laeve

Chorion

Umbilical aa.

Umbilical aa., v.

Decidua capsularis and parietalis

Amnion

Umbilical ring

Uterine musculature coat
(myometrium)

Portal v.

Decidua basalis

Umbilical v.

Uteroplacental aa.

Celiac trunk

Attachment
of umbilical cord

Inf. vena cava

Chorionic villi

Ductus venosus
(ARANTIUS)

Placental septum

Right atrium

Intervillous
placental space

Foramen ovale

Uterine vv.

Marginal sinus of placenta

Pulmonary trunk

Serous coat of perimetrium (uterus)

Sup. vena cava

Margin of placenta

Ascending aorta

Int. uterine orifice

Ductus arteriosus (BOTALLO)

Left atrium

Uterovesical fossa

Posterior lip
of ext. orifice of uterus

Ant. lip, uterine orifice

Rectouterine pouch
(of DOUGLAS)

Amniotic cavity

Vagina

Fig. 98. Schematic representation of fetal circulation. The position of the fetus does not represent the normal position at the end of pregnancy. Oxygenated blood, red; venous blood, blue; mixed blood, violet.

Thoracic Viscera – Thymus

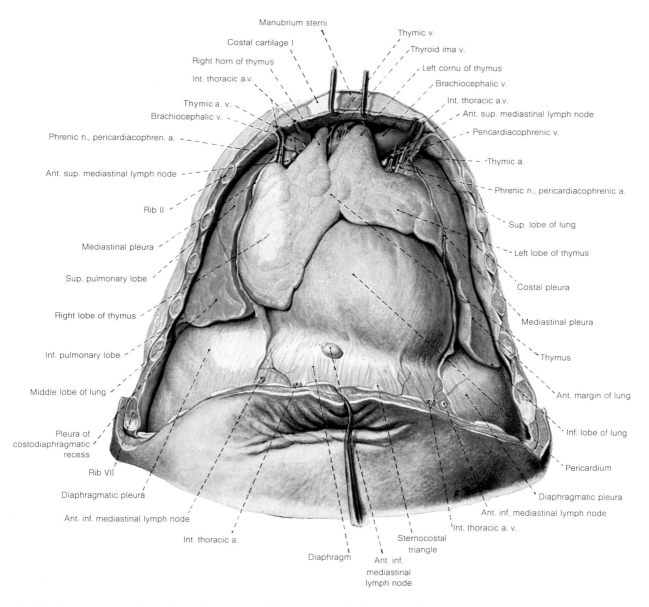

Manubrium sterni

Costal cartilage I

Right horn of thymus

Int. thoracic a.v.

Thymic a. v.

Brachiocephalic v.

Phrenic n., pericardiacophren. a.

Ant. sup. mediastinal lymph node

Rib II

Mediastinal pleura

Sup. pulmonary lobe

Right lobe of thymus

Inf. pulmonary lobe

Middle lobe of lung

Pleura of costodiaphragmatic recess

Rib VII

Diaphragmatic pleura

Ant. inf. mediastinal lymph node

Int. thoracic a.

Diaphragm

Ant. inf. mediastinal lymph node

Sternocostal triangle

Int. thoracic a. v.

Ant. inf. mediastinal lymph node

Diaphragmatic pleura

Pericardium

Inf. lobe of lung

Ant. margin of lung

Thymus

Mediastinal pleura

Costal pleura

Left lobe of thymus

Sup. lobe of lung

Phrenic n., pericardiacophrenic a.

Thymic a.

Pericardiacophrenic v.

Ant. sup. mediastinal lymph node

Int. thoracic a.v.

Brachiocephalic v.

Left cornu of thymus

Thyroid ima v.

Thymic v.

Fig. 99. Thoracic viscera of a newborn after removal of the anterior wall of the thorax. Ventral view. The relatively large thymus lies over the pericardium. (From PERNKOPF: Atlas der topographischen und angewandten Anatomie des Menschen, Vol. 2, 2nd ed. [Ed. H. FERNER]. Urban & Schwarzenberg, Munich–Vienna–Baltimore 1980.)

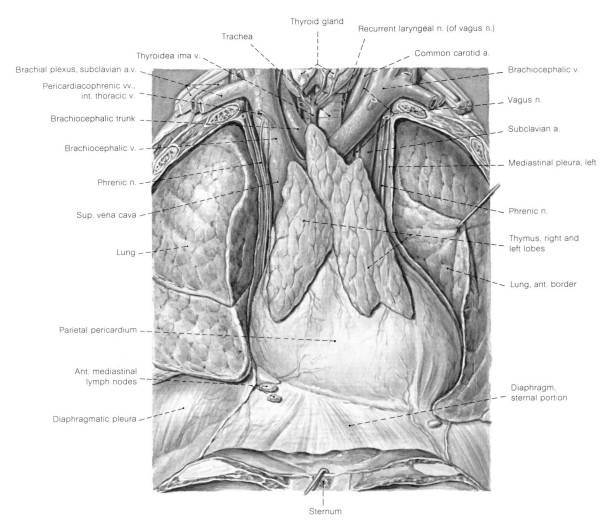

Thyroid gland

Trachea

Recurrent laryngeal n. (of vagus n.)

Thyroidea ima v.

Common carotid a.

Brachial plexus, subclavian a.v.

Brachiocephalic v.

Pericardiacophrenic vv.,
int. thoracic v.

Vagus n.

Brachiocephalic trunk

Subclavian a.

Brachiocephalic v.

Mediastinal pleura, left

Phrenic n.

Phrenic n.

Sup. vena cava

Thymus, right and
left lobes

Lung

Lung, ant. border

Parietal pericardium

Ant. mediastinal
lymph nodes

Diaphragm,
sternal portion

Diaphragmatic pleura

Sternum

Fig. 100. Thymus of a young boy *in situ.* Ventral view. The anterior chest wall is put aside after cutting the ribs and intercostal musculature. The costal and mediastinal pleura were partially removed to expose the closed pericardium. In the cervical region and the upper thorax, the lower part of the thyroid with its vessels, the trachea, and the large vessel trunks may be seen. The lungs have been pulled aside to expose the thymus.

72

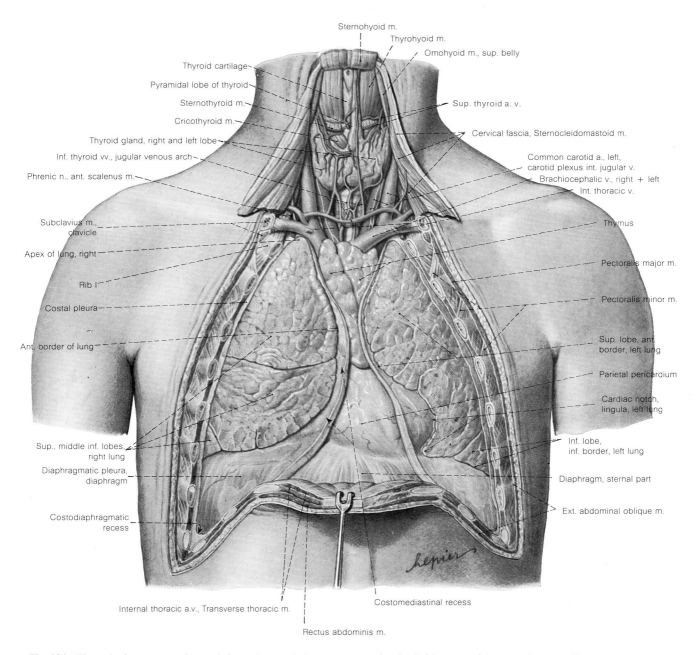

Sternohyoid m.

Thyrohyoid m.

Omohyoid m., sup. belly

Thyroid cartilage

Pyramidal lobe of thyroid

Sternothyroid m.

Cricothyroid m.

Sup. thyroid a. v.

Thyroid gland, right and left lobe

Cervical fascia, Sternocleidomastoid m.

Inf. thyroid vv., jugular venous arch

Common carotid a., left, carotid plexus int. jugular v.

Phrenic n., ant. scalenus m.

Brachiocephalic v., right + left

Int. thoracic v.

Subclavius m., clavicle

Thymus

Apex of lung, right

Pectoralis major m.

Rib I

Pectoralis minor m.

Costal pleura

Ant. border of lung

Sup. lobe, ant. border, left lung

Parietal pericardium

Cardiac notch, lingula, left lung

Sup., middle inf. lobes, right lung

Inf. lobe, inf. border, left lung

Diaphragmatic pleura, diaphragm

Diaphragm, sternal part

Costodiaphragmatic recess

Ext. abdominal oblique m.

Internal thoracic a.v., Transverse thoracic m.

Costomediastinal recess

Rectus abdominis m.

Fig. 101. Thoracic viscera *in situ.* Ventral view. The costal pleura was opened on both sides. Part of the ventral chest wall was dissected out. Large vascular trunks and the thyroid gland were exposed in the superior aperture of the thorax and neck.

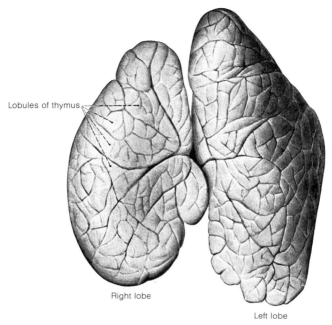

Fig. 102. Thymus of a 2-year old child. Ventral view.

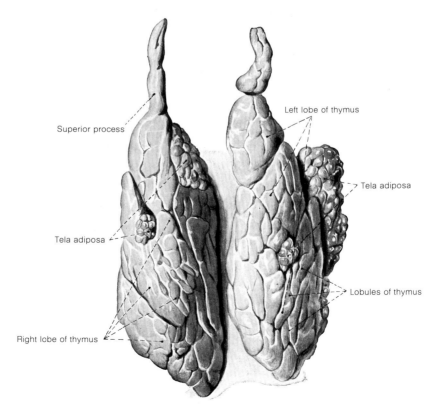

Fig. 103. Thymus gland, well preserved for this age, of a 24-year old man. Some of the underlying fat was removed. Ventral view.

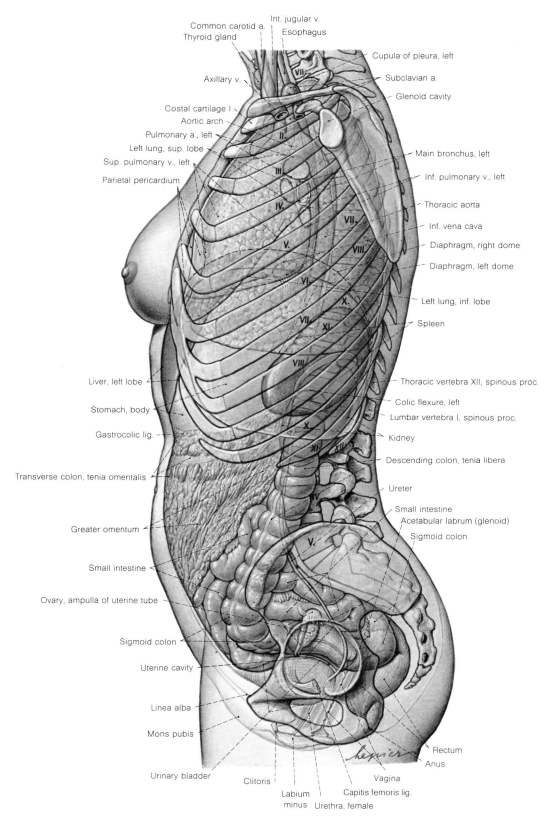

Common carotid a.
Thyroid gland
Int. jugular v.
Esophagus
Cupula of pleura, left
Subclavian a.
Glenoid cavity
Axillary v.
Costal cartilage I
Aortic arch
Pulmonary a., left
Left lung, sup. lobe
Sup. pulmonary v., left
Parietal pericardium
Main bronchus, left
Inf. pulmonary v., left
Thoracic aorta
Inf. vena cava
Diaphragm, right dome
Diaphragm, left dome
Left lung, inf. lobe
Spleen
Liver, left lobe
Stomach, body
Gastrocolic lig.
Transverse colon, tenia omentalis
Greater omentum
Small intestine
Ovary, ampulla of uterine tube
Sigmoid colon
Uterine cavity
Linea alba
Mons pubis
Urinary bladder
Thoracic vertebra XII, spinous proc.
Colic flexure, left
Lumbar vertebra I, spinous proc.
Kidney
Descending colon, tenia libera
Ureter
Small intestine
Acetabular labrum (glenoid)
Sigmoid colon
Rectum
Anus
Clitoris
Labium minus
Urethra, female
Vagina
Capitis femoris lig.

Fig. 104. Phantom silhouettes of the skeleton with the chest and abdominal organs of a woman. Designed to facilitate the development of a concept of relationships in x-ray diagnosis. Left side view. A part of the capitis femoris ligament is shown in the acetabular fossa. The urethra, vagina, and uterus are shown in a mediosagittal section. (From TANDLER and PERNKOPF.)

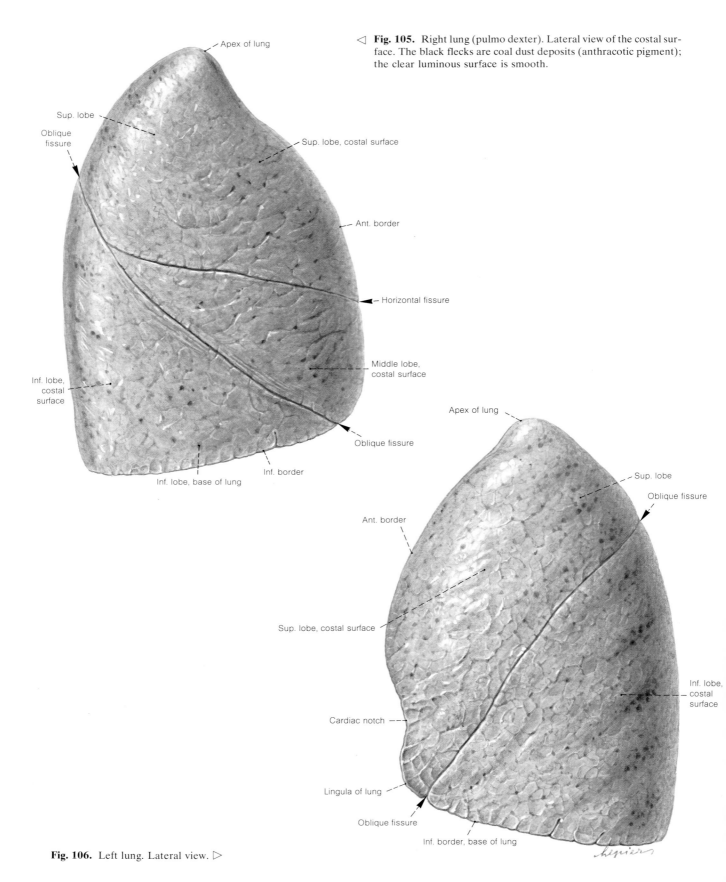

Apex of lung

◁ **Fig. 105.** Right lung (pulmo dexter). Lateral view of the costal surface. The black flecks are coal dust deposits (anthracotic pigment); the clear luminous surface is smooth.

Sup. lobe

Oblique fissure

Sup. lobe, costal surface

Ant. border

Horizontal fissure

Inf. lobe, costal surface

Middle lobe, costal surface

Oblique fissure

Inf. lobe, base of lung

Inf. border

Apex of lung

Sup. lobe

Oblique fissure

Ant. border

Sup. lobe, costal surface

Inf. lobe, costal surface

Cardiac notch

Lingula of lung

Oblique fissure

Inf. border, base of lung

Fig. 106. Left lung. Lateral view. ▷

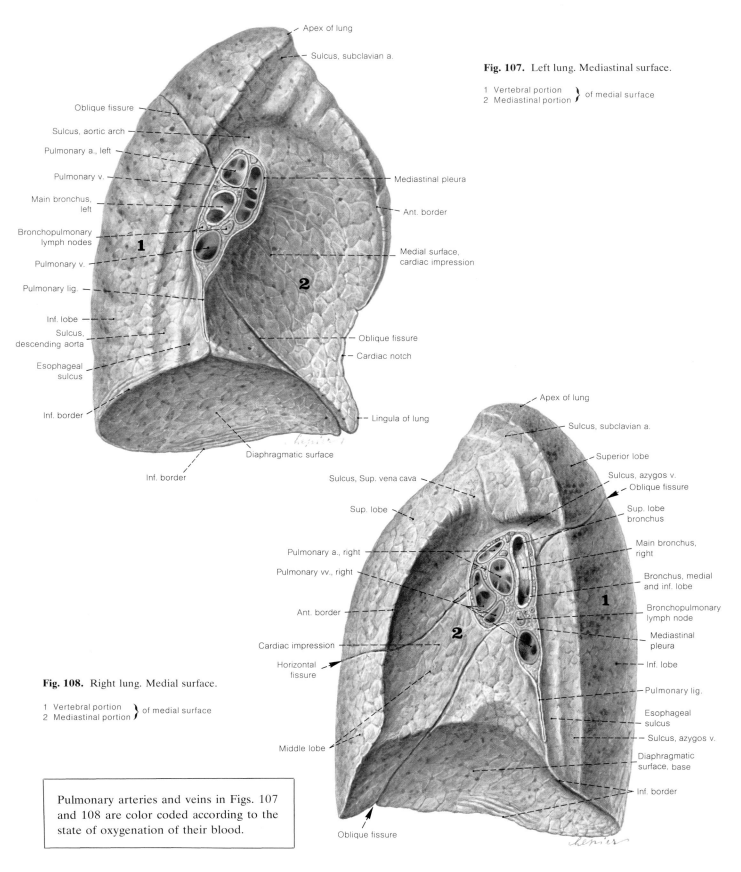

Apex of lung

Sulcus, subclavian a.

Fig. 107. Left lung. Mediastinal surface.

1 Vertebral portion } of medial surface
2 Mediastinal portion }

Oblique fissure

Sulcus, aortic arch

Pulmonary a., left

Pulmonary v.

Main bronchus, left

Bronchopulmonary lymph nodes

Pulmonary v.

Pulmonary lig.

Inf. lobe

Sulcus, descending aorta

Esophageal sulcus

Inf. border

Inf. border

Mediastinal pleura

Ant. border

Medial surface, cardiac impression

Oblique fissure

Cardiac notch

Lingula of lung

Diaphragmatic surface

Apex of lung

Sulcus, subclavian a.

Superior lobe

Sulcus, azygos v.

Oblique fissure

Sup. lobe bronchus

Main bronchus, right

Bronchus, medial and inf. lobe

Bronchopulmonary lymph node

Mediastinal pleura

Inf. lobe

Pulmonary lig.

Esophageal sulcus

Sulcus, azygos v.

Diaphragmatic surface, base

Inf. border

Sulcus, Sup. vena cava

Sup. lobe

Pulmonary a., right

Pulmonary vv., right

Ant. border

Cardiac impression

Horizontal fissure

Middle lobe

Oblique fissure

Fig. 108. Right lung. Medial surface.

1 Vertebral portion } of medial surface
2 Mediastinal portion }

Pulmonary arteries and veins in Figs. 107 and 108 are color coded according to the state of oxygenation of their blood.

77

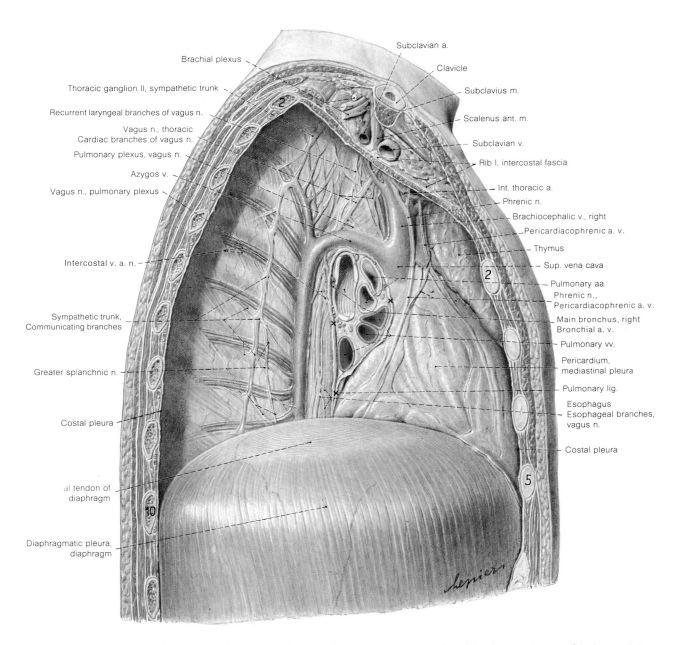

Fig. 109. Right pleural cavity after removal of the chest wall and the right lung. × × × = cut edge of the pleura at the root of the lung and the pulmonary ligament. Note: Pulmonary artery = blue; pulmonary vein = red.

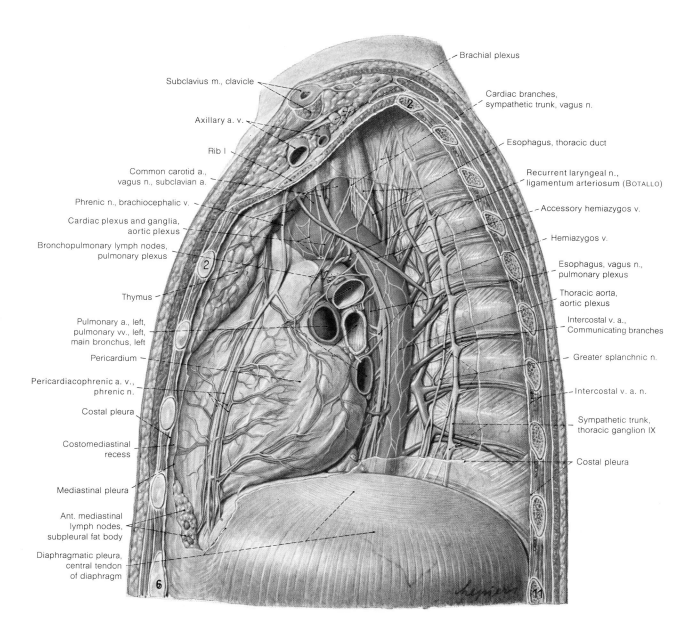

Brachial plexus

Cardiac branches,
sympathetic trunk, vagus n.

Esophagus, thoracic duct

Recurrent laryngeal n.,
ligamentum arteriosum (BOTALLO)

Accessory hemiazygos v.

Hemiazygos v.

Esophagus, vagus n.,
pulmonary plexus

Thoracic aorta,
aortic plexus

Intercostal v. a.,
Communicating branches

Greater splanchnic n.

Intercostal v. a. n.

Sympathetic trunk,
thoracic ganglion IX

Costal pleura

Subclavius m., clavicle

Axillary a. v.

Rib I

Common carotid a.,
vagus n., subclavian a.

Phrenic n., brachiocephalic v.

Cardiac plexus and ganglia,
aortic plexus

Bronchopulmonary lymph nodes,
pulmonary plexus

Thymus

Pulmonary a., left,
pulmonary vv., left,
main bronchus, left

Pericardium

Pericardiacophrenic a. v.,
phrenic n.

Costal pleura

Costomediastinal
recess

Mediastinal pleura

Ant. mediastinal
lymph nodes,
subpleural fat body

Diaphragmatic pleura,
central tendon
of diaphragm

Fig. 110. Left pleural cavity after the removal of the chest wall and left lung. A large part of the mediastinal and costal portions of the pleura and a smaller part of the diaphragmatic pleura were removed. The pericardium was left intact.

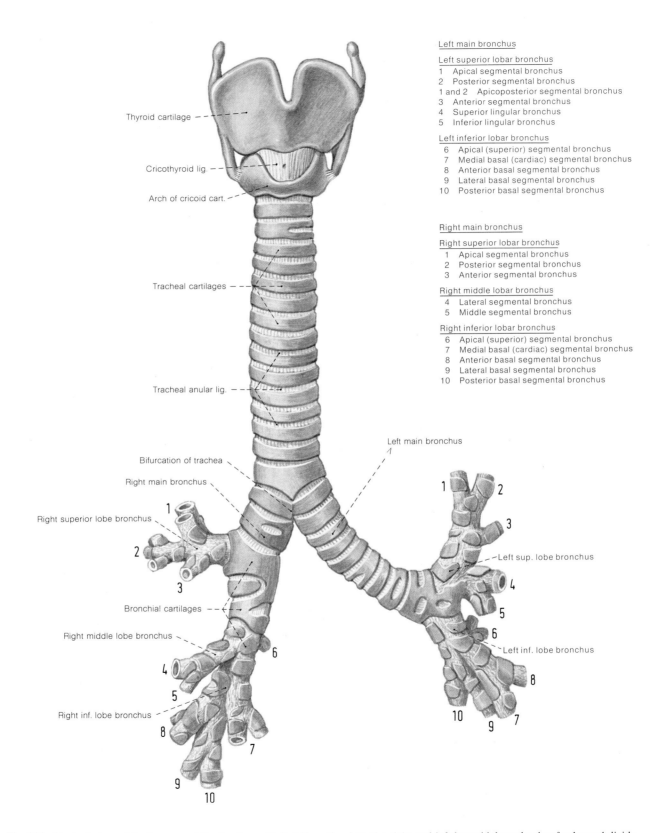

Left main bronchus

Left superior lobar bronchus
1 Apical segmental bronchus
2 Posterior segmental bronchus
1 and 2 Apicoposterior segmental bronchus
3 Anterior segmental bronchus
4 Superior lingular bronchus
5 Inferior lingular bronchus

Left inferior lobar bronchus
6 Apical (superior) segmental bronchus
7 Medial basal (cardiac) segmental bronchus
8 Anterior basal segmental bronchus
9 Lateral basal segmental bronchus
10 Posterior basal segmental bronchus

Right main bronchus

Right superior lobar bronchus
1 Apical segmental bronchus
2 Posterior segmental bronchus
3 Anterior segmental bronchus

Right middle lobar bronchus
4 Lateral segmental bronchus
5 Middle segmental bronchus

Right inferior lobar bronchus
6 Apical (superior) segmental bronchus
7 Medial basal (cardiac) segmental bronchus
8 Anterior basal segmental bronchus
9 Lateral basal segmental bronchus
10 Posterior basal segmental bronchus

Thyroid cartilage

Cricothyroid lig.

Arch of cricoid cart.

Tracheal cartilages

Tracheal anular lig.

Left main bronchus

Bifurcation of trachea

Right main bronchus

Right superior lobe bronchus

Left sup. lobe bronchus

Bronchial cartilages

Left inf. lobe bronchus

Right middle lobe bronchus

Right inf. lobe bronchus

Fig. 111. Ventral view of the larynx and the trachea with its bifurcation into the right and left bronchial trunks that further subdivide. The numbers 1–10 designate the division of the lobar bronchi (the secondary divisions) into the bronchial segments (the tertiary divisions). (See Figs. 117–120: Bronchopulmonary segments.)

Left main bronchus

Left superior lobar bronchus
1 Apical segmental bronchus
2 Posterior segmental bronchus
1 and 2 Apicoposterior segmental bronchus
3 Anterior segmental bronchus
4 Superior lingular bronchus
5 Inferior lingular bronchus

Left inferior lobar bronchus
6 Apical (superior) segmental bronchus
7 Medial basal (cardiac) segmental bronchus
8 Anterior basal segmental bronchus
9 Lateral basal segmental bronchus
10 Posterior basal segmental bronchus

Right main bronchus

Right superior lobar bronchus
1 Apical segmental bronchus
2 Posterior segmental bronchus
3 Anterior segmental bronchus

Right middle lobar bronchus
4 Lateral segmental bronchus
5 Middle segmental bronchus

Right inferior lobar bronchus
6 Apical (superior) segmental bronchus
7 Medial basal (cardiac) segmental bronchus
8 Anterior basal segmental bronchus
9 Lateral basal segmental bronchus
10 Posterior basal segmental bronchus

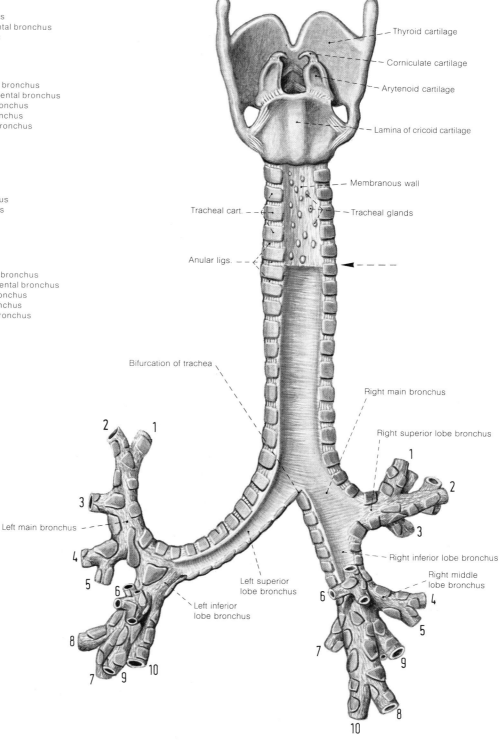

Fig. 112. Dorsal view of the larynx, trachea, and its bifurcation and the further division into lobar bronchi (3 on right, 2 on left), and the bronchial segments 1–10. Below the arrow (←), the superficial layer of the membranous wall is removed so that the muscular layer is visible with its horizontal or oblique interlacing fibers of muscle bundles. Observe the slight expansion of the air passage about the middle of its length.

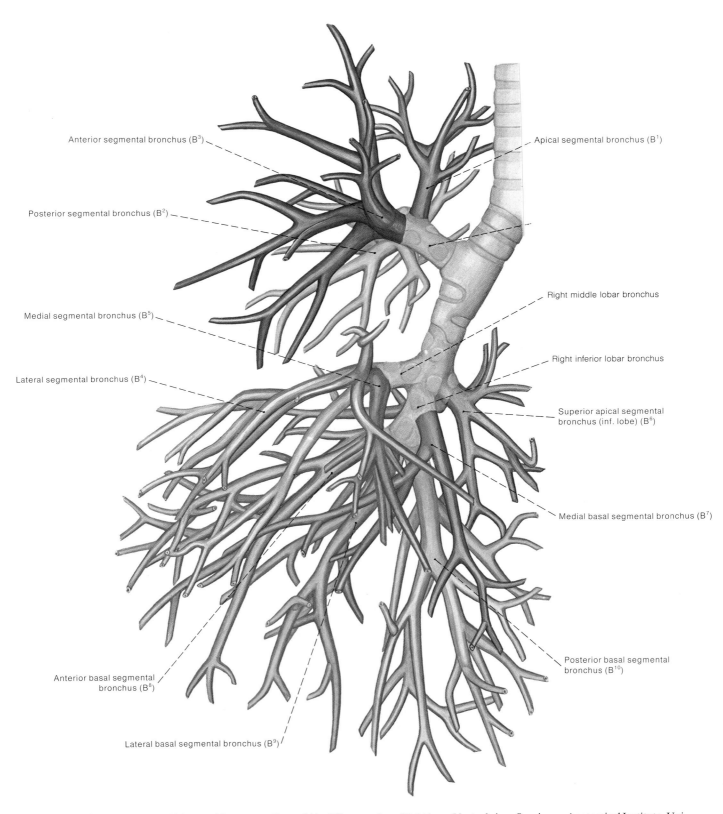

Anterior segmental bronchus (B³)

Posterior segmental bronchus (B²)

Medial segmental bronchus (B⁵)

Lateral segmental bronchus (B⁴)

Apical segmental bronchus (B¹)

Right middle lobar bronchus

Right inferior lobar bronchus

Superior apical segmental bronchus (inf. lobe) (B⁶)

Medial basal segmental bronchus (B⁷)

Anterior basal segmental bronchus (B⁸)

Lateral basal segmental bronchus (B⁹)

Posterior basal segmental bronchus (B¹⁰)

Fig. 113. Tracheobronchial tree with segmental bronchi in different colors. Right lung. Ventral view. Specimen: Anatomical Institute, University of Vienna. (From PERNKOPF: Atlas der topographischen und angewandten Anatomie des Menschen, Vol. 2, 2nd ed. [Ed. H. FERNER]. Urban & Schwarzenberg, Munich–Vienna–Baltimore 1980.)

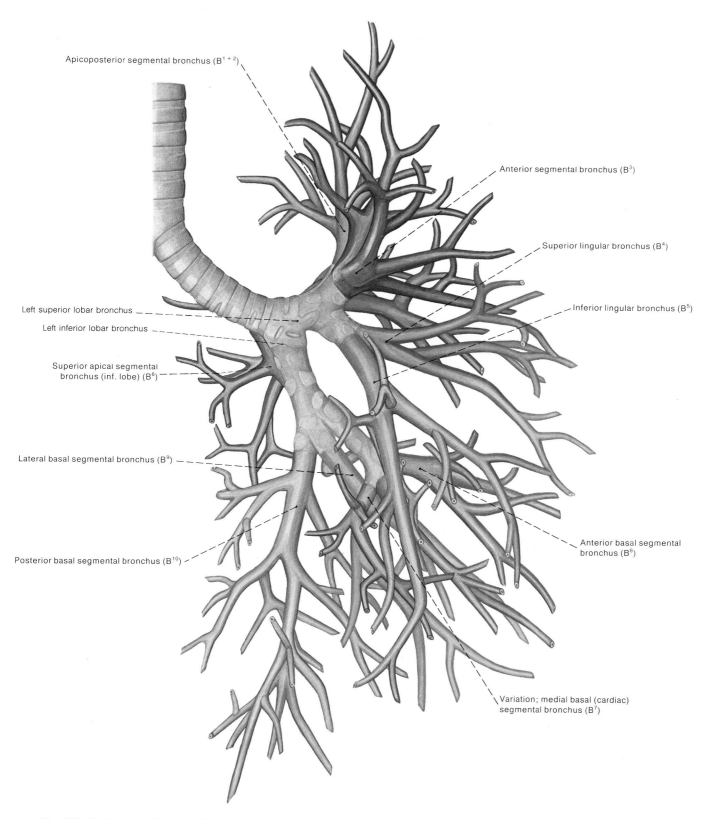

Apicoposterior segmental bronchus (B^{1+2})

Anterior segmental bronchus (B^3)

Superior lingular bronchus (B^4)

Left superior lobar bronchus

Left inferior lobar bronchus

Inferior lingular bronchus (B^5)

Superior apical segmental bronchus (inf. lobe) (B^6)

Lateral basal segmental bronchus (B^9)

Anterior basal segmental bronchus (B^8)

Posterior basal segmental bronchus (B^{10})

Variation; medial basal (cardiac) segmental bronchus (B^7)

Fig. 114. Tracheobronchial tree with segmental bronchi in different colors. Left lung. Ventral view. Specimen: Anatomical Institute, University of Vienna. (From PERNKOPF: Atlas der topographischen und angewandten Anatomie des Menschen, Vol. 2, 2nd ed. [Ed. H. FERNER]. Urban & Schwarzenberg, Munich–Vienna–Baltimore 1980.)

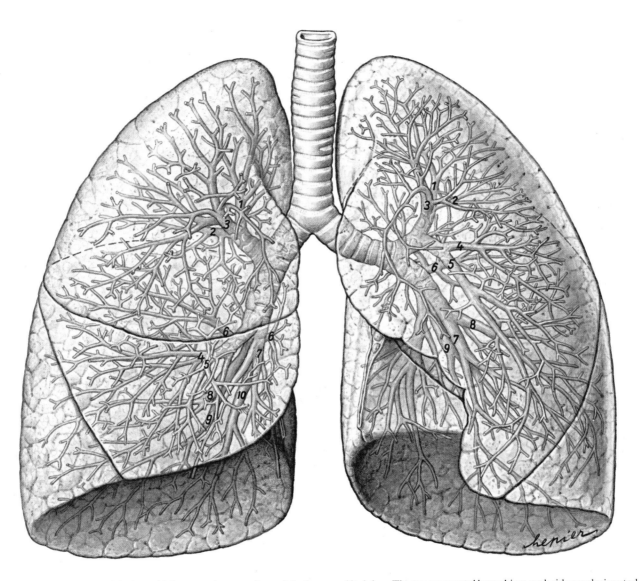

Fig. 115. Projection of the bronchial tree on the outer form of the lungs and its lobes. The ten segmental bronchi on each side are designated with different colors and numbered 1–10. The phantom diagrams are useful for orientation in identifying bronchial segments in x-ray views of the lungs.

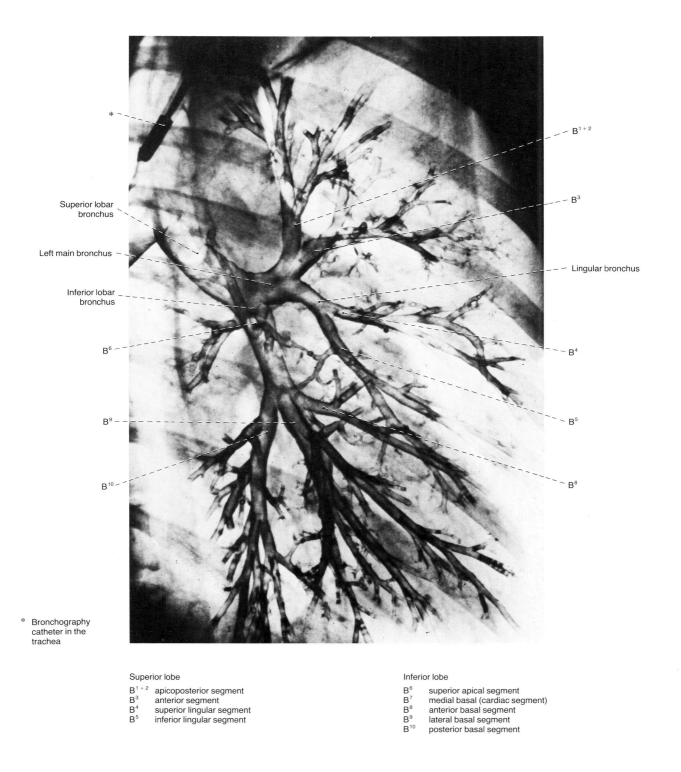

* — B^{1+2}

— B^3

Superior lobar
bronchus

Left main bronchus —

— Lingular bronchus

Inferior lobar
bronchus

B^6 —

— B^4

B^9 —

— B^5

B^{10} —

— B^8

* Bronchography
catheter in the
trachea

Superior lobe		Inferior lobe	
B^{1+2}	apicoposterior segment	B^6	superior apical segment
B^3	anterior segment	B^7	medial basal (cardiac segment)
B^4	superior lingular segment	B^8	anterior basal segment
B^5	inferior lingular segment	B^9	lateral basal segment
		B^{10}	posterior basal segment

Fig. 116. Bronchogram of left lung. From the superior lobar bronchus of the left lung there originate the segmental bronchi B^1 and B^2 (mostly with a common trunk) supplying an apicoposterior pulmonary segment. Due to the space requirements of the heart in the left side of the thorax, the segmental bronchi of the lingula are arranged on top of each other (B^4 = superior lingular bronchius, B^5 = inferior lingular bronchus); in contrast, the segments of the middle lobe of the right lung lie side by side (B^4 = lateral segmental bronchus, B^5 = medial basal segmental bronchus). One segmental bronchus, B^7 (medial basal segmental bronchus) is mostly missing on the left side. (Original: PD Dr. W. S. Rau, Zentrum Radiologie im Klinikum der Universität Freiburg i. Brsg.)

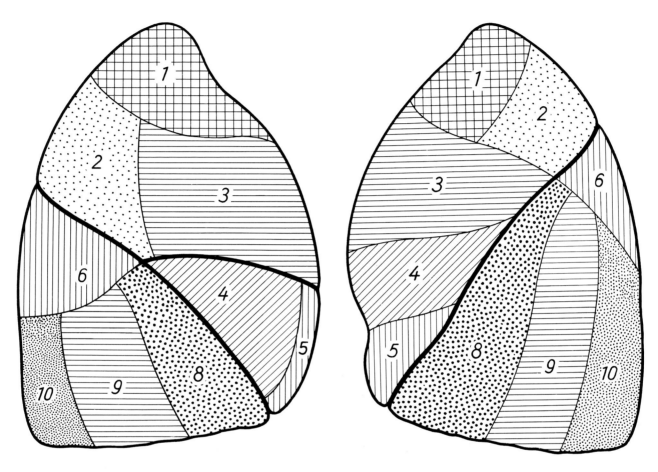

Fig. 117. The bronchopulmonary segments of the right lung. Lateral aspect.

Fig. 118. The bronchopulmonary segments of the left lung. Lateral aspect.

right lung

Superior lobe
1 Apical
2 Posterior
3 Anterior

Middle lobe
4 Lateral
5 Medial

Inferior lobe
6 Superior (apical)
8 Anterior basal
9 Lateral basal
10 Posterior basal

left lung

Superior lobe
1 Apical[1])
2 Posterior[1])
3 Anterior
4 Superior (lingular)
5 Inferior (lingular)

Inferior lobe
6 Superior (apical)
8 Anterior basal
9 Lateral basal
10 Posterior basal

[1]) 1 and 2 = Common apicoposterior segment.

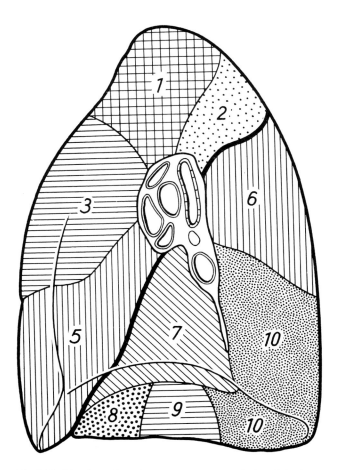 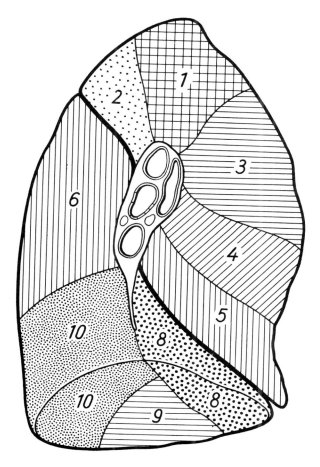

Fig. 119. The bronchopulmonary segments of the right lung. Medial aspect.

Fig. 120. The bronchopulmonary segments of the left lung. Medial aspect. Segment 7 can be found in the left lung only as an exception.

right lung

Superior lobe		Inferior lobe	
1	Apical	6	Superior (apical)
2	Posterior	7	Medial basal
3	Anterior		(cardiac)
		8	Anterior basal
Middle lobe		9	Lateral basal
4	Lateral	10	Posterior basal
5	Medial		

left lung

Superior lobe		Inferior lobe	
1	Apical[1]	6	Superior (apical)
2	Posterior[1]	(7)	Medial basal
3	Anterior	8	Anterior basal
4	Superior (lingular)	9	Lateral basal
5	Inferior (lingular)	10	Posterior basal

[1]) 1 and 2 = Common apicoposterior segment.

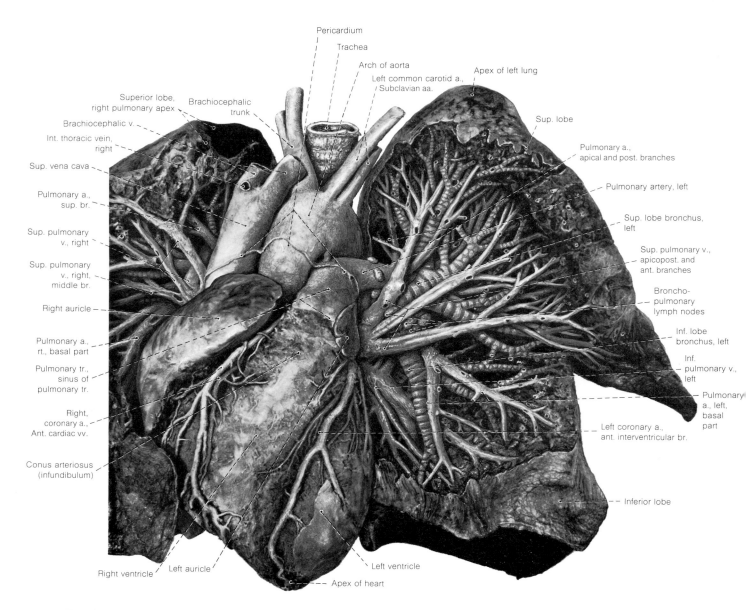

Pericardium

Trachea

Arch of aorta

Left common carotid a.,
Subclavian aa.

Apex of left lung

Superior lobe,
right pulmonary apex

Brachiocephalic
trunk

Brachiocephalic v.

Int. thoracic vein,
right

Sup. vena cava

Pulmonary a.,
sup. br.

Sup. pulmonary
v., right

Sup. pulmonary
v., right,
middle br.

Right auricle

Pulmonary a.,
rt., basal part

Pulmonary tr.,
sinus of
pulmonary tr.

Right,
coronary a.,
Ant. cardiac vv.

Conus arteriosus
(infundibulum)

Sup. lobe

Pulmonary a.,
apical and post. branches

Pulmonary artery, left

Sup. lobe bronchus,
left

Sup. pulmonary v.,
apicopost. and
ant. branches

Broncho-
pulmonary
lymph nodes

Inf. lobe
bronchus, left

Inf.
pulmonary v.,
left

Pulmonary
a., left,
basal
part

Left coronary a.,
ant. interventricular br.

Inferior lobe

Right ventricle

Left auricle

Left ventricle

Apex of heart

Fig. 121. Heart-lung preparation. Ventral view. Coronary vessels, heart-lung vessels, the bronchial tree, as well as some lymph nodes in the region of the left lung.

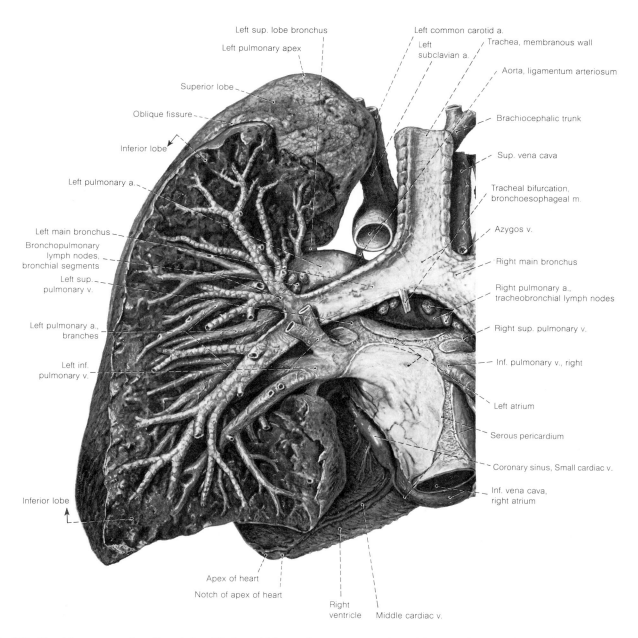

Left sup. lobe bronchus

Left pulmonary apex

Superior lobe

Oblique fissure

Inferior lobe

Left pulmonary a.

Left main bronchus

Bronchopulmonary
lymph nodes,
bronchial segments

Left sup.
pulmonary v.

Left pulmonary a.,
branches

Left inf.
pulmonary v.

Inferior lobe

Apex of heart

Notch of apex of heart

Right
ventricle

Middle cardiac v.

Left common carotid a.

Left
subclavian a.

Trachea, membranous wall

Aorta, ligamentum arteriosum

Brachiocephalic trunk

Sup. vena cava

Tracheal bifurcation,
bronchoesophageal m.

Azygos v.

Right main bronchus

Right pulmonary a.,
tracheobronchial lymph nodes

Right sup. pulmonary v.

Inf. pulmonary v., right

Left atrium

Serous pericardium

Coronary sinus, Small cardiac v.

Inf. vena cava,
right atrium

Fig. 122. Heart-lung preparation. Dorsal view. The bronchial tree, the coronary vessels, and the heart-lung vessels as well as the regional lymph nodes.

Figs. 123–126. Lung boundaries (red) and pleural boundaries (blue) in projection on the ribs, sternum, and vertebral column. Note the difference in the outline of the lung and the pleural borders. They are farthest apart in the region of the axillary line (hand's breadth).

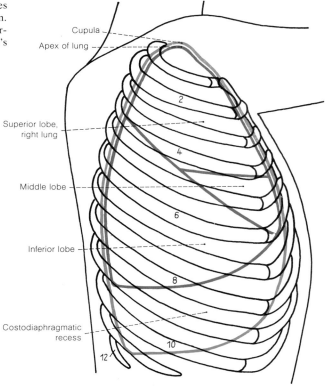

Cupula

Apex of lung

Superior lobe, right lung

Middle lobe

Inferior lobe

Costodiaphragmatic recess

Fig. 123. Lateral view from the right.

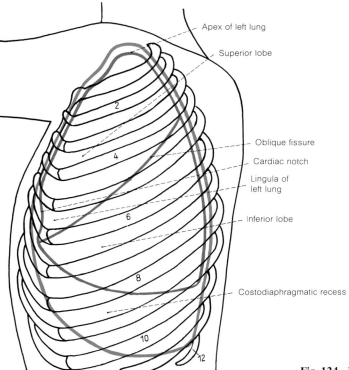

Apex of left lung

Superior lobe

Oblique fissure

Cardiac notch

Lingula of left lung

Inferior lobe

Costodiaphragmatic recess

Fig. 124. Lateral view from the left.

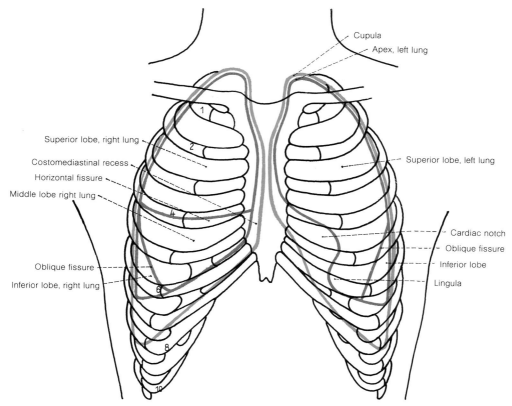

Cupula
Apex, left lung
Superior lobe, right lung
Costomediastinal recess
Horizontal fissure
Middle lobe right lung
Superior lobe, left lung
Cardiac notch
Oblique fissure
Inferior lobe
Lingula
Oblique fissure
Inferior lobe, right lung

Fig. 125. Ventral view.

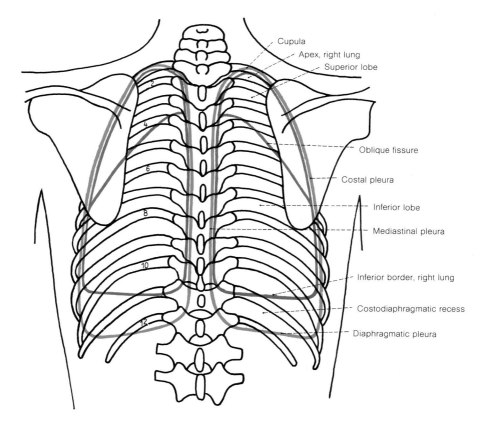

Cupula
Apex, right lung
Superior lobe
Oblique fissure
Costal pleura
Inferior lobe
Mediastinal pleura
Inferior border, right lung
Costodiaphragmatic recess
Diaphragmatic pleura

Fig. 126. Dorsal view.

Figs. 127–129. Schematic transverse sections through the thorax. Pleura: red, pericardium: blue.

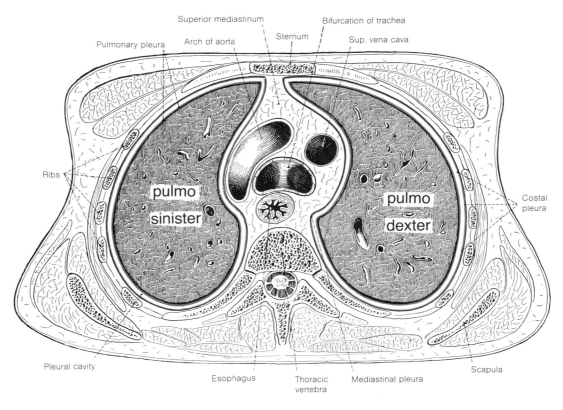

Fig. 127. Section at the level of the bifurcation of the trachea.

Pleural recesses.

Niches that are formed by the parietal pleura and into which the lungs can extend during maximal inspiration (complementary spaces):
Costodiaphragmatic recess between diaphragm and thoracic wall.
Costomediastinal recess between costal pleura and mediastinal pleura (left deeper than right).

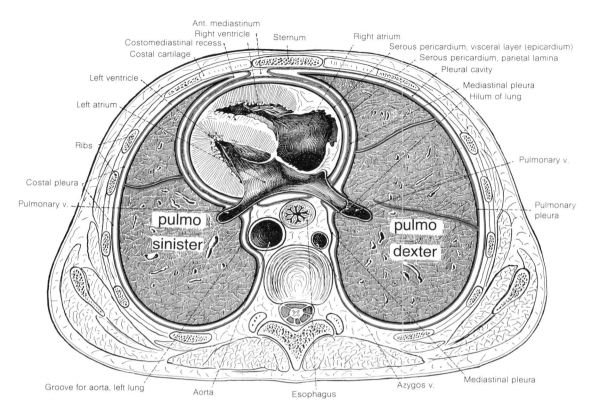

Fig. 128. Section at the level of the hilum of the lung.

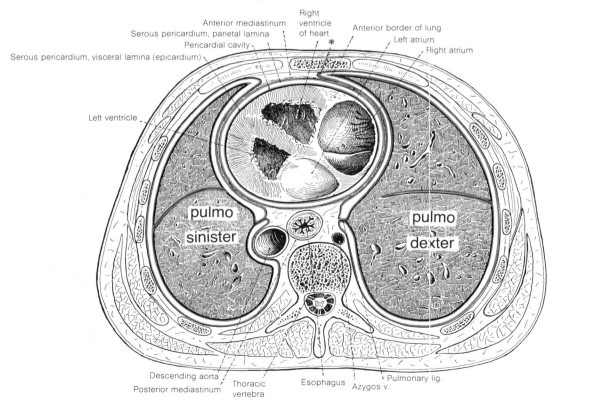

Fig. 129. Section caudal to the hilum of the lung at the level of the pulmonary ligaments. * Costomediastinal sinus.

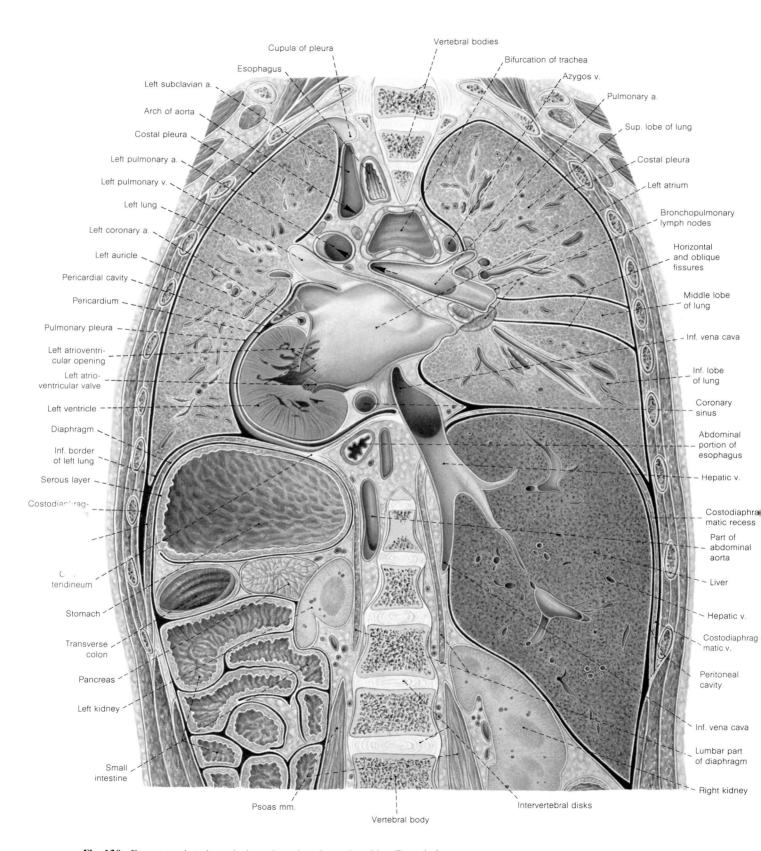

Cupula of pleura

Vertebral bodies

Esophagus

Bifurcation of trachea

Left subclavian a.

Azygos v.

Arch of aorta

Pulmonary a.

Costal pleura

Sup. lobe of lung

Left pulmonary a.

Costal pleura

Left pulmonary v.

Left atrium

Left lung

Bronchopulmonary lymph nodes

Left coronary a.

Horizontal and oblique fissures

Left auricle

Pericardial cavity

Middle lobe of lung

Pericardium

Pulmonary pleura

Inf. vena cava

Left atrioventri-cular opening

Inf. lobe of lung

Left atrio-ventricular valve

Coronary sinus

Left ventricle

Diaphragm

Abdominal portion of esophagus

Inf. border of left lung

Hepatic v.

Serous layer

Costodiaphrag-matic recess

Costodiaphrag-...

Part of abdominal aorta

C. tendineum

Liver

Stomach

Hepatic v.

Transverse colon

Costodiaphrag-matic v.

Pancreas

Peritoneal cavity

Left kidney

Inf. vena cava

Lumbar part of diaphragm

Small intestine

Right kidney

Psoas mm.

Intervertebral disks

Vertebral body

Fig. 130. Frozen section through thoracic and peritoneal cavities. Dorsal view.

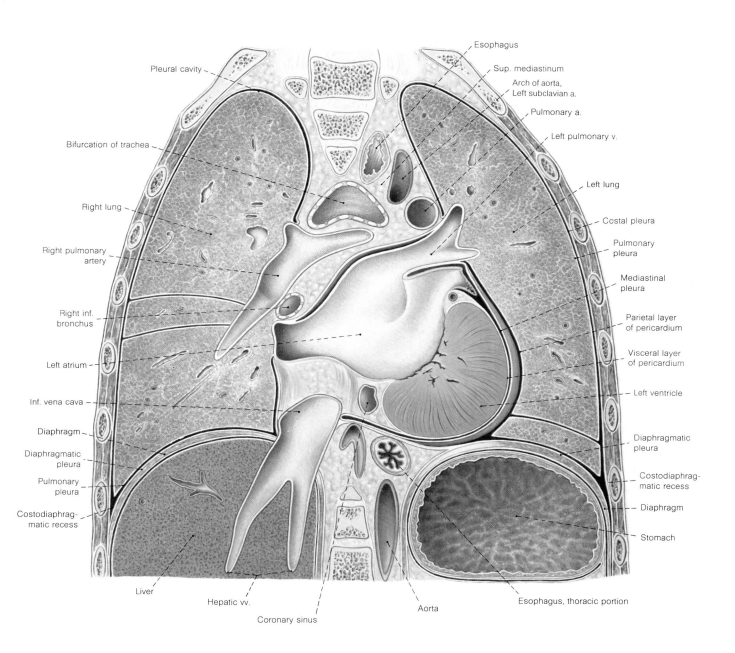

Fig. 131. Schematic view of pleura and pericardium. Frontal section. Ventral view. Pleura red, pericardium blue.

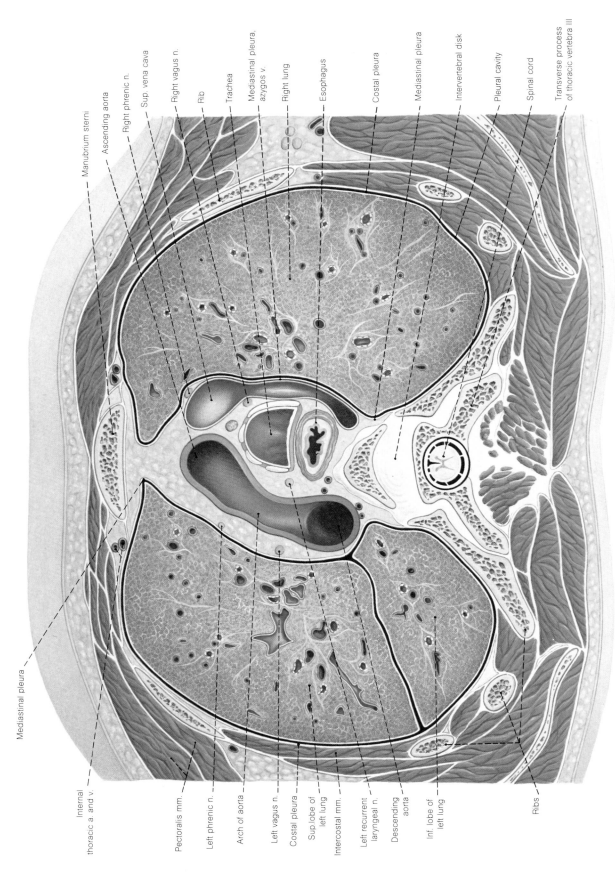

Manubrium sterni

Ascending aorta

Right phrenic n.

Sup. vena cava

Right vagus n.

Rib

Trachea

Mediastinal pleura, azygos v.

Right lung

Esophagus

Costal pleura

Mediastinal pleura

Intervertebral disk

Pleural cavity

Spinal cord

Transverse process of thoracic vertebra III

Mediastinal pleura

Internal thoracic a. and v.

Pectoralis mm.

Left phrenic n.

Arch of aorta

Left vagus n.

Costal pleura

Sup. lobe of left lung

Intercostal mm.

Left recurrent laryngeal n.

Descending aorta

Inf. lobe of left lung

Ribs

Fig. 132. Horizontal section through the cranial portion of the thoracic cavity at the level of the intervertebral disk between the 3rd and 4th thoracic vertebrae. Cranial view of the caudal sectional plane. Shown are the pleural sacs, lungs, viscera, vessels and nerves in the superior mediastinum. The arched end piece of the azygos vein running toward the superior vena cava is shown almost in its entire length. The arch of the aorta is sectional so that the convexity of the arch is located above the sectional plane.

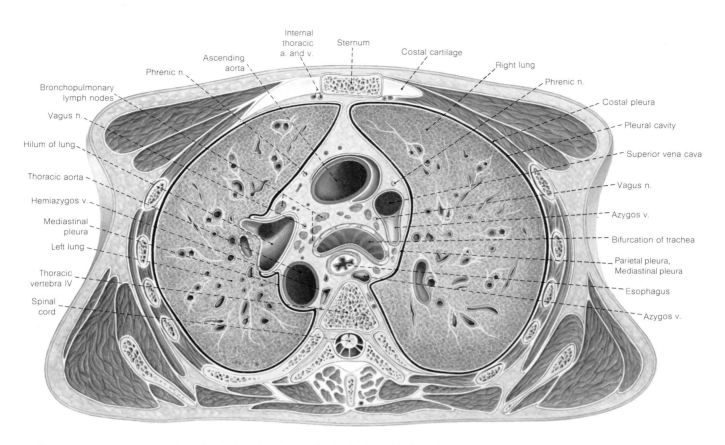

Fig. 133. Transverse section through the thoracic cavity at the level of the 4th thoracic vertebra.

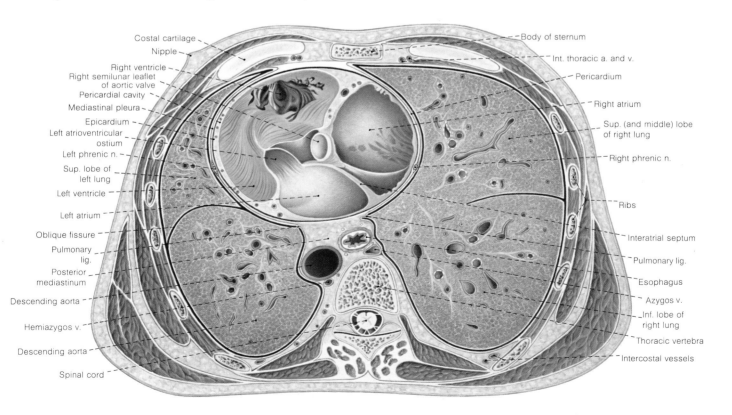

Fig. 134. Transverse section through the thoracic cavity at the level of the nipples.

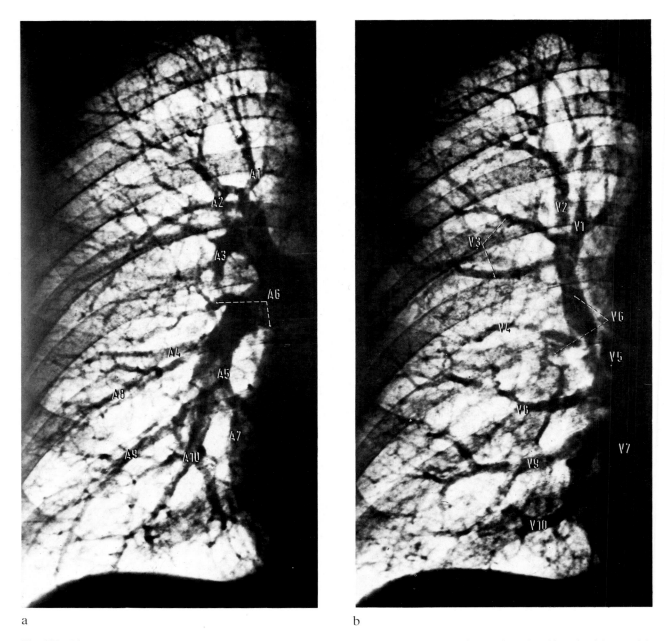

a   b

Fig. 135. Right pulmonary angiogram. Injection of a radioopaque medium through a catheter which was introduced into the right ventricle of the heart via the brachial vein, superior vena cava, and right atrium. Arterial phase (Fig. 135 a) and, after passage of the contrast medium through the pulmonary capillaries, venous phase (Fig. 135 b). The arteries run parallel to the bronchi and divide dichotomously. The segmental tributaries to the veins run more horizontally and combine further into an almost monopodial main axis. (Originals: PD Dr. W. S. Rau, Zentrum Radiologie am Klinikum der Universität Freiburg i. Brsg.)

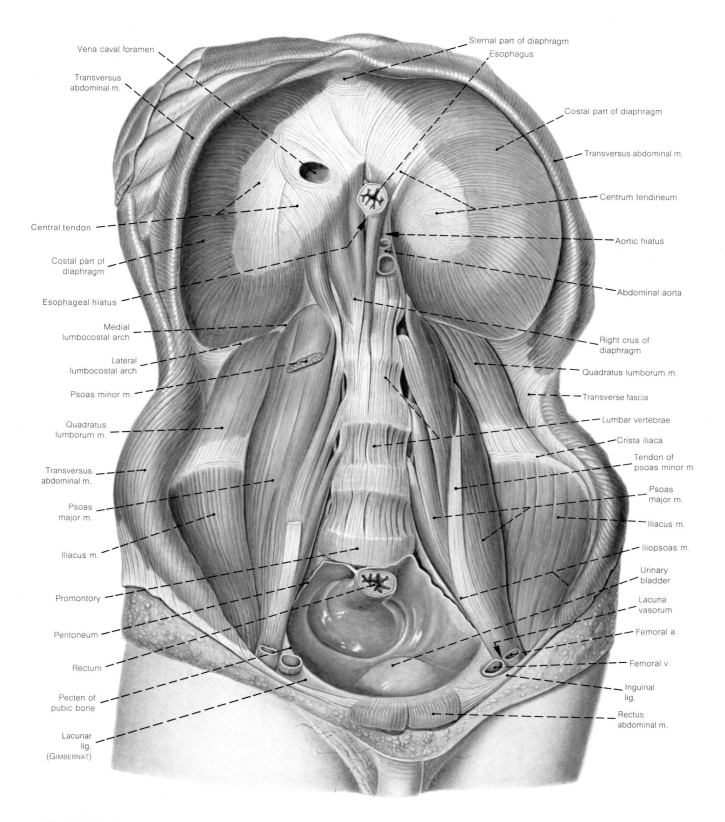

Fig. 136. Diaphragm and muscles of the posterior abdominal wall. Anterior abdominal wall opened, flat abdominal muscles reflected. Contents of the abdominal cavity removed. The thorax is extended backward so as to permit observation of the diaphragmatic dome from the inside. Lumbar spinal column in extreme lordosis. On the left side of the picture, a portion of the psoas minor muscle has been removed.

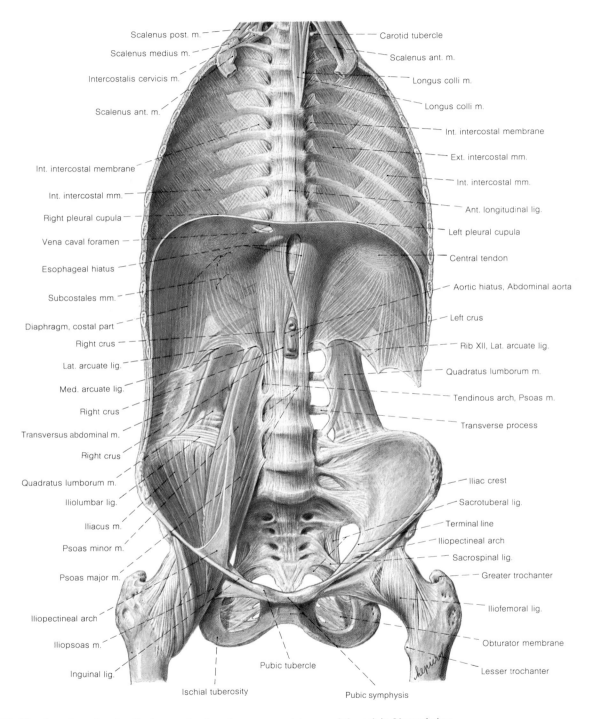

Scalenus post. m.

Scalenus medius m.

Intercostalis cervicis m.

Scalenus ant. m.

Int. intercostal membrane

Int. intercostal mm.

Right pleural cupula

Vena caval foramen

Esophageal hiatus

Subcostales mm.

Diaphragm, costal part

Right crus

Lat. arcuate lig.

Med. arcuate lig.

Right crus

Transversus abdominal m.

Right crus

Quadratus lumborum m.

Iliolumbar lig.

Iliacus m.

Psoas minor m.

Psoas major m.

Iliopectineal arch

Iliopsoas m.

Inguinal lig.

Ischial tuberosity

Pubic tubercle

Carotid tubercle

Scalenus ant. m.

Longus colli m.

Longus colli m.

Int. intercostal membrane

Ext. intercostal mm.

Int. intercostal mm.

Ant. longitudinal lig.

Left pleural cupula

Central tendon

Aortic hiatus, Abdominal aorta

Left crus

Rib XII, Lat. arcuate lig.

Quadratus lumborum m.

Tendinous arch, Psoas m.

Transverse process

Iliac crest

Sacrotuberal lig.

Terminal line

Iliopectineal arch

Sacrospinal lig.

Greater trochanter

Iliofemoral lig.

Obturator membrane

Lesser trochanter

Pubic symphysis

Fig. 137. The thoracic cavity, the diaphragm, the dorsal psoas musculature, and the pelvis. Ventral view.

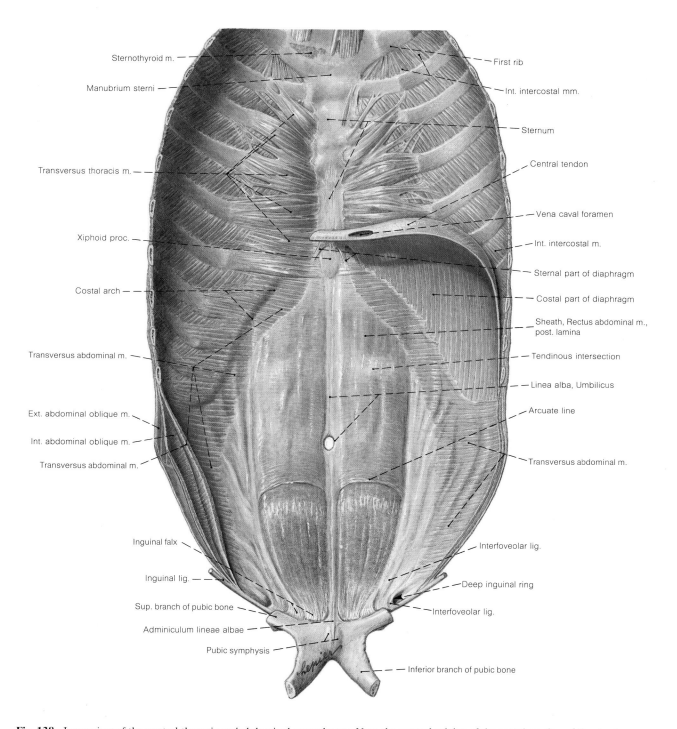

Sternothyroid m.

Manubrium sterni

Transversus thoracis m.

Xiphoid proc.

Costal arch

Transversus abdominal m.

Ext. abdominal oblique m.

Int. abdominal oblique m.

Transversus abdominal m.

Inguinal falx

Inguinal lig.

Sup. branch of pubic bone

Adminiculum lineae albae

Pubic symphysis

First rib

Int. intercostal mm.

Sternum

Central tendon

Vena caval foramen

Int. intercostal m.

Sternal part of diaphragm

Costal part of diaphragm

Sheath, Rectus abdominal m., post. lamina

Tendinous intersection

Linea alba, Umbilicus

Arcuate line

Transversus abdominal m.

Interfoveolar lig.

Deep inguinal ring

Interfoveolar lig.

Inferior branch of pubic bone

Fig. 138. Inner view of the ventral thoracic and abdominal musculature. Note the ventral origins of the costal portion of the diaphragm.

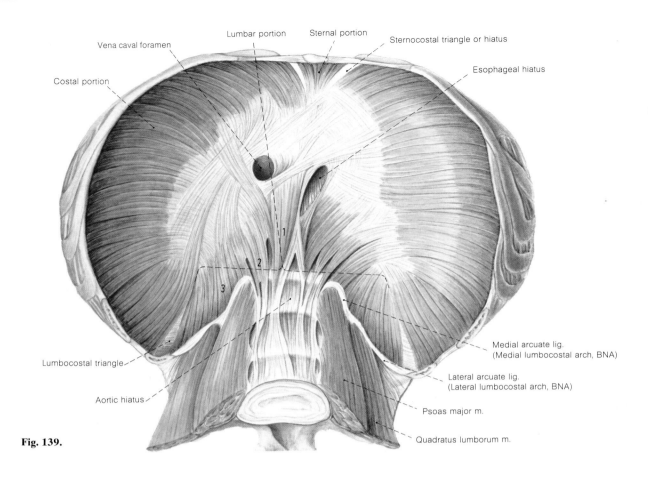

Fig. 139.

Diaphragm

Name	Origin		Insertion
Sternal portion	Inner surface of xiphoid process		In the central tendon: *vena caval foramen* In the lumbar portion: the *esophageal hiatus*
Costal portion	Inner surface of 6 caudal ribs (cartilages)		
Lumbar portion	Medial crus + intermediate crus (tendinous)	Ventral surface of lumbar vertebrae 2–4 (tendon), between the component of both sides: *hiatus aortica*	
	Lateral crus	Transverse process of lumbar vertebra 1 (2); medial and lateral lumbar costal arches	

Nerve: Phrenic nerve from the cervical plexus C 4 (3–5)

Function: Respiratory muscle (diaphragmatic breathing) produces inspiration, sustains abdominal muscular pressure

Name	Origin	Insertion
Quadratus lumborum muscle 4-sided muscle in dorsal wall of abdomen	Internal lip of crest of ilium; iliolumbar ligament	12th rib (medial border); transverse processes of upper 4 lumbar vertebrae

Nerve: Branches of 12th thoracic and upper 3 lumbar nerves (T 12; L 1–4)

Function: Depresses and fixes last rib (expiration); abducts or bends trunk to same side, when acting unilaterally

◁ **Fig. 139.** Ventral view of diaphragm. 1. Medial crus. 2. Intermediate crus. 3. Lateral crus.

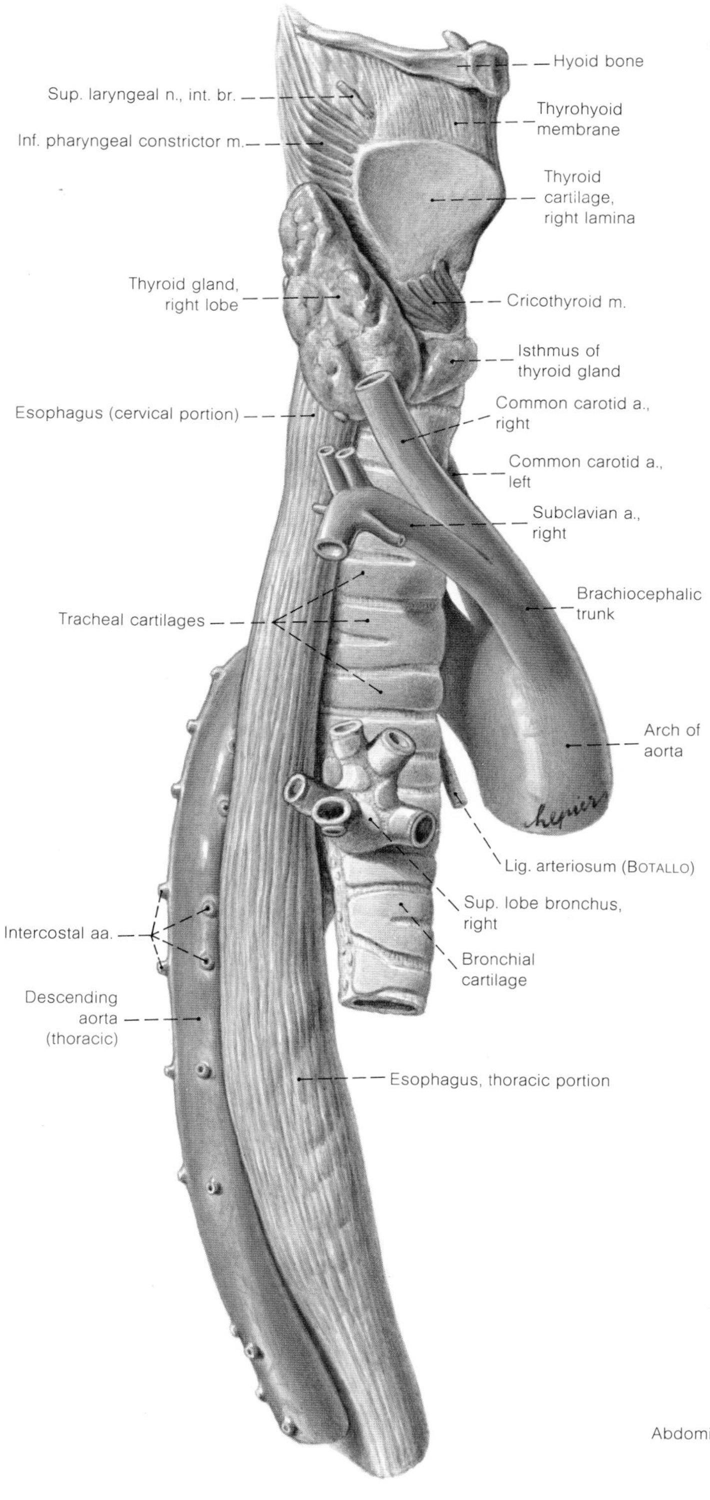

Sup. laryngeal n., int. br.

Inf. pharyngeal constrictor m.

Thyroid gland, right lobe

Esophagus (cervical portion)

Tracheal cartilages

Intercostal aa.

Descending aorta (thoracic)

Hyoid bone

Thyrohyoid membrane

Thyroid cartilage, right lamina

Cricothyroid m.

Isthmus of thyroid gland

Common carotid a., right

Common carotid a., left

Subclavian a., right

Brachiocephalic trunk

Arch of aorta

Lig. arteriosum (BOTALLO)

Sup. lobe bronchus, right

Bronchial cartilage

Esophagus, thoracic portion

Common carotid artery, right

Subclavian a., right

Esophagus

Brachiocephalic trunk

Right main bronchus

Right sup. lobe of bronchus

Trachea

Common carotid a., left

Subclavian a., left

Aortic arch

Lig. arteriosum (BOTALLO)

Tracheal bifurcation

Left main bronchus

Descending aorta (thoracic)

Esophagus (thoracic portion), muscle layer

Diaphragm, central tendon

Inf. vena cava opening

Diaphragm, lumbar part, right crus

Inf. phrenic aa.

Aortic hiatus

Celiac trunk

Abdominal aorta (descending)

Esophageal hiatus

Esophagus, abdominal part

Cardia

Diaphragm, lumbar part, left crus

Fig. 140. The air and food passageways in the cervical and thoracic regions and their relationship to neighboring organs (aorta, bronchi, trachea etc.). View from the right.

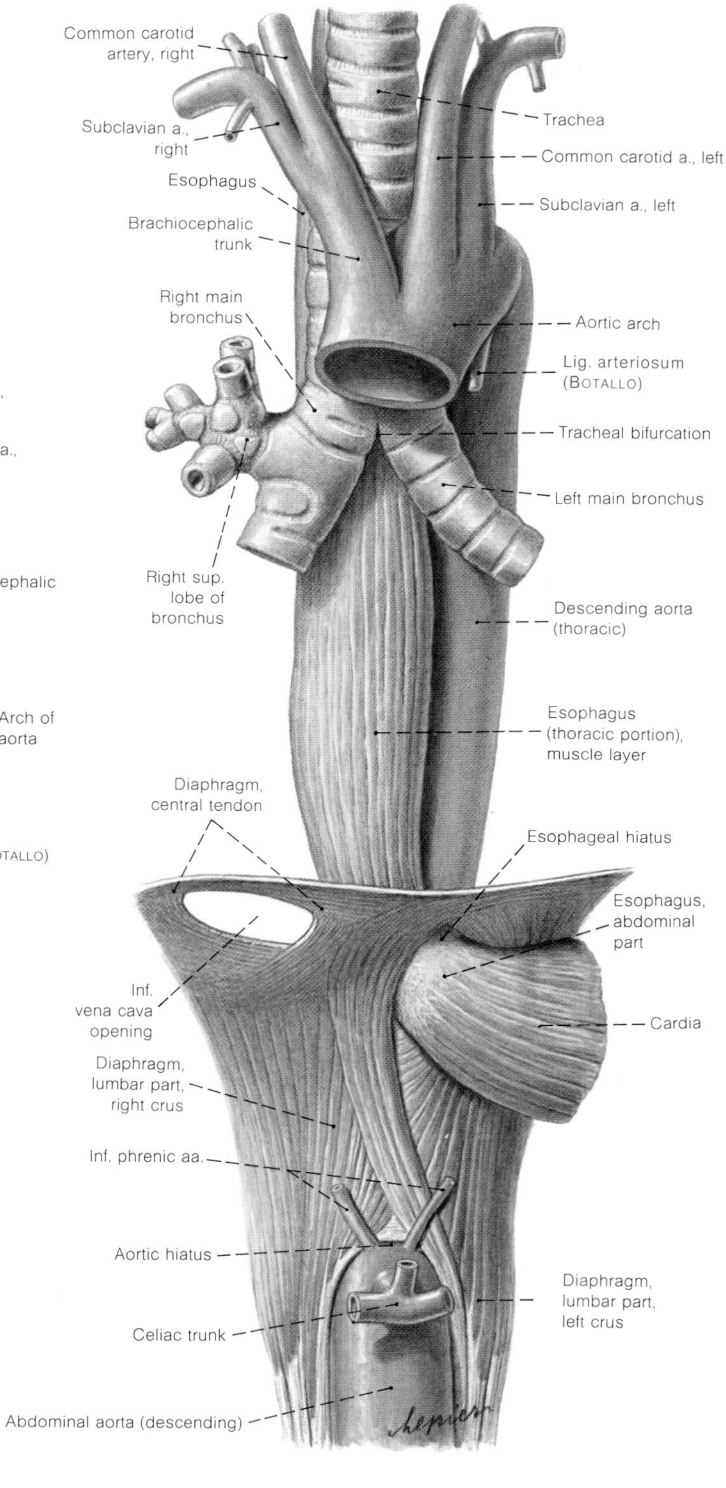

Fig. 141. Ventral view of lower esophagus, trachea, aorta, and part of the stomach and diaphragm, with a large opening for the inferior vena cava.

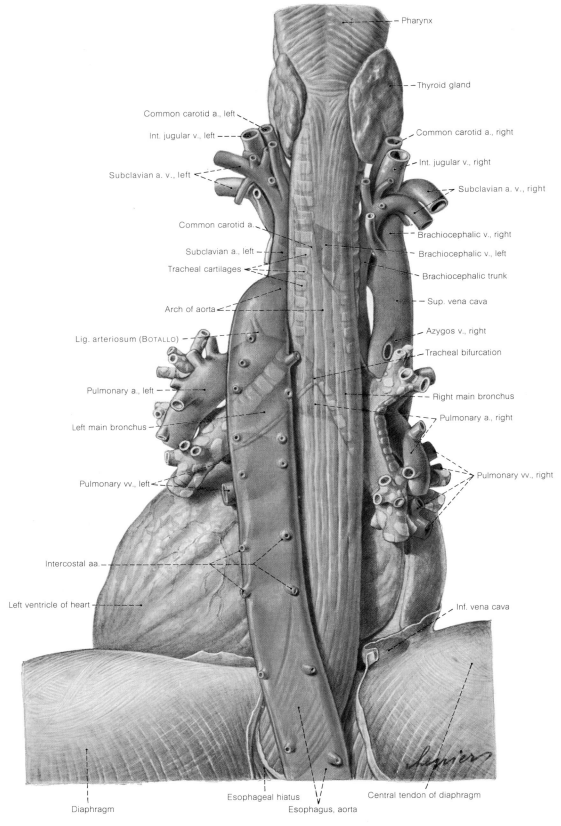

Pharynx

Thyroid gland

Common carotid a., left

Int. jugular v., left

Common carotid a., right

Int. jugular v., right

Subclavian a. v., left

Subclavian a. v., right

Common carotid a.

Brachiocephalic v., right

Subclavian a., left

Brachiocephalic v., left

Tracheal cartilages

Brachiocephalic trunk

Sup. vena cava

Arch of aorta

Azygos v., right

Lig. arteriosum (BOTALLO)

Tracheal bifurcation

Pulmonary a., left

Right main bronchus

Left main bronchus

Pulmonary a., right

Pulmonary vv., right

Pulmonary vv., left

Intercostal aa.

Inf. vena cava

Left ventricle of heart

Diaphragm

Esophageal hiatus

Central tendon of diaphragm

Esophagus, aorta

Fig. 142. Dorsal view of the esophagus. Its relative position is seen to the thyroid, trachea and its branches, to the heart and vessels near the heart, to the thoracic aorta, and to the diaphragm.

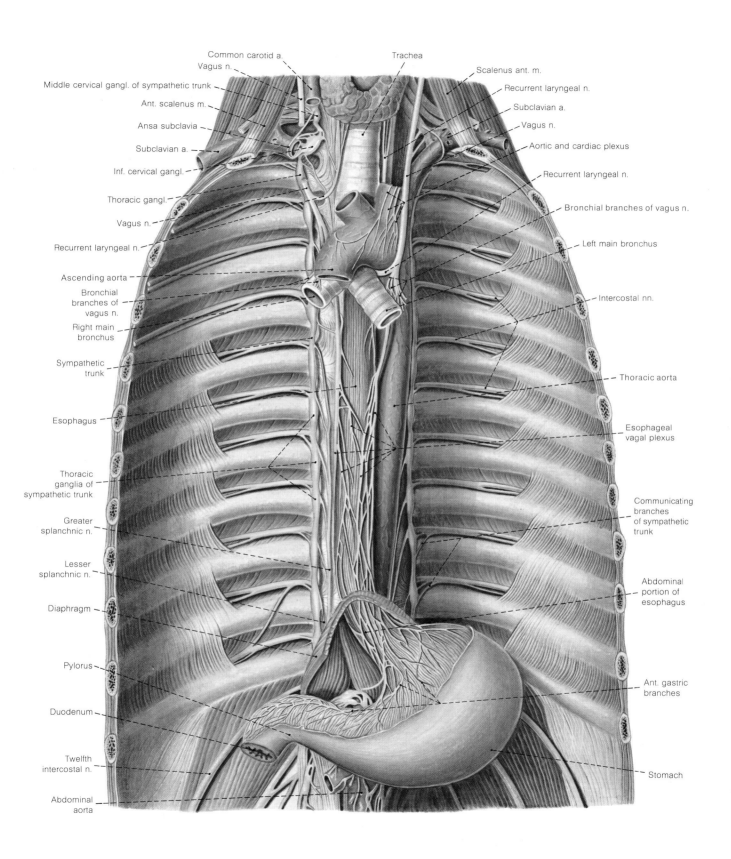

Fig. 143. Esophagus with esophageal plexus, vagus nerves and sympathetic trunk. Ventral view.

Trunk

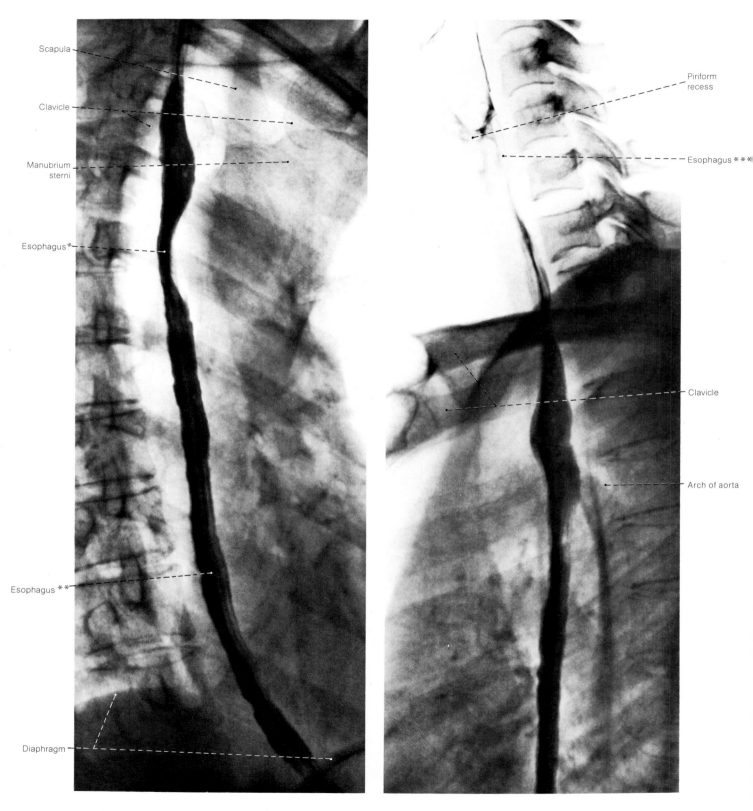

Fig. 144. Roentgenograms of esophagus (right and left antero-oblique projections). (From L. WICKE: Atlas der Röntgenanatomie, 2nd ed. Urban & Schwarzenberg, Munich–Vienna–Baltimore 1980.) * 2nd esophageal narrowing caused by the arch of the aorta. ** retrocardial portion of esophagus. *** proximal esophagus sphincter (1st narrowing).

Anterior Abdominal Wall

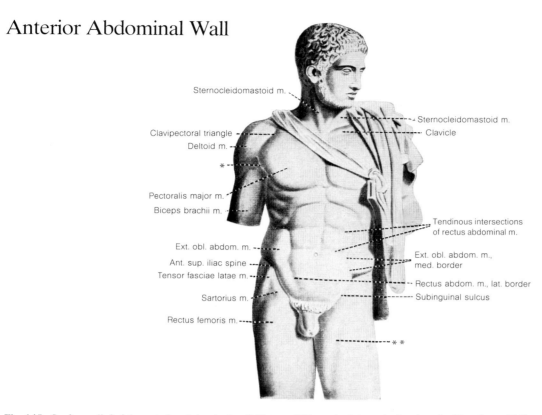

Sternocleidomastoid m.

Clavipectoral triangle
Deltoid m.

*

Pectoralis major m.
Biceps brachii m.

Ext. obl. abdom. m.
Ant. sup. iliac spine
Tensor fasciae latae m.

Sartorius m.

Rectus femoris m.

Sternocleidomastoid m.
Clavicle

Tendinous intersections
of rectus abdominal m.

Ext. obl. abdom. m.,
med. border

Rectus abdom. m., lat. border
Subinguinal sulcus

**

Fig. 145. Surface relief of the anterior abdominal wall. Statue of Diomede. * Anterior border of axillary fossa. ** Groove medial to the sartorius m. (From Benninghoff/Goerttler: Lehrbuch der Anatomie des Menschen, Vol. 1, 13th ed. [Eds. H. Ferner and J. Staubesand]. Urban & Schwarzenberg, Munich–Vienna–Baltimore 1980.)

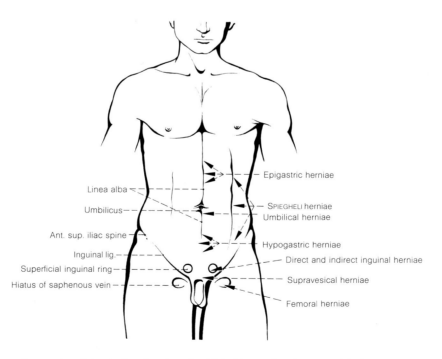

Linea alba
Umbilicus

Ant. sup. iliac spine

Inguinal lig.
Superficial inguinal ring
Hiatus of saphenous vein

Epigastric herniae

Spiegheli herniae
Umbilical herniae

Hypogastric herniae

Direct and indirect inguinal herniae

Supravesical herniae

Femoral herniae

Fig. 146. Herniation sites on the anterior abdominal wall and on the thigh (hiatus of saphenous vein). (From Benninghoff/Goerttler: Lehrbuch der Anatomie des Menschen, Vol. 1, 13th ed. [Eds. H. Ferner and J. Staubesand]. Urban & Schwarzenberg, Munich–Vienna–Baltimore 1980.)

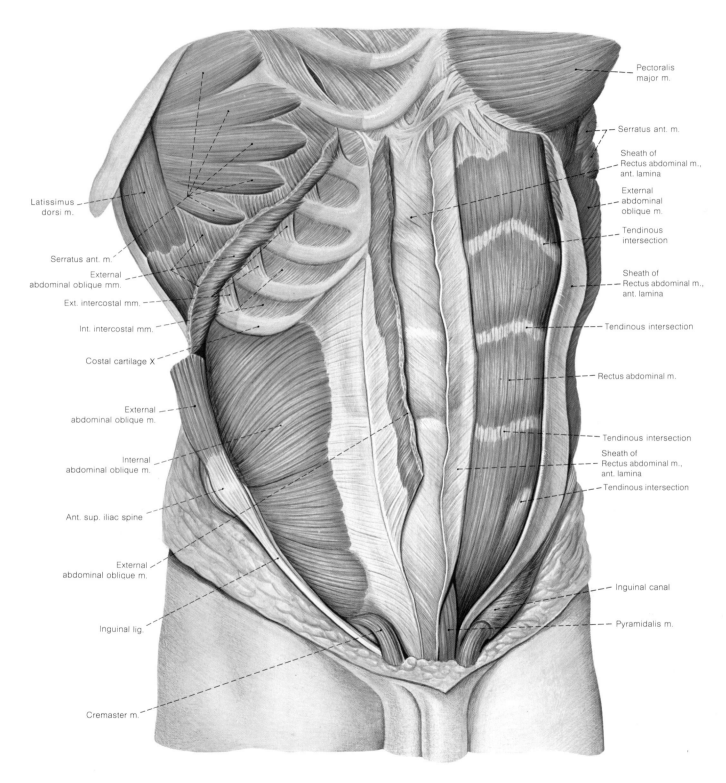

Pectoralis major m.

Serratus ant. m.

Sheath of Rectus abdominal m., ant. lamina

External abdominal oblique m.

Tendinous intersection

Sheath of Rectus abdominal m., ant. lamina

Tendinous intersection

Rectus abdominal m.

Tendinous intersection

Sheath of Rectus abdominal m., ant. lamina

Tendinous intersection

Inguinal canal

Pyramidalis m.

Latissimus dorsi m.

Serratus ant. m.

External abdominal oblique mm.

Ext. intercostal mm.

Int. intercostal mm.

Costal cartilage X

External abdominal oblique m.

Internal abdominal oblique m.

Ant. sup. iliac spine

External abdominal oblique m.

Inguinal lig.

Cremaster m.

Fig. 147. Abdominal musculature seen from ventral and right. On the left, the outer layer of the rectus sheath has been opened along its midline, the rectus abdominal and pyramidalis muscles are exposed. On the right, the external oblique abdominal muscle has been cut (T-section) in order to display the internal oblique abdominal muscle.

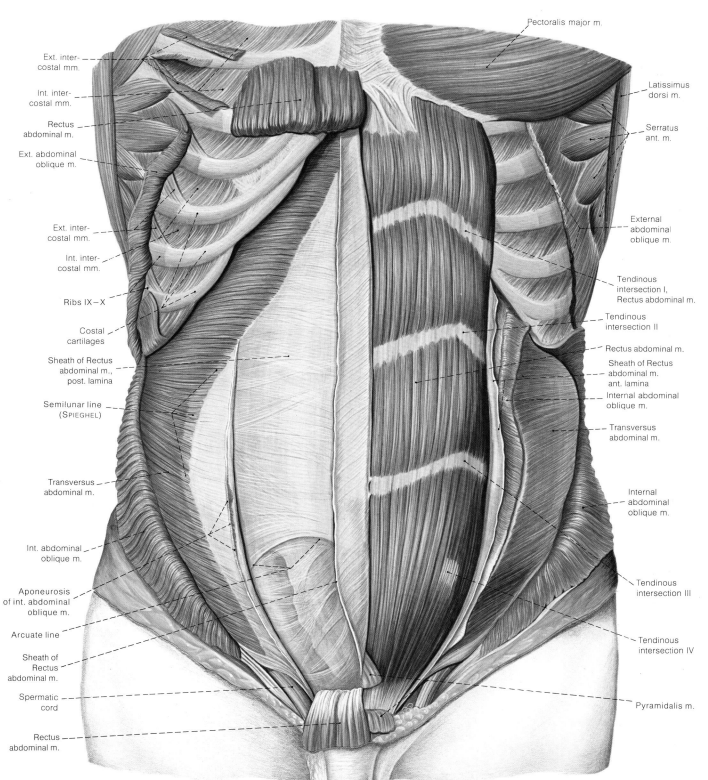

Pectoralis major m.

Ext. inter-costal mm.

Int. inter-costal mm.

Rectus abdominal m.

Ext. abdominal oblique m.

Ext. inter-costal mm.

Int. inter-costal mm.

Ribs IX–X

Costal cartilages

Sheath of Rectus abdominal m., post. lamina

Semilunar line (SPIEGHEL)

Transversus abdominal m.

Int. abdominal oblique m.

Aponeurosis of int. abdominal oblique m.

Arcuate line

Sheath of Rectus abdominal m.

Spermatic cord

Rectus abdominal m.

Latissimus dorsi m.

Serratus ant. m.

External abdominal oblique m.

Tendinous intersection I, Rectus abdominal m.

Tendinous intersection II

Rectus abdominal m.

Sheath of Rectus abdominal m. ant. lamina

Internal abdominal oblique m.

Transversus abdominal m.

Internal abdominal oblique m.

Tendinous intersection III

Tendinous intersection IV

Pyramidalis m.

Fig. 148. Deep layers of the abdominal muscles. On the left, the pyramidalis muscle is cut in order to display the tendon of the exposed rectus abdominal muscle; the obliquus inferius abdominal muscle is cut. On the right, the rectus abdominal and obliquus inferius abdominal muscles are sectioned in order to display the posterior layer of the rectus sheath with the arcuate line as well as the semilunar line.

109

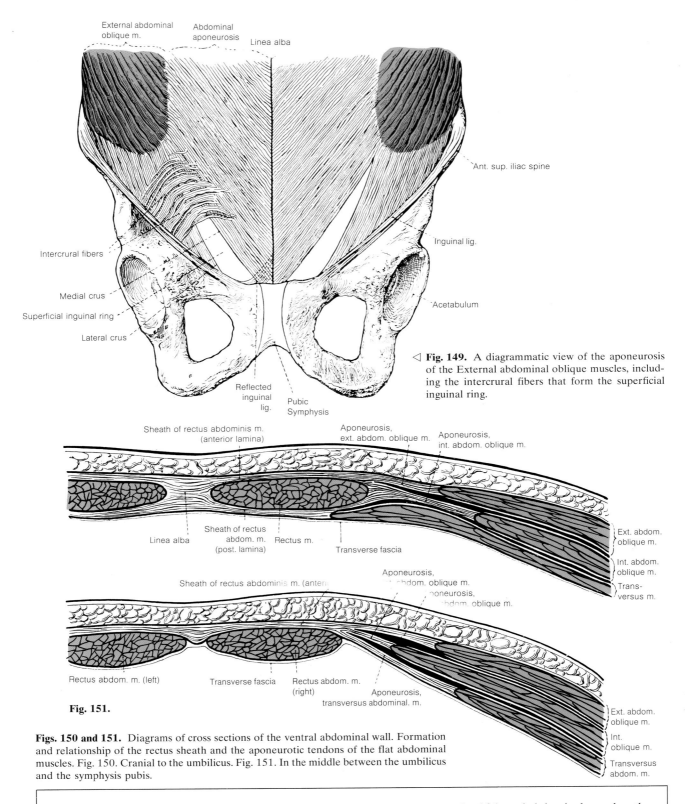

Fig. 149. A diagrammatic view of the aponeurosis of the External abdominal oblique muscles, including the intercrural fibers that form the superficial inguinal ring.

Fig. 151.

Figs. 150 and 151. Diagrams of cross sections of the ventral abdominal wall. Formation and relationship of the rectus sheath and the aponeurotic tendons of the flat abdominal muscles. Fig. 150. Cranial to the umbilicus. Fig. 151. In the middle between the umbilicus and the symphysis pubis.

NOTE: The rectus sheath above the linea arcuata is made up of the aponeurosis of 3 broad abdominal muscles: the m. obliquus ext. and half of the m. obliquus int. form the ventral layer; the other half of the m. obliquus internus and the m. transversus abdominis form the dorsal layer. Below the linea arcuata, all 3 aponeuroses pass ventral to the m. rectus; the dorsal wall of the sheath is formed here by only the fascia transversalis.

Straight Muscles of the Abdomen (Figs. 147, 148, 150, 151)

Name	Origin	Insertion
1. Rectus abdominal muscle Contains 3 or 4 tendinous intersections	5th to 7th cartilage, xiphoid process	Cranial border of the pubis between the pubic tubercle and the symphysis
Nerves: Middle and caudal intercostal nerves (T 7 – T 12) (rarely upper lumbar nerves)		
Function: Flexes the vertebral column; pulls the sternum toward the pubis (antagonist of long back muscles); tenses anterior abdominal wall; and assists in compressing the abdominal contents		
2. Pyramidalis muscle (inconstant)	Ventral surface of pubis and anterior pubic ligament	Linea alba cranial to symphysis
Nerve: Branch of 12th thoracic nerve		
Function: Tenses the linea alba. The size of the triangular muscle varies		

Flat Muscles of the Abdomen (Figs. 147, 148, 150, 151)

Name	Origin	Insertion
1. External abdominal oblique muscle Course of the fibers from lateral-cranial toward the medial-caudal	Flesh digitations from lower 8 ribs. The dorsal border is free	On external lip of iliac crest, on the inguinal ligament and outer layer of the rectus sheath
Nerve: Intercostal nerves, branches of lumbar plexus (iliohypogastric and ilioinguinal nerves)		
Function: Maintains abdominal pressure to keep viscera in position; forces viscera up to elevate diaphragm during expiration; increases abdominal pressure to initiate and aid the rectum in evacuation of its contents; both sides flex vertebral column; one side bends it laterally and rotates it		
2. Internal abdominal oblique muscle Course of fibers at right angles to the External Oblique	Intermediate lip of iliac crest; thoracolumbar fascia; lateral two-thirds of inguinal ligament	Fleshy digitations to lower 3 ribs (9–12), the linea alba, aponeurosis helps in formation of rectus sheath (see Figs. 150, 151)
Nerve: Same as above		
Function: Same as for External, but rotates toward the same side, supports the External of the opposing side, bends the body laterally		
3. Cremaster muscle	Caudal fibers of the Internal oblique muscle (often from Transverse abdominal muscle)	Goes with the spermatic cord to the testis
Nerve: Genital branch of the genitofemoral nerve		
Function: Supports and elevates the testis		
4. Transversus abdominal muscle	1. *Costal:* Deep surface of costal cartilages of lower 6 ribs 2. *Vertebral:* The thoracolumbar fascia from the transverse processes of the lumbar vertebrae 3. *Pelvic:* Internal lip of iliac crest, lateral third of inguinal ligament	Aponeurosis helps form rectus sheath; attaches to xiphoid process and linea alba; helps form falx inguinalis which attaches to superior border of the pubis and pectineal line
Nerve: Intercostal nerves, branches of lumbar plexus (iliohypogastric, ilioinguinal, genitofemoral nerves)		
Function: Contraction and expansion of abdominal wall, and maintains abdominal pressure to keep viscera in position		

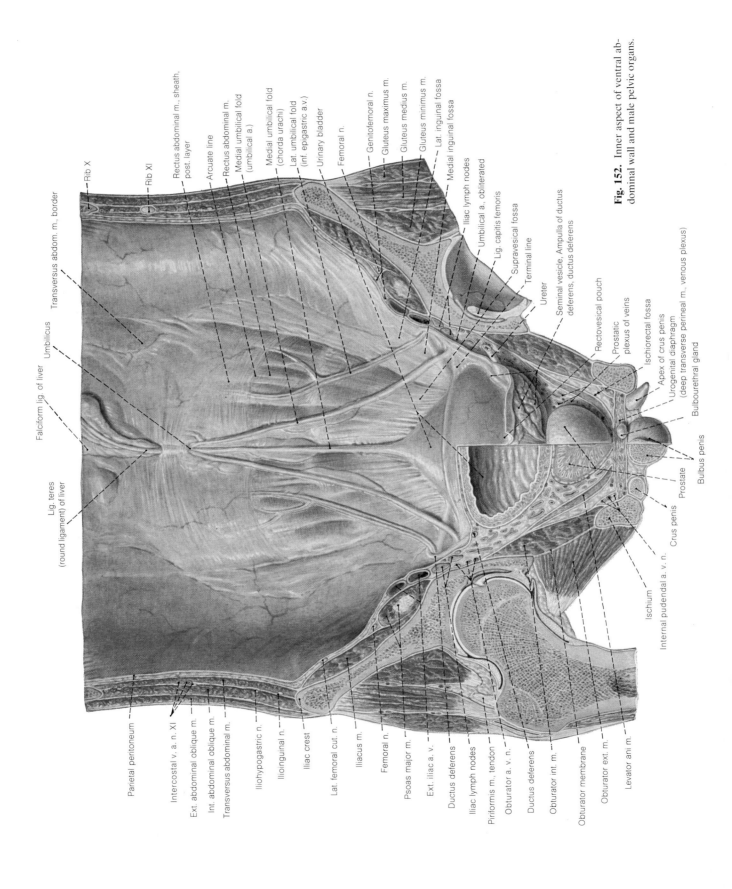

Rib X

Rib XI

Rectus abdominal m., sheath, post. layer

Arcuate line

Rectus abdominal m.

Medial umbilical fold (umbilical a.)

Medial umbilical fold (chorda urachi)

Lat. umbilical fold (inf. epigastric a.v.)

Urinary bladder

Femoral n.

Genitofemoral n.

Gluteus maximus m.

Gluteus medius m.

Gluteus minimus m.

Lat. inguinal fossa

Medial inguinal fossa

Iliac lymph nodes

Umbilical a., obliterated

Lig. capitis femoris

Supravesical fossa

Terminal line

Ureter

Seminal vesicle, Ampulla of ductus deferens, ductus deferens

Rectovesical pouch

Prostatic plexus of veins

Ischiorectal fossa

Apex of crus penis

Urogenital diaphragm (deep transverse perineal m., venous plexus)

Bulbourethral gland

Bulbus penis

Prostate

Crus penis

Internal pudendal a. v. n.

Ischium

Levator ani m.

Obturator ext. m.

Obturator membrane

Obturator int. m.

Ductus deferens

Obturator a. v. n.

Iliac lymph nodes

Ductus deferens

Piriformis m., tendon

Ext. iliac a. v.

Psoas major m.

Femoral n.

Iliacus m.

Lat. femoral cut. n.

Iliac crest

Ilioinguinal n.

Iliohypogastric n.

Transversus abdominal m.

Int. abdominal oblique m.

Ext. abdominal oblique m.

Intercostal v. a. n. XI

Parietal peritoneum

Lig. teres (round ligament) of liver

Falciform lig. of liver

Umbilicus

Transversus abdom. m., border

Fig. 152. Inner aspect of ventral abdominal wall and male pelvic organs.

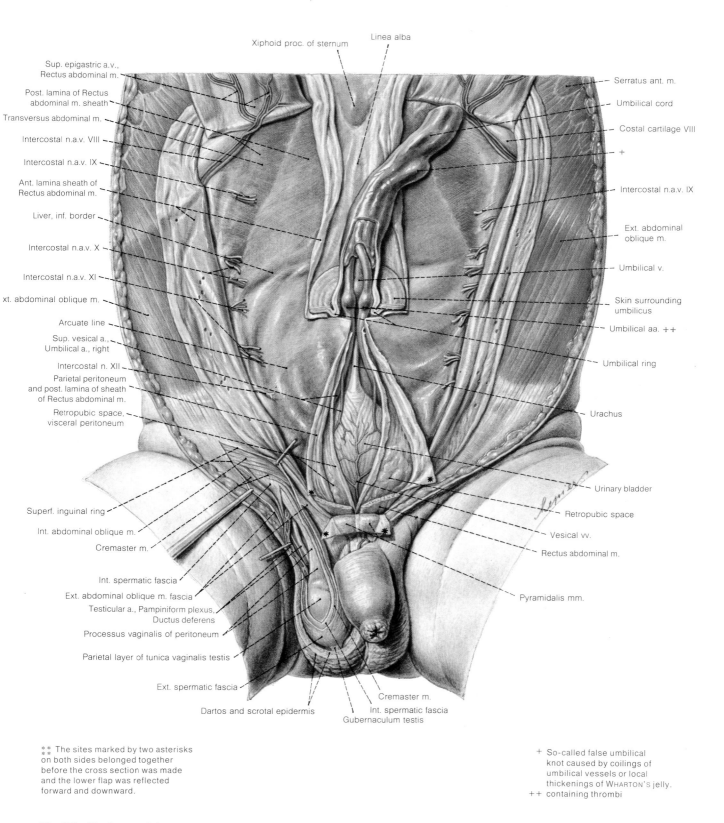

Xiphoid proc. of sternum

Linea alba

Sup. epigastric a.v., Rectus abdominal m.

Post. lamina of Rectus abdominal m. sheath

Transversus abdominal m.

Intercostal n.a.v. VIII

Intercostal n.a.v. IX

Ant. lamina sheath of Rectus abdominal m.

Liver, inf. border

Intercostal n.a.v. X

Intercostal n.a.v. XI

xt. abdominal oblique m.

Arcuate line

Sup. vesical a., Umbilical a., right

Intercostal n. XII

Parietal peritoneum and post. lamina of sheath of Rectus abdominal m.

Retropubic space, visceral peritoneum

Superf. inguinal ring

Int. abdominal oblique m.

Cremaster m.

Int. spermatic fascia

Ext. abdominal oblique m. fascia

Testicular a., Pampiniform plexus, Ductus deferens

Processus vaginalis of peritoneum

Parietal layer of tunica vaginalis testis

Ext. spermatic fascia

Dartos and scrotal epidermis

Gubernaculum testis

Int. spermatic fascia

Cremaster m.

Serratus ant. m.

Umbilical cord

Costal cartilage VIII

+

Intercostal n.a.v. IX

Ext. abdominal oblique m.

Umbilical v.

Skin surrounding umbilicus

Umbilical aa. ++

Umbilical ring

Urachus

Urinary bladder

Retropubic space

Vesical vv.

Rectus abdominal m.

Pyramidalis mm.

** The sites marked by two asterisks on both sides belonged together before the cross section was made and the lower flap was reflected forward and downward.

+ So-called false umbilical knot caused by coilings of umbilical vessels or local thickenings of WHARTON's jelly.
++ containing thrombi

Fig. 153. The layers of the ventral abdominal wall of a newborn. Insertion of the umbilical cord and passage of its vessels at the navel. Between the navel and symphysis, the bladder and urachus are visible. In the right inguinal region, the contents of the inguinal canal, as well as the various layers of the testis, are exposed.

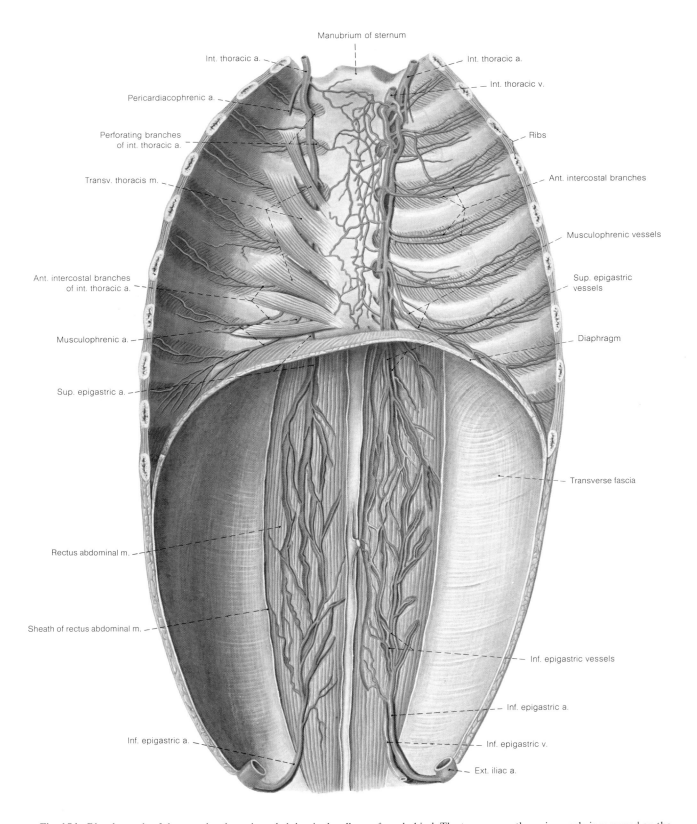

Manubrium of sternum

Int. thoracic a.

Pericardiacophrenic a.

Perforating branches
of int. thoracic a.

Transv. thoracis m.

Ant. intercostal branches
of int. thoracic a.

Musculophrenic a.

Sup. epigastric a.

Rectus abdominal m.

Sheath of rectus abdominal m.

Inf. epigastric a.

Int. thoracic a.

Int. thoracic v.

Ribs

Ant. intercostal branches

Musculophrenic vessels

Sup. epigastric
vessels

Diaphragm

Transverse fascia

Inf. epigastric vessels

Inf. epigastric a.

Inf. epigastric v.

Ext. iliac a.

Fig. 154. Blood vessels of the anterior thoracic and abdominal wall seen from behind. The transversus thoracis muscle is removed on the right side in order to expose the internal thoracic vessels. Branches and anastomoses of the superior and inferior epigastric vessels are shown within the rectus abdominal muscle.

Upper and Lower Abdominal Cavity

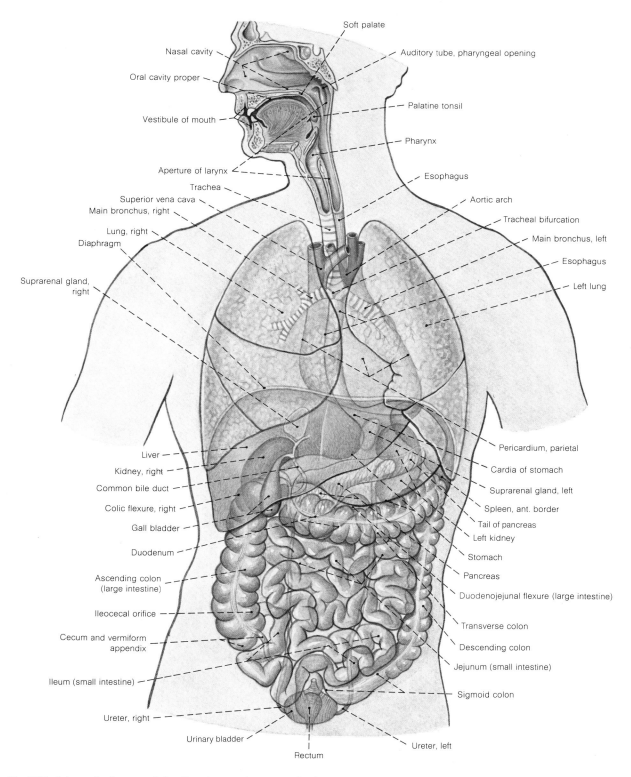

Soft palate

Nasal cavity

Oral cavity proper

Auditory tube, pharyngeal opening

Palatine tonsil

Vestibule of mouth

Pharynx

Aperture of larynx

Esophagus

Trachea

Aortic arch

Superior vena cava

Main bronchus, right

Tracheal bifurcation

Lung, right

Main bronchus, left

Diaphragm

Esophagus

Suprarenal gland, right

Left lung

Pericardium, parietal

Liver

Cardia of stomach

Kidney, right

Suprarenal gland, left

Common bile duct

Spleen, ant. border

Colic flexure, right

Tail of pancreas

Gall bladder

Left kidney

Duodenum

Stomach

Ascending colon (large intestine)

Pancreas

Duodenojejunal flexure (large intestine)

Ileocecal orifice

Transverse colon

Cecum and vermiform appendix

Descending colon

Jejunum (small intestine)

Ileum (small intestine)

Sigmoid colon

Ureter, right

Urinary bladder

Ureter, left

Rectum

Fig. 155. Schematic diagram of the digestive, respiratory, and urinary systems.

115

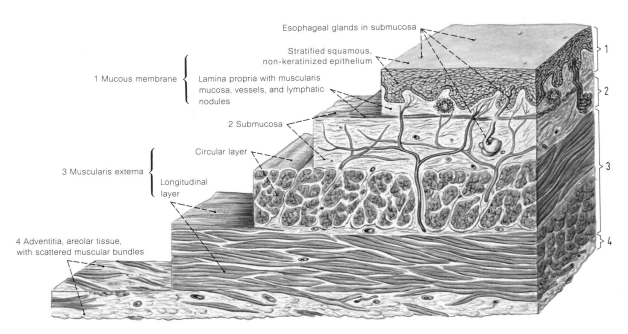

1 Mucous membrane {

Esophageal glands in submucosa

Stratified squamous,
non-keratinized epithelium

Lamina propria with muscularis
mucosa, vessels, and lymphatic
nodules

2 Submucosa

Circular layer

3 Muscularis externa {

Longitudinal
layer

4 Adventitia, areolar tissue,
with scattered muscular bundles

Fig. 156. Layers of the esophageal wall: for rapid transportation of food and liquids to the stomach.

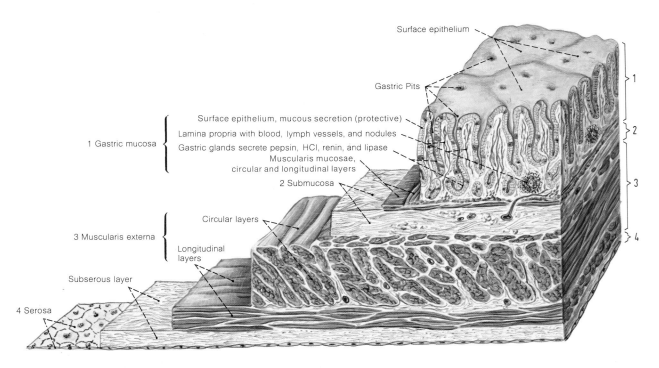

Surface epithelium

Gastric Pits

1 Gastric mucosa {

Surface epithelium, mucous secretion (protective)

Lamina propria with blood, lymph vessels, and nodules

Gastric glands secrete pepsin, HCl, renin, and lipase

Muscularis mucosae,
circular and longitudinal layers

2 Submucosa

Circular layers

3 Muscularis externa {

Longitudinal
layers

Subserous layer

4 Serosa

Fig. 157. Layers of the stomach wall (fundus): for secretion of enzymes and hydrochloric acid to promote digestion.

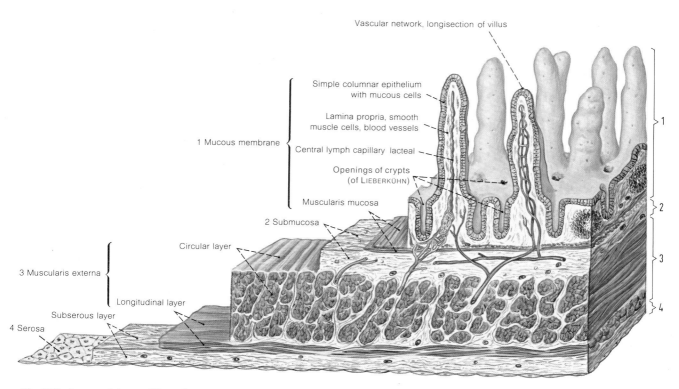

Vascular network, longisection of villus

Simple columnar epithelium with mucous cells

Lamina propria, smooth muscle cells, blood vessels

1 Mucous membrane

Central lymph capillary lacteal

Openings of crypts (of LIEBERKÜHN)

Muscularis mucosa

2 Submucosa

Circular layer

3 Muscularis externa

Longitudinal layer

Subserous layer

4 Serosa

Fig. 158. Layers of the small intestine: Large surface provided by villi for absorption of required nutriments. The solitary lymph follicles in the lamina propria of the mucous membrane (not labeled). In the stroma of both sectioned villi are shown the central chyle vessels (lacteal) or the villous capillaries.

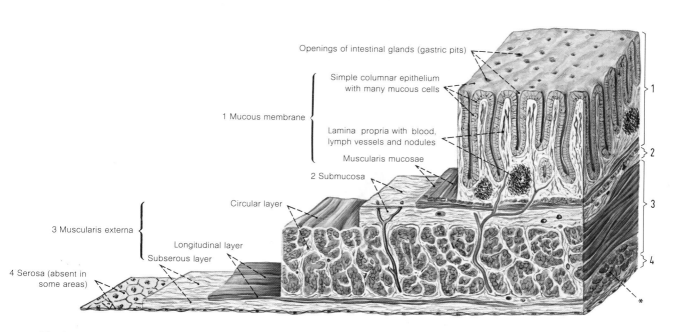

Openings of intestinal glands (gastric pits)

Simple columnar epithelium with many mucous cells

1 Mucous membrane

Lamina propria with blood, lymph vessels and nodules

Muscularis mucosae

2 Submucosa

Circular layer

3 Muscularis externa

Longitudinal layer

Subserous layer

4 Serosa (absent in some areas)

Fig. 159. Layers of the large intestine: Modified for absorption of water and regulation of consistency. In the region of the retroperitoneum, the tunica serosa is supplanted by the tunica adventitia. * Tenia coli, thickening of longitudinal musculature.

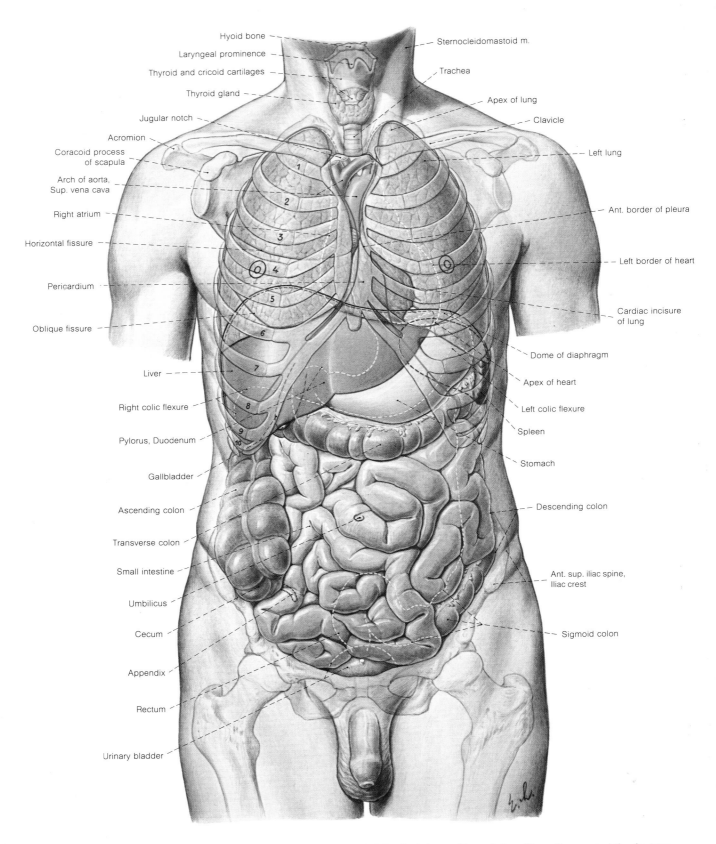

Fig. 160. Sagittal projection areas and contact surfaces of thoracic and abdominal viscera. Ventral view. (From Pernkopf: Atlas der topographischen und angewandten Anatomie des Menschen, Vol. 2, 2nd ed. [Ed. H. Ferner]. Urban & Schwarzenberg, Munich–Vienna–Baltimore 1980.)

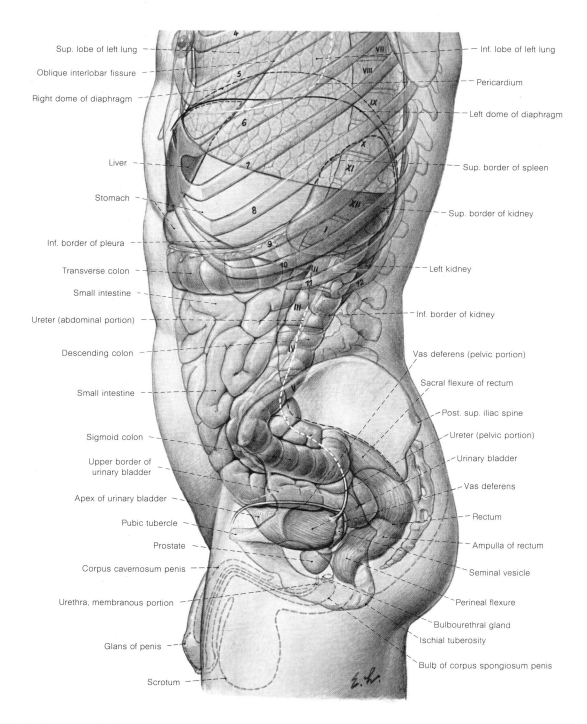

Fig. 161. Left lateral projection areas and contact surfaces of abdominal viscera. Broken lines indicate completed contours. (From PERN-KOPF: Atlas der topographischen und angewandten Anatomie des Menschen, Vol. 2, 2nd ed. [Ed. H. FERNER]. Urban & Schwarzenberg, Munich–Vienna–Baltimore 1980.)

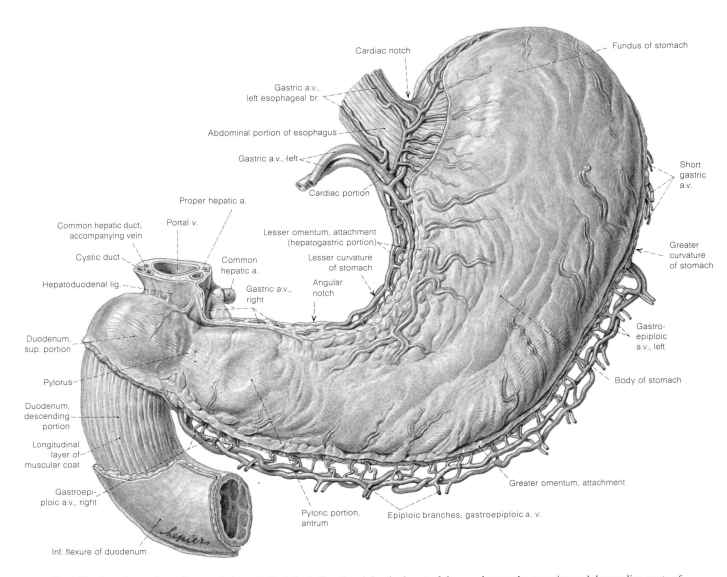

Cardiac notch

Fundus of stomach

Gastric a.v.,
left esophageal br.

Abdominal portion of esophagus

Gastric a.v., left

Cardiac portion

Short
gastric
a.v.

Proper hepatic a.

Common hepatic duct,
accompanying vein

Portal v.

Lesser omentum, attachment
(hepatogastric portion)

Greater
curvature
of stomach

Cystic duct

Common
hepatic a.

Lesser curvature
of stomach

Hepatoduodenal lig.

Gastric a.v.,
right

Angular
notch

Duodenum,
sup. portion

Gastro-
epiploic
a.v., left

Pylorus

Body of stomach

Duodenum,
descending
portion

Longitudinal
layer of
muscular coat

Gastroepi-
ploic a.v., right

Greater omentum, attachment

Pyloric portion,
antrum

Epiploic branches, gastroepiploic a. v.

Inf. flexure of duodenum

Fig. 162. Anterior surface of stomach (ventriculus), including the abdominal part of the esophagus, the superior and descending parts of the duodenum, as well as the blood vessels of the stomach. In the region of the descending part of the duodenum, one sees the longitudinal musculature, because the covering fat and connective tissue with the transverse mesocolon were removed.

Figs. 164 and 165. Schematic representation of the arterial blood supply of the stomach. (After EL-EISHI, H. I., S. F. AYOUB and ▷ M. ABD-EL-KHALEK: The arterial supply of the human stomach. Acta anat. 86, 1973.)

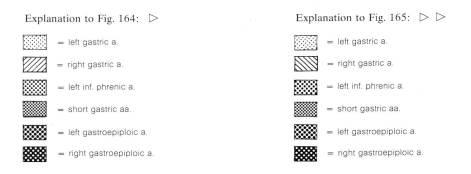

Explanation to Fig. 164: ▷

= left gastric a.

= right gastric a.

= left inf. phrenic a.

= short gastric aa.

= left gastroepiploic a.

= right gastroepiploic a.

Explanation to Fig. 165: ▷ ▷

= left gastric a.

= right gastric a.

= left inf. phrenic a.

= short gastric aa.

= left gastroepiploic a.

= right gastroepiploic a.

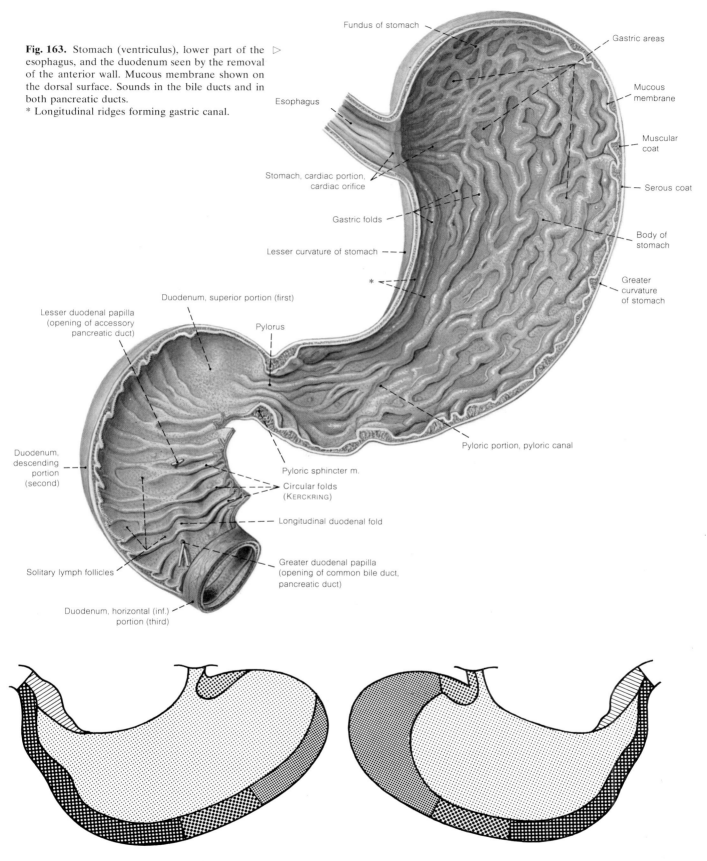

Fig. 163. Stomach (ventriculus), lower part of the ▷ esophagus, and the duodenum seen by the removal of the anterior wall. Mucous membrane shown on the dorsal surface. Sounds in the bile ducts and in both pancreatic ducts.
* Longitudinal ridges forming gastric canal.

Fundus of stomach

Gastric areas

Mucous membrane

Muscular coat

Serous coat

Esophagus

Body of stomach

Stomach, cardiac portion, cardiac orifice

Gastric folds

Greater curvature of stomach

Lesser curvature of stomach

*

Duodenum, superior portion (first)

Lesser duodenal papilla (opening of accessory pancreatic duct)

Pylorus

Pyloric portion, pyloric canal

Duodenum, descending portion (second)

Pyloric sphincter m.

Circular folds (KERCKRING)

Longitudinal duodenal fold

Solitary lymph follicles

Greater duodenal papilla (opening of common bile duct, pancreatic duct)

Duodenum, horizontal (inf.) portion (third)

Fig. 164. Ventral view of the stomach.

Fig. 165. Dorsal view of the stomach.

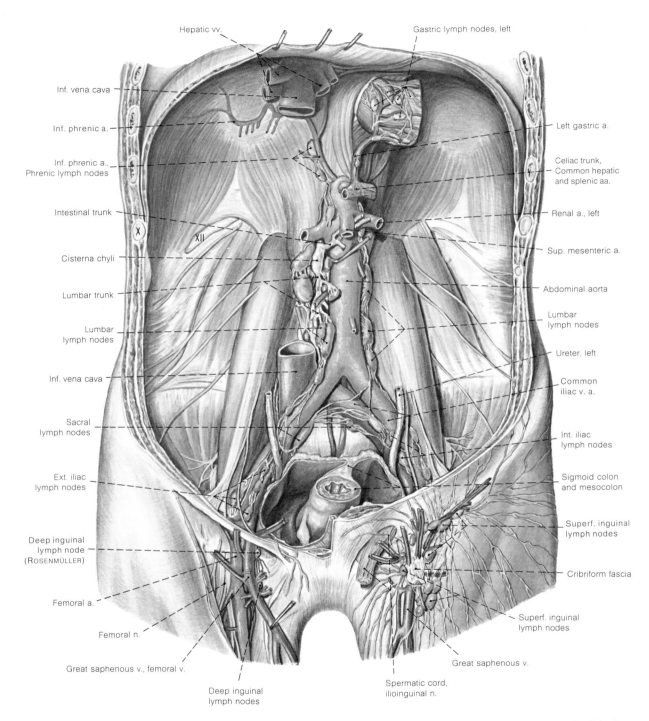

Hepatic vv.

Gastric lymph nodes, left

Inf. vena cava

Inf. phrenic a.

Left gastric a.

Inf. phrenic a.,
Phrenic lymph nodes

Celiac trunk,
Common hepatic
and splenic aa.

Intestinal trunk

Renal a., left

Cisterna chyli

Sup. mesenteric a.

Lumbar trunk

Abdominal aorta

Lumbar
lymph nodes

Lumbar
lymph nodes

Inf. vena cava

Ureter, left

Sacral
lymph nodes

Common
iliac v. a.

Ext. iliac
lymph nodes

Int. iliac
lymph nodes

Deep inguinal
lymph node
(ROSENMÜLLER)

Sigmoid colon
and mesocolon

Femoral a.

Superf. inguinal
lymph nodes

Femoral n.

Cribriform fascia

Great saphenous v., femoral v.

Superf. inguinal
lymph nodes

Deep inguinal
lymph nodes

Spermatic cord,
ilioinguinal n.

Great saphenous v.

Fig. 166. The lymphatic plexus and lymph nodes of the dorsal abdominal wall and their connections with the lymph vessels of the lower extremity. (Compare with Figs. 246 and 248.)

Fig. 167. Lymph nodes and lymph vessels of stomach, pancreas and porta hepatis. ▷

Fig. 168. Lymphatic vessels and lymph nodes of the mesentery of the ileum, injected with India ink. ▷

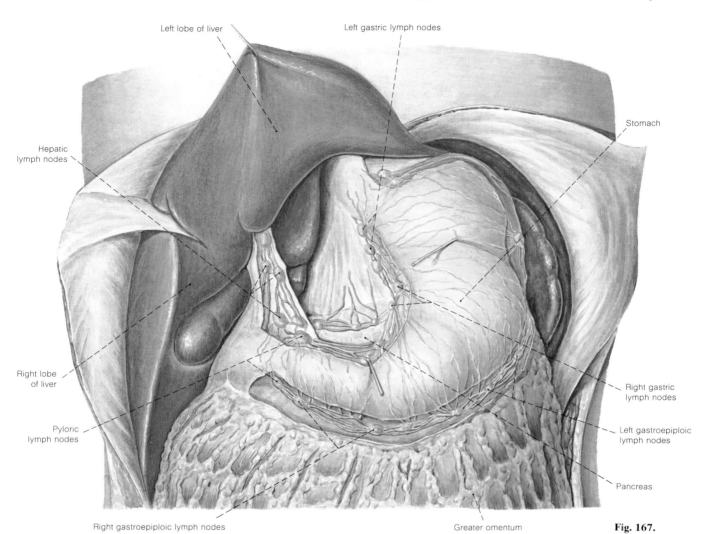

Left lobe of liver

Left gastric lymph nodes

Stomach

Hepatic
lymph nodes

Right lobe
of liver

Right gastric
lymph nodes

Pyloric
lymph nodes

Left gastroepiploic
lymph nodes

Pancreas

Right gastroepiploic lymph nodes

Greater omentum

Fig. 167.

Mesenteric lymph nodes

Root of mesentery

Mesenteric
lymph nodes

Mesenteric lymph nodes

Small intestine

Lymph vessels

Fig. 168.

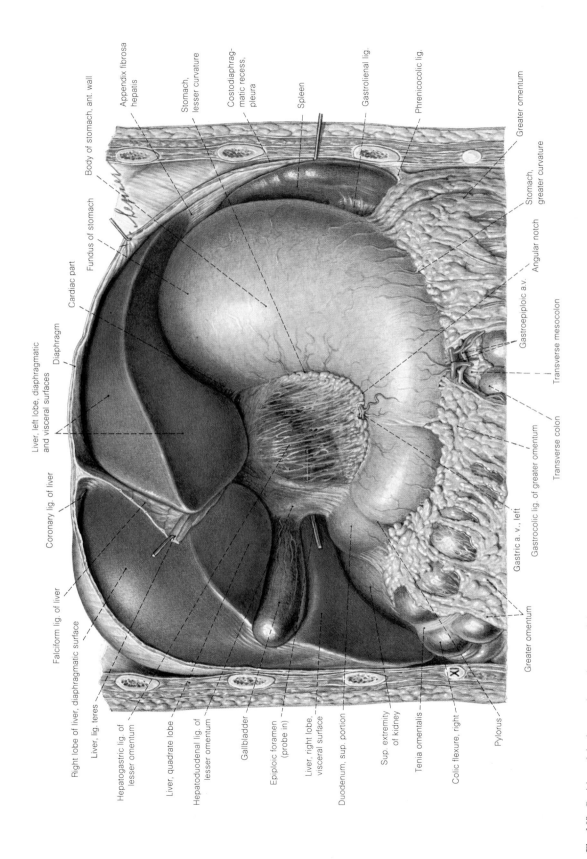

Fig. 169. Position of the intraperitoneal organs of the upper abdomen. Liver with gallbladder, stomach, and spleen. Liver pulled up, sound in the epiploic foramen and vestibule of the omental bursa, the lesser omentum taut, stomach full. Gastric vessels on lesser and greater curvature of stomach partly exposed.

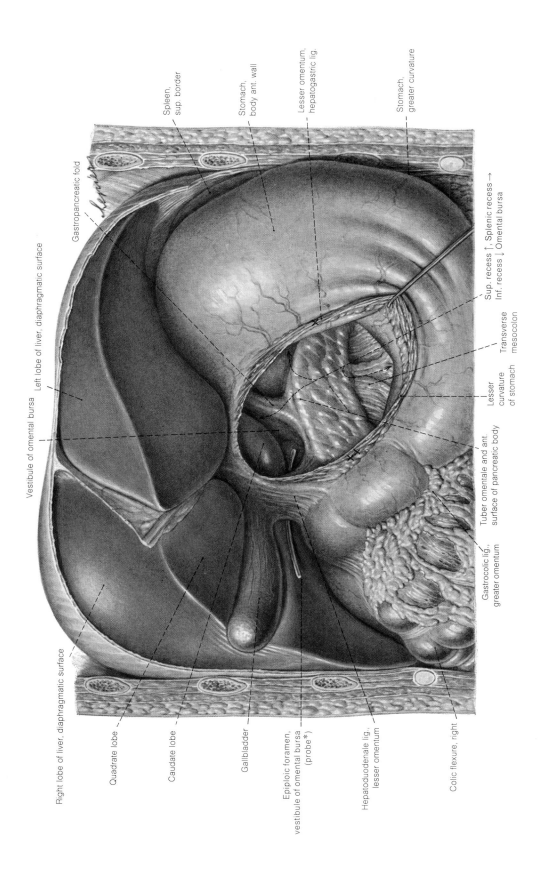

Right lobe of liver, diaphragmatic surface

Quadrate lobe

Caudate lobe

Gallbladder

Epiploic foramen,
vestibule of omental bursa
(probe*)

Hepatoduodenale lig.,
lesser omentum

Colic flexure, right

Gastropancreatic fold

Spleen,
sup. border

Stomach,
body ant. wall

Lesser omentum,
hepatogastric lig.

Stomach,
greater curvature

Vestibule of omental bursa

Left lobe of liver, diaphragmatic surface

Sup. recess ↑, Splenic recess →
Inf. recess ↓ Omental bursa

Transverse
mesocolon

Lesser
curvature
of stomach

Tuber omentale and ant.
surface of pancreatic body

Gastrocolic lig.,
greater omentum

Fig. 170. Organs of the abdominal cavity. The liver is held upward so that the visceral surface and gallbladder are clearly seen. The stomach is pulled downward toward the left with a hook in the lesser curvature. The omental bursa is opened after cutting the hepatogastric ligament of the lesser omentum. Looking on the omental bursa there are the vestibule of the omental bursa (under the caudate lobe of the liver) and the adjoining principle part of the omental bursa. The boundary forms the gastropancreatic folds. The arrows point in the direction of the 3 recesses of the omental bursa. A sound (*) is introduced into the epiploic foramen. Its point reaches the vestibule of the omental bursa and lies between the caudate lobe of the liver and the tuber omentale of the pancreas. ×, × × = expanded incision of the hepatogastric ligament.

125

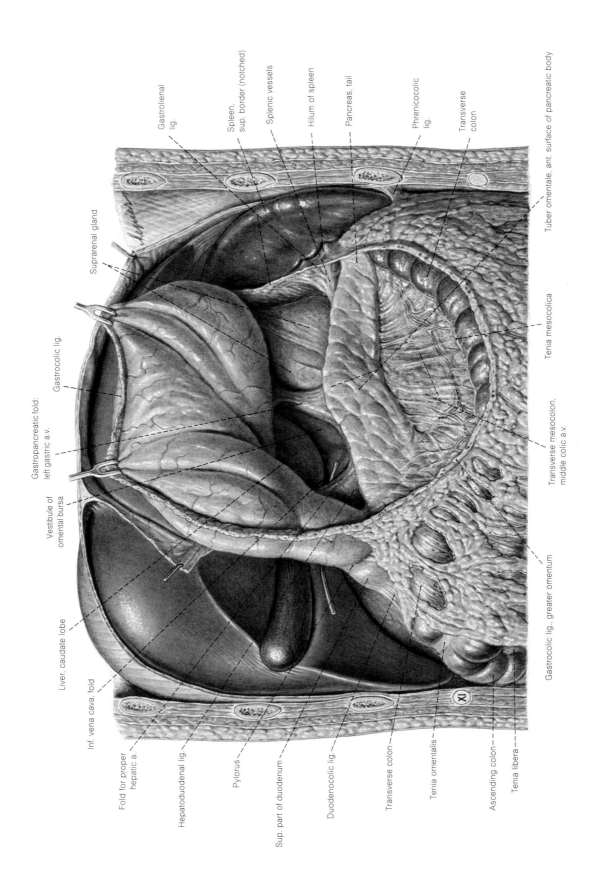

Gastrolienal lig.

Spleen, sup. border (notched)

Splenic vessels

Hilum of spleen

Pancreas, tail

Phrenicocolic lig.

Transverse colon

Tuber omentale, ant. surface of pancreatic body

Suprarenal gland

Gastropancreatic fold: left gastric a.v.

Gastrocolic lig.

Vestibule of omental bursa

Liver, caudate lobe

Inf. vena cava, fold

Fold for proper hepatic a.

Hepatoduodenal lig.

Pylorus

Sup. part of duodenum

Duodenocolic lig.

Transverse colon

Tenia omentalis

Ascending colon

Tenia libera

Gastrocolic lig., greater omentum

Transverse mesocolon, middle colic a.v.

Tenia mesocolica

Fig. 171. Intraperitoneal organs of the abdominal viscera. The gastrocolic ligament, on the greater curvature of the stomach, was cut through and the stomach pulled upward, revealing the omental bursa. It extends upward to the caudate lobe of the liver; toward the left to the hilus of the spleen; downward in adults after the secondary fusion of the 4 layers of the greater omentum to the transverse colon. Before the fusion of the 4 layers of the greater omentum, the omental bursa extends to the lower part of the greater omentum. The fusion can take place at different levels.

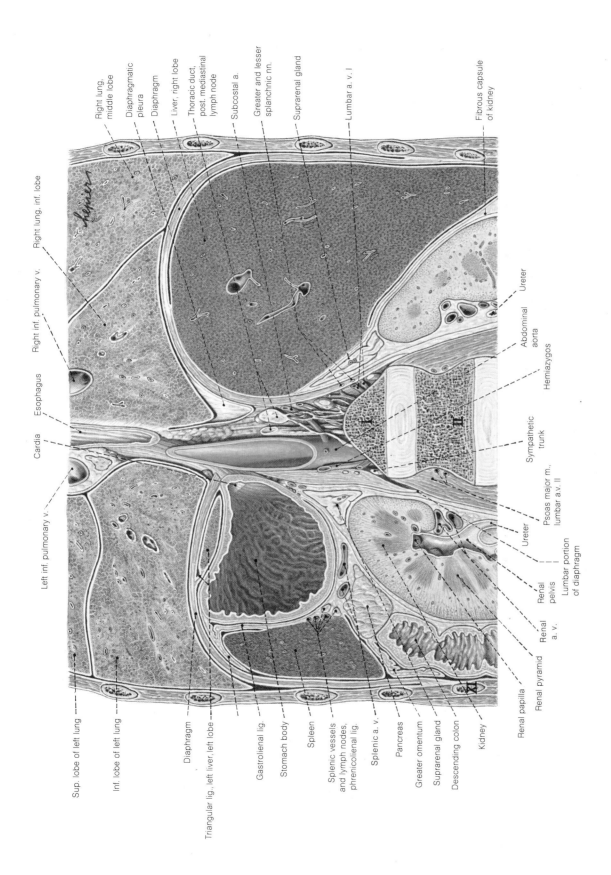

Right lung, middle lobe
Diaphragmatic pleura
Diaphragm
Liver, right lobe
Thoracic duct, post. mediastinal lymph node
Subcostal a.
Greater and lesser splanchnic nn.
Suprarenal gland
Lumbar a. v. I
Fibrous capsule of kidney

Right lung, inf. lobe
Right inf. pulmonary v.
Esophagus
Cardia
Left inf. pulmonary v.

Ureter
Abdominal aorta
Hemiazygos
Sympathetic trunk
Ureter
Psoas major m.., lumbar a.v. II
Lumbar portion of diaphragm
Renal pelvis
Renal a. v.

Sup. lobe of left lung
Inf. lobe of left lung
Diaphragm
Triangular lig., left liver, left lobe
Gastrolienal lig.
Stomach body
Spleen
Splenic vessels and lymph nodes, phrenicolienal lig.
Splenic a. v.
Pancreas
Greater omentum
Suprarenal gland
Descending colon
Kidney
Renal papilla
Renal pyramid

Fig. 172. Frontal longitudinal section through the trunk. View of anterior segment from the dorsal aspect. Aorta crosses the esophagus. In the lower part of the picture, the first 2 lumbar vertebrae were cut (lumbar lordosis!). In the region of the thoracic cavity, one sees between the two lungs, the posterior mediastinum with esophagus which is cut axially and seems conspicuously dilated. Abdominal aorta has a diagonal cut at the angular crossing of both organs (esophagus and aorta). Caudal to the diaphragm, in the region of the abdominal cavity, one sees a small part of the esophagus (pars abdominalis) which passes to the left as it empties via the cardiac orifice into the cardiac portion of the stomach. XI = sawcut of 11th rib.

127

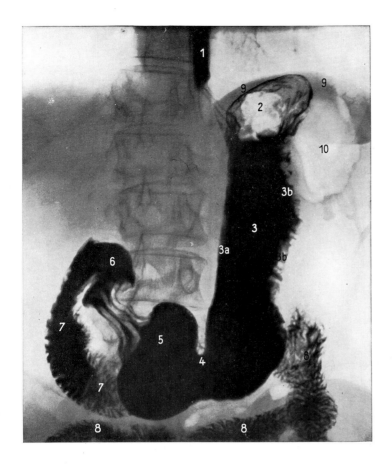

Fig. 173. X-ray film of lower esophagus, stomach, duodenum and the upper loops of the jejunum. Anterior-posterior view.

1 Esophagus, caudal end filled with contrast medium. Cardiac orifice of stomach closed. The medium-filled creases between folds are visible in the empty part of the cardia and fundus.
2 Fundus of stomach with bubble of air.
3 Body of stomach
3 a Lesser curvature of stomach
3 b Greater curvature of stomach, with gastric folds and creases silhouetted
4 Angular notch with peristaltic constriction
5 Pyloric antrum expanded preceding an ejection of stomach contents into:
6 Bulb of duodenum
7 Descending part of duodenum with circular plicae
8 Jejunum
9 Left dome of diaphragm
10 Air orgas-filled left colic flexure

1 Esophagus
2 Air space in fundus of stomach
3 Constriction at angular notch
4 Constriction at pyloric antrum
5 Pylorus (in Fig. 174: closed; Fig. 175: beginning to open)
6 Bulb of duodenum

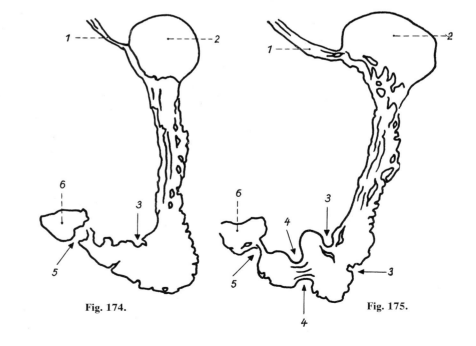

Fig. 174.

Fig. 175.

Figs. 174 and 175. The mucous membrane topography of the stomach from the x-ray picture of a standing subject. These figures show the consecutive waves of peristalsis. The longitudinal line and the dentated boundary of the curvature conform to the mucous membrane topography.

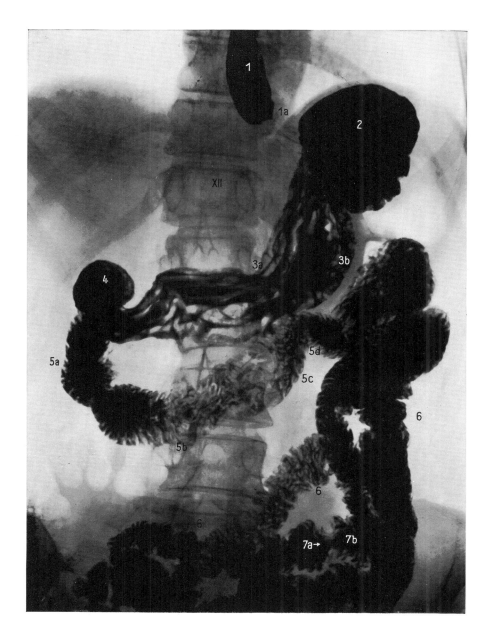

XII = twelfth thoracic vertebra

1 Esophagus. la. Cardia closed, contrast medium in creases of mucous membrane
2 Fundus of stomach (filled)
3 a Lesser curvature of stomach with longitudinal mucosal folds
3 b Greater curvature with gastric folgs and areas
4 Duodenal bulb, superior part of duodenum

5 a Descending part of duodenum
5 b Horizontal part of duodenum
5 c Ascending part of duodenum
5 d Duodenojejunal flexure
6 Jejunum with circular plicae
7 Peristaltic contraction wave from 7 a to 7 b

Fig. 176. X-ray picture of gastrointestinal tract: Lower third of the esophagus, stomach, duodenum, and jejunum. Most of contrast medium has left the stomach. Sagittal exposure. (See also Fig. 162.)

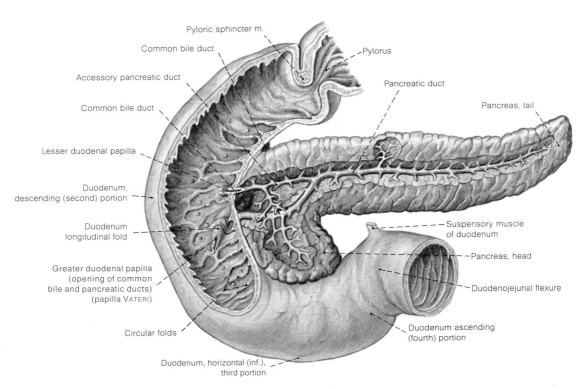

Pyloric sphincter m.

Common bile duct

Accessory pancreatic duct

Common bile duct

Lesser duodenal papilla

Duodenum;
descending (second) portion

Duodenum
longitudinal fold

Greater duodenal papilla
(opening of common
bile and pancreatic ducts)
(papilla VATERI)

Circular folds

Duodenum, horizontal (inf.),
third portion

Pylorus

Pancreatic duct

Pancreas, tail

Suspensory muscle
of duodenum

Pancreas, head

Duodenojejunal flexure

Duodenum ascending
(fourth) portion

Fig. 177. The pylorus of the stomach, duodenum, and pancreas. Ventral view. The anterior wall of the pylorus and the upper part of the duodenum were removed. The larger ducts of the pancreas were revealed by splitting the pancreas along the ventral surface.

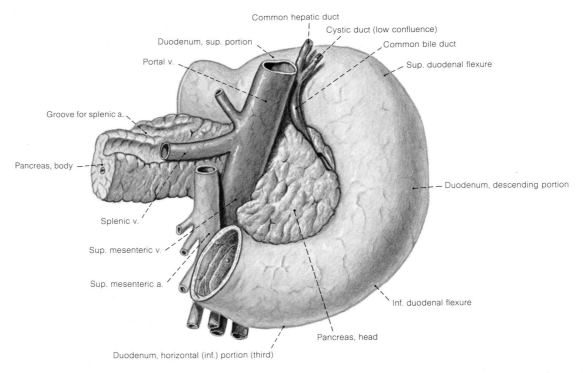

Common hepatic duct

Duodenum, sup. portion

Cystic duct (low confluence)

Common bile duct

Portal v.

Sup. duodenal flexure

Groove for splenic a.

Pancreas, body

Duodenum, descending portion

Splenic v.

Sup. mesenteric v.

Sup. mesenteric a.

Inf. duodenal flexure

Duodenum, horizontal (inf.) portion (third)

Pancreas, head

Fig. 178. Head and body of pancreas with bile duct (ductus choledochus) and blood vessels: portal vein, splenic vein (v. lienalis), superior mesenteric artery and vein. Dorsal view.

130

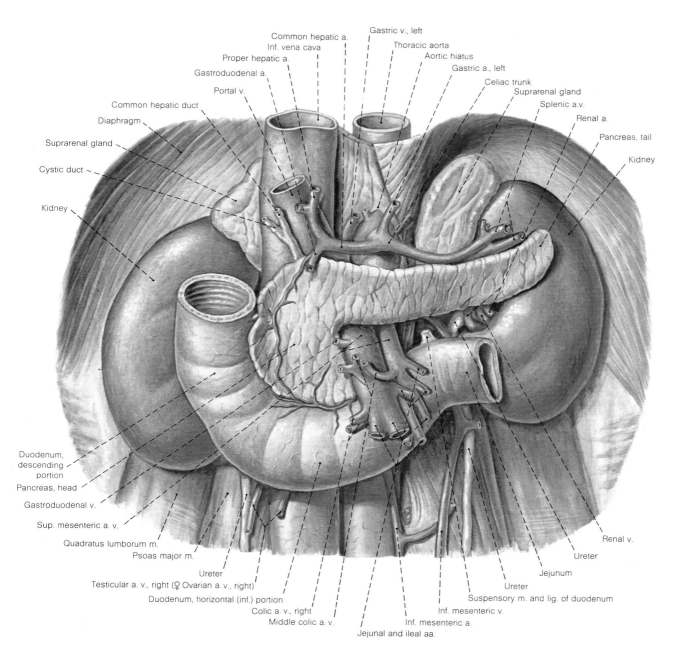

Common hepatic a.
Inf. vena cava
Proper hepatic a.
Gastroduodenal a.
Portal v.
Common hepatic duct
Diaphragm
Suprarenal gland
Cystic duct
Kidney
Gastric v., left
Thoracic aorta
Aortic hiatus
Gastric a., left
Celiac trunk
Suprarenal gland
Splenic a.v.
Renal a.
Pancreas, tail
Kidney
Duodenum, descending portion
Pancreas, head
Gastroduodenal v.
Sup. mesenteric a. v.
Quadratus lumborum m.
Psoas major m.
Ureter
Testicular a. v., right (♀ Ovarian a. v., right)
Duodenum, horizontal (inf.) portion
Colic a. v., right
Middle colic a. v.
Jejunal and ileal aa.
Inf. mesenteric a.
Inf. mesenteric v.
Suspensory m. and lig. of duodenum
Ureter
Jejunum
Ureter
Renal v.

Fig. 179. The retroperitoneal structures of the upper abdomen (pancreas and duodenum). Ventral view.

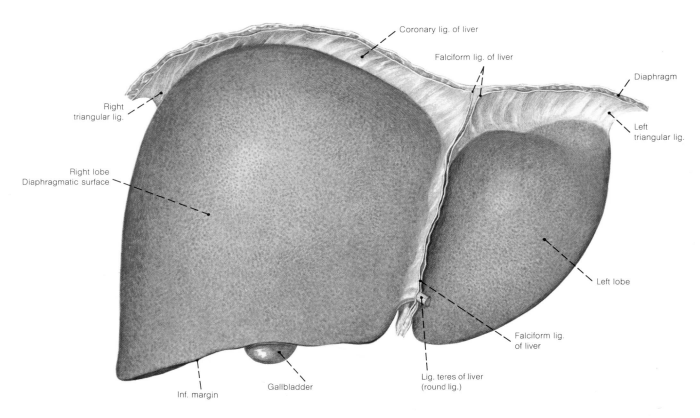

Fig. 180. Ventral surface of the liver (hepar) with a part of the diaphragm.

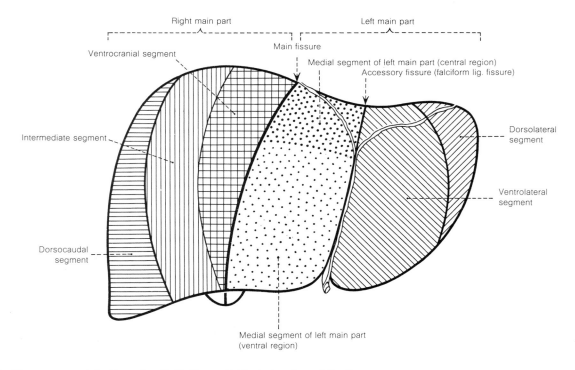

Fig. 181. The segments of the liver after C. H. HJORTSJÖ. Ventral surface of the liver.

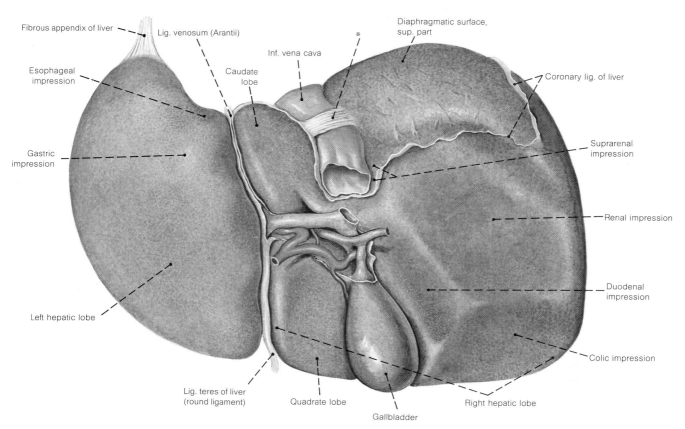

Fig. 182. Dorsal (visceral) surface of the liver. Porta hepatis and adhesion of the liver with the diaphragm area without peritoneal covering (bare area). * So-called ligament of the vena cava.

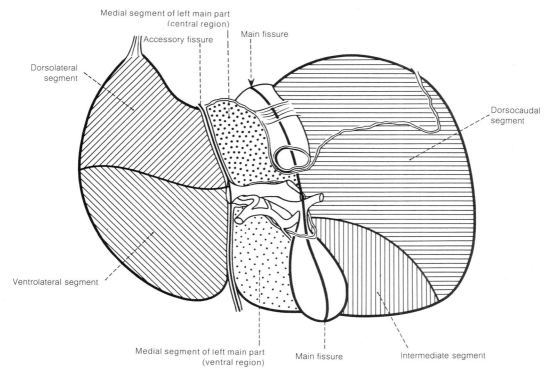

Fig. 183. The segments of the liver after C. H. HJORTSJÖ. Dorsal surface of the liver.

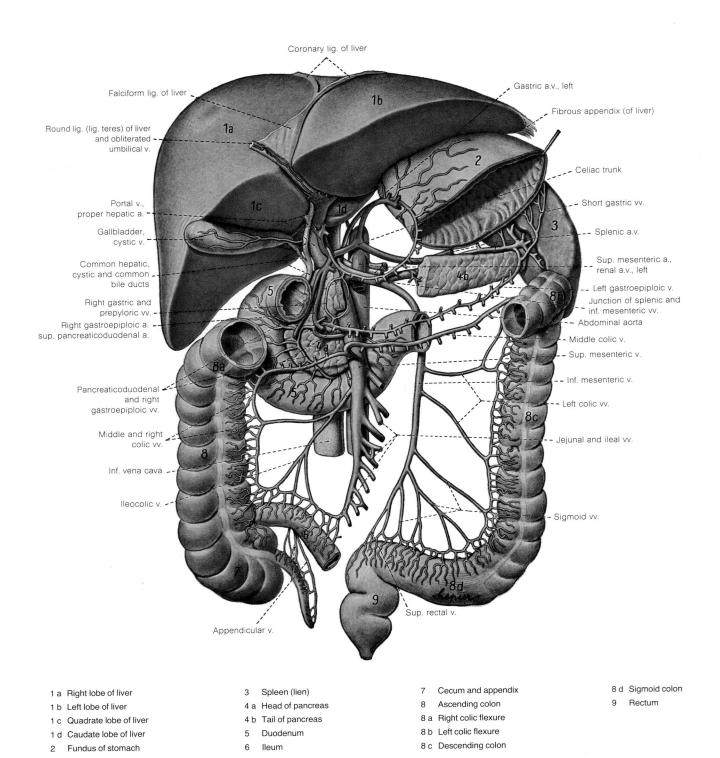

Coronary lig. of liver

Falciform lig. of liver

Round lig. (lig. teres) of liver and obliterated umbilical v.

Gastric a.v., left

Fibrous appendix (of liver)

Celiac trunk

Short gastric vv.

Portal v., proper hepatic a.

Splenic a.v.

Gallbladder, cystic v.

Sup. mesenteric a., renal a.v., left

Common hepatic, cystic and common bile ducts

Left gastroepiploic v.

Right gastric and prepyloric vv.

Junction of splenic and inf. mesenteric vv.

Right gastroepiploic a. sup. pancreaticoduodenal a.

Abdominal aorta

Middle colic v.

Sup. mesenteric v.

Inf. mesenteric v.

Pancreaticoduodenal and right gastroepiploic vv.

Left colic vv.

Middle and right colic vv.

Jejunal and ileal vv.

Inf. vena cava

Ileocolic v.

Sigmoid vv.

Sup. rectal v.

Appendicular v.

1 a Right lobe of liver	3 Spleen (lien)	7 Cecum and appendix	8 d Sigmoid colon
1 b Left lobe of liver	4 a Head of pancreas	8 Ascending colon	9 Rectum
1 c Quadrate lobe of liver	4 b Tail of pancreas	8 a Right colic flexure	
1 d Caudate lobe of liver	5 Duodenum	8 b Left colic flexure	
2 Fundus of stomach	6 Ileum	8 c Descending colon	

Fig. 184. The roots of the portal vein. Arrow indicates junction of superior mesenteric vein with the splenic (lienal) vein to form the portal vein.

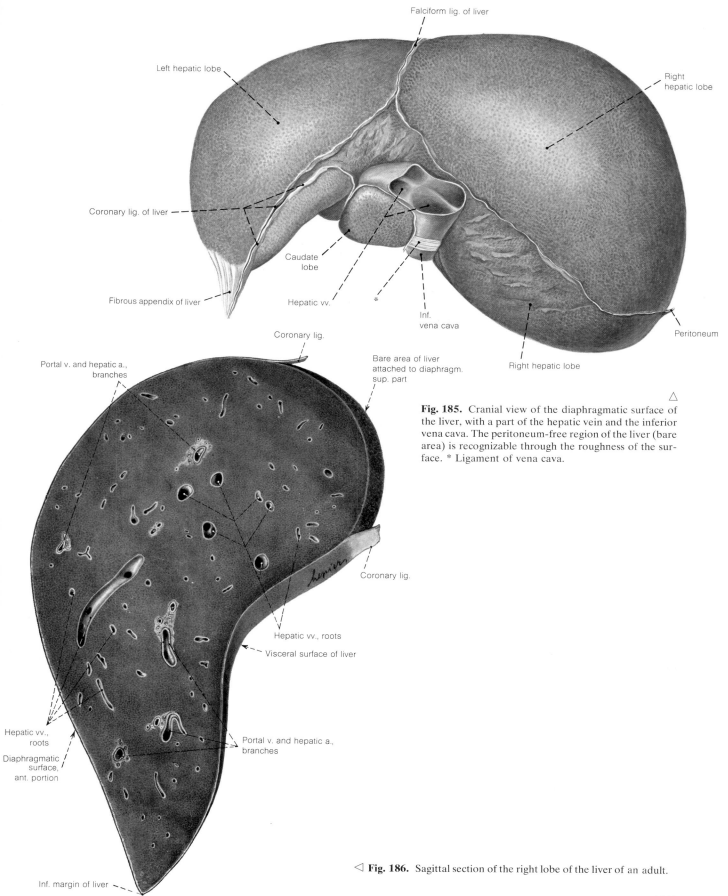

Falciform lig. of liver

Left hepatic lobe

Right hepatic lobe

Coronary lig. of liver

Caudate lobe

Hepatic vv.

*

Inf. vena cava

Fibrous appendix of liver

Peritoneum

Right hepatic lobe

Coronary lig.

Bare area of liver attached to diaphragm. sup. part

Portal v. and hepatic a., branches

Fig. 185. Cranial view of the diaphragmatic surface of the liver, with a part of the hepatic vein and the inferior vena cava. The peritoneum-free region of the liver (bare area) is recognizable through the roughness of the surface. * Ligament of vena cava.

Coronary lig.

Hepatic vv., roots

Visceral surface of liver

Hepatic vv., roots

Diaphragmatic surface, ant. portion

Portal v. and hepatic a., branches

Inf. margin of liver

◁ **Fig. 186.** Sagittal section of the right lobe of the liver of an adult.

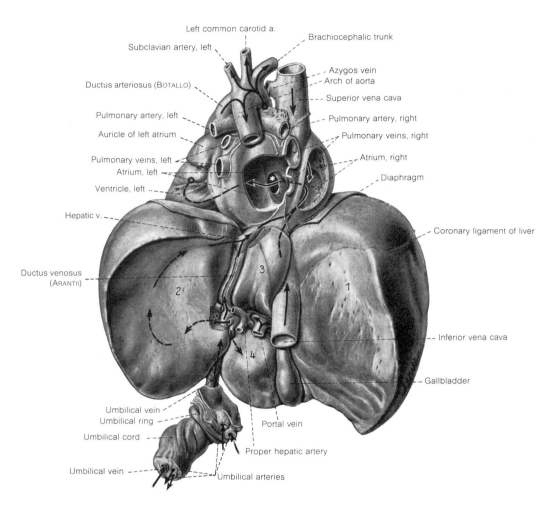

Fig. 187. Fetal circulation. Relationship of the fetal liver and heart with the umbilical vein and the ductus venosus (ARANTII) on the visceral surface of the liver. The arrows indicate direction of the blood flow.
1 Right lobe; 2 Left lobe; 3 Caudate lobe; 4 Quadrate lobe.* foramen ovale.

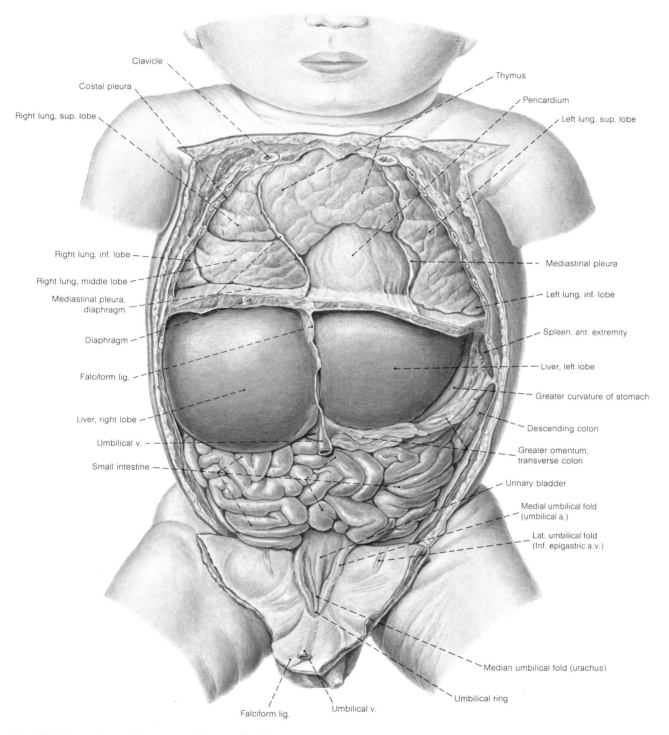

Clavicle

Costal pleura

Right lung, sup. lobe

Thymus

Pericardium

Left lung, sup. lobe

Right lung, inf. lobe

Right lung, middle lobe

Mediastinal pleura, diaphragm

Diaphragm

Falciform lig.

Liver, right lobe

Umbilical v.

Small intestine

Mediastinal pleura

Left lung, inf. lobe

Spleen, ant. extremity

Liver, left lobe

Greater curvature of stomach

Descending colon

Greater omentum, transverse colon

Urinary bladder

Medial umbilical fold (umbilical a.)

Lat. umbilical fold (Inf. epigastric a.v.)

Median umbilical fold (urachus)

Umbilical ring

Falciform lig.

Umbilical v.

Fig. 188. Liver of the newborn *in situ*. The ventral wall is widely opened and, for the most part, removed. The lower part of the abdominal wall is seen as a triangular flap; the umbilical folds, which come together at the navel, are visible. Note the size of the liver. Its weight, in relation to the total body weight of the newborn, is about double that of an adult's.

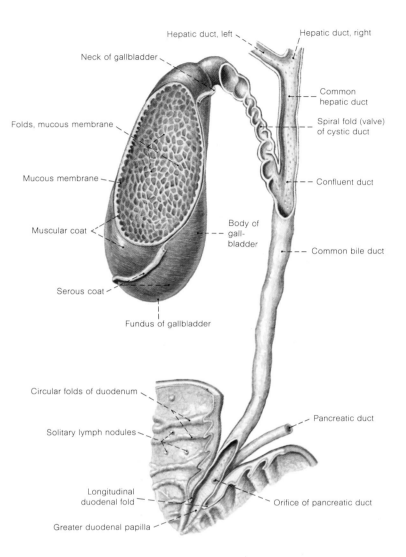

Hepatic duct, left

Hepatic duct, right

Neck of gallbladder

Common hepatic duct

Folds, mucous membrane

Spiral fold (valve) of cystic duct

Mucous membrane

Confluent duct

Muscular coat

Body of gall-bladder

Common bile duct

Serous coat

Fundus of gallbladder

Circular folds of duodenum

Solitary lymph nodules

Pancreatic duct

Longitudinal duodenal fold

Orifice of pancreatic duct

Greater duodenal papilla

Fig. 189. Gallbladder (vesica fellea), the extrahepatic biliary tract, and the junction of the common bile duct (ductus choledochus) with the duodenum. The longitudinal plica of the duodenum is split so that the orifices of the excretory ducts of the liver and pancreas are both seen.

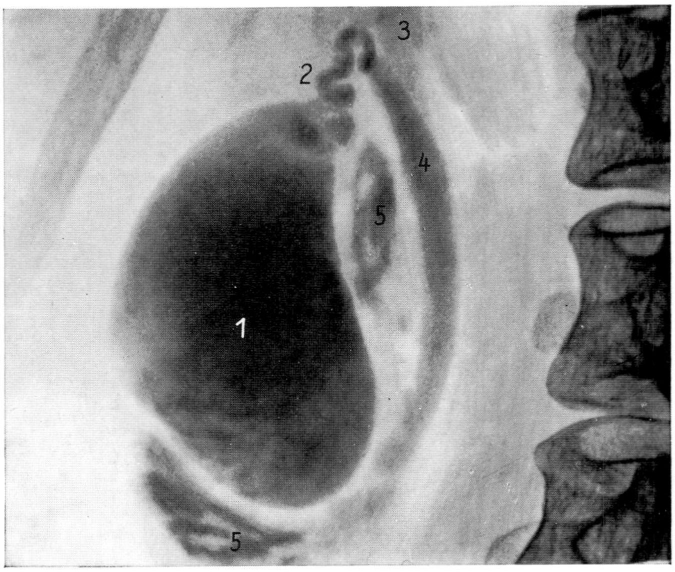

1 Body and fundus of the gallbladder
2 Neck of gallbladder and cystic duct with spiral folds
3 Common hepatic duct
4 Union of common hepatic and cystic ducts to form common bile duct
5 Contrast medium in duodenum

Fig. 190. X-ray film of a gallbladder and the extrahepatic bile duct, full of contrast medium.

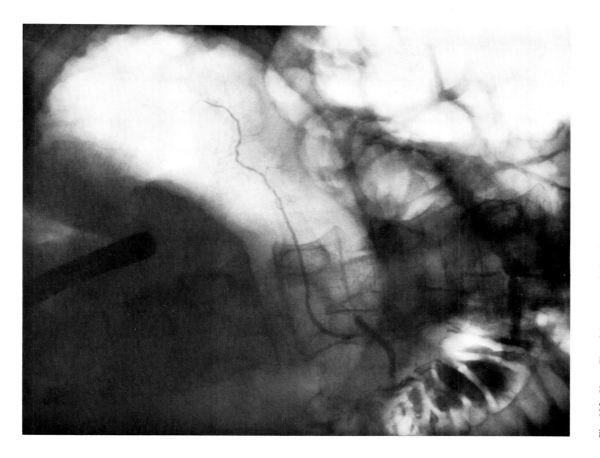

Fig. 192. X-ray film of the pancreatic duct in its entire length. Due to air filling of the stomach all details of the pancreatic ducts up to the second order are visible. (Original: Prof. Dr. J. ALTARAS, Zentrum für Radiologie am Klinikum der Universität Giessen.)

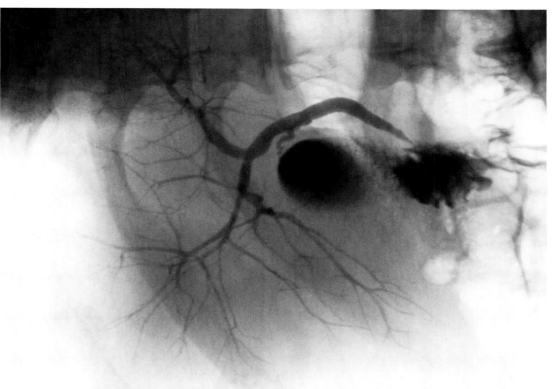

Fig. 191. X-ray film of the extrahepatic and intrahepatic bile passages and of the gallbladder. Retrograde filling with contrast medium. (Original: Prof. Dr. J. ALTARAS, Zentrum für Radiologie am Klinikum der Universität Giessen.)

Figs. 193–195. Variations in the course and the union of the cystic and common hepatic ducts to the common bile duct (ductus choledochus) and their orifices in the duodenal papilla on the dorsal wall of the descending part of the duodenum. Diagram with a window in part of the descending duodenum at the level of the greater duodenal papilla. Liver and gallbladder are pushed up.

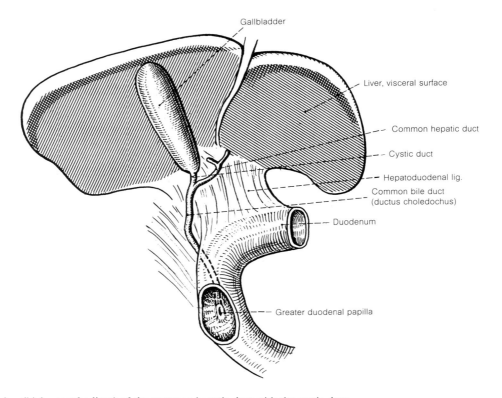

Gallbladder

Liver, visceral surface

Common hepatic duct

Cystic duct

Hepatoduodenal lig.

Common bile duct (ductus choledochus)

Duodenum

Greater duodenal papilla

Fig. 193. The union (high near the liver) of the common hepatic duct with the cystic duct.

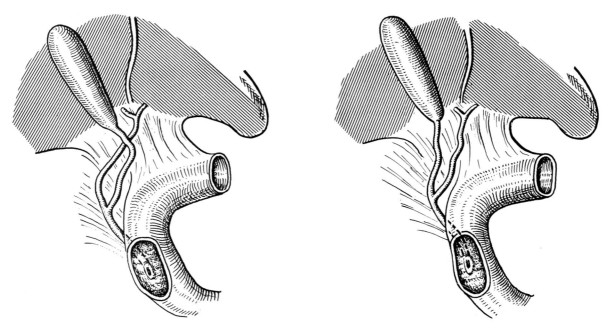

Fig. 194. Lower union (near the duodenum) of cystic and hepatic ducts after the ducts cross each other.

Fig. 195. Late union (near duodenum) of both ducts.

Figs. 196–201. Variations in the openings of the excretory ducts of the liver and pancreas.

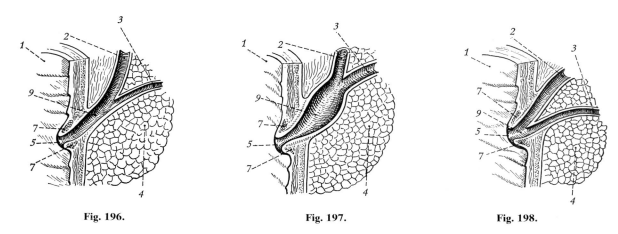

Fig. 196.   Fig. 197.   Fig. 198.

Fig. 196. Long terminal hepatopancreatic duct.
Fig. 197. Ampullary-like expansion of the long terminal hepatopancreatic duct.
Fig. 198. Short, terminal hepatopancreatic duct.

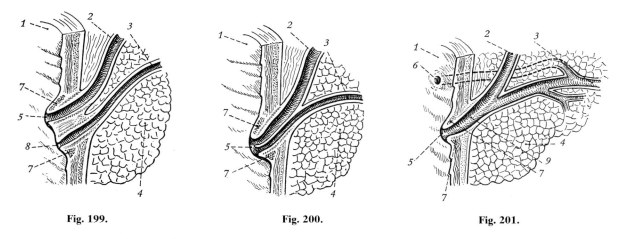

Fig. 199.   Fig. 200.   Fig. 201.

Fig. 199. Common hepatic and pancreatic ducts open separately on single, partially divided papilla.
Fig. 200. Single opening, but hepatopancreatic ducts separated by a septum.
Fig. 201. Well-developed accessory pancreatic opening into lesser duodenal papilla, and long terminal hepatopancreatic duct opening into greater duodenal papilla.

1 Duodenum
2 Common bile duct (ductus choledochus)
3 Pancreatic duct
4 Pancreas
5 Greater duodenal papilla
6 Lesser duodenal papilla, accessory pancreatic duct
7 Sphincter of the ductus choledochus
8 Pancreatic duct opening in divided papilla
9 Hepatopancreatic duct

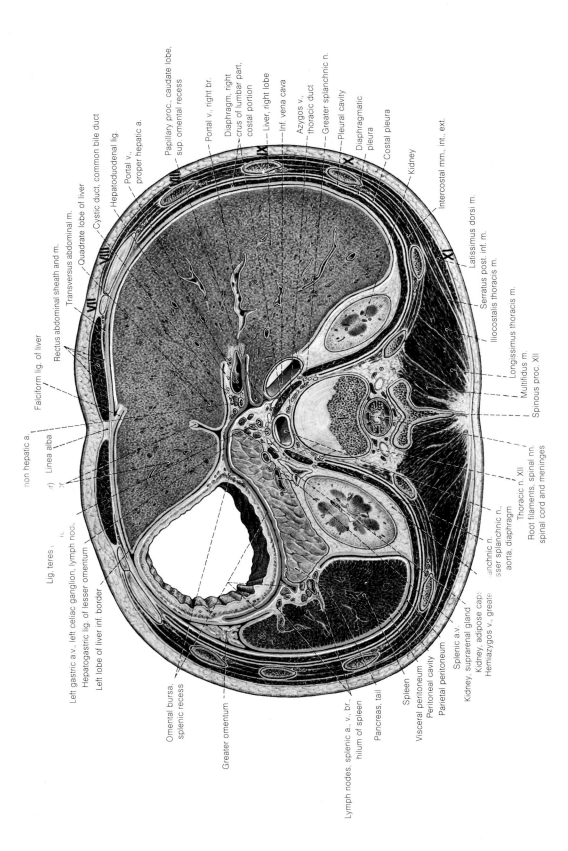

Fig. 202. Transverse cut of the abdominal viscera. A sliced preparation at the level of the intervertebral disk between the thoracic vertebra XII and lumbar I. The stomach remained in an expanded condition during the preparation. The contents were then removed. The hepatoduodenal and hepatogastric ligaments unite to form the lesser omentum.
The light red (pink) line = the peritoneum of the greater peritoneal cavity. ⎫
The dark red line = the peritoneum of the omental bursa. ⎬ Both spaces are thin slits, since the organs normally fill the abdominal cavity.
⎭
Note the different positions of the kidneys: The left is higher, Th XI–L II; the right, Th XII–L III, is lower. I = 1st lumbar vertebra; VII–XII = ribs

Non hepatic a.

Lig. teres

r) Linea alba
r)

Omental bursa,
splenic recess

Greater omentum

Left gastric a.v., left celiac ganglion, lymph node
Hepatogastric lig. of lesser omentum
Left lobe of liver inf. border

Lymph nodes, splenic a., v., br.,
hilum of spleen

Pancreas, tail

Spleen
Visceral peritoneum
Peritoneal cavity
Parietal peritoneum
Splenic a.v.
Kidney, suprarenal gland
Kidney, adipose caps.
Hemiazygos v., greater

Falciform lig. of liver
Rectus abdominal sheath and m.
Transversus abdominal m.
Quadrate lobe of liver
Cystic duct, common bile duct
Hepatoduodenal lig.
Portal v.,
proper hepatic a.
Papillary proc., caudate lobe,
sup. omental recess
Portal v., right br.
Diaphragm, right
crus of lumbar part,
costal portion
Liver, right lobe
Inf. vena cava
Azygos v.,
thoracic duct
Greater splanchnic n.
Pleural cavity
Diaphragmatic
pleura
Costal pleura
Kidney

Intercostal mm., int., ext.

Latissimus dorsi m.
Serratus post. inf. m.
Iliocostalis thoracis m.
Longissimus thoracis m.
Multifidus m.
Spinous proc. XII

Thoracic n. XII
Root filaments, spinal nn.
spinal cord and meninges
anchnic n.
sser splanchnic n.,
aorta, diaphragm

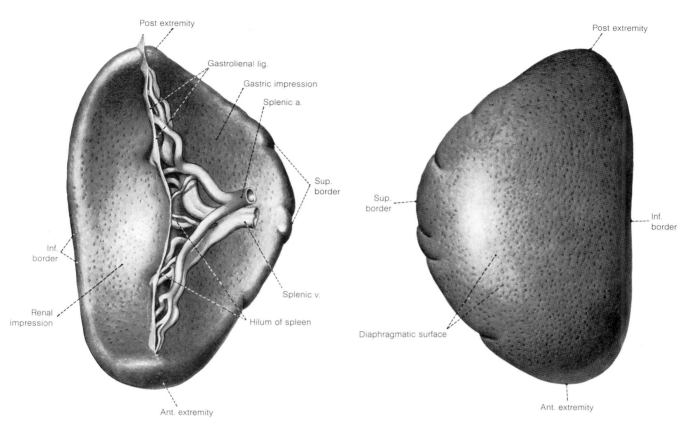

Post extremity

Gastrolienal lig.

Gastric impression

Splenic a.

Sup.
border

Inf.
border

Renal
impression

Splenic v.

Hilum of spleen

Ant. extremity

Fig. 203. Spleen (lien). Visceral surface.

Post extremity

Sup.
border

Inf.
border

Diaphragmatic surface

Ant. extremity

Fig. 204. Spleen. Diaphragmatic surface.

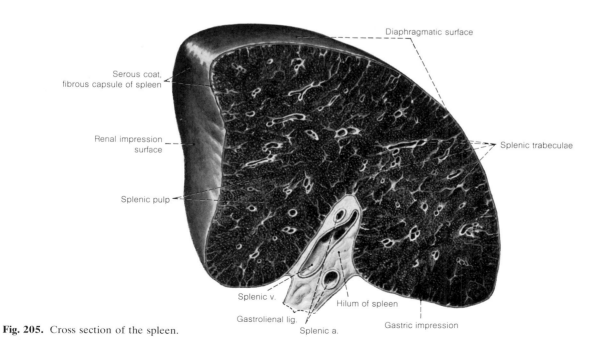

Diaphragmatic surface

Serous coat,
fibrous capsule of spleen

Renal impression
surface

Splenic trabeculae

Splenic pulp

Splenic v.

Hilum of spleen

Gastrolienal lig.

Gastric impression

Splenic a.

Fig. 205. Cross section of the spleen.

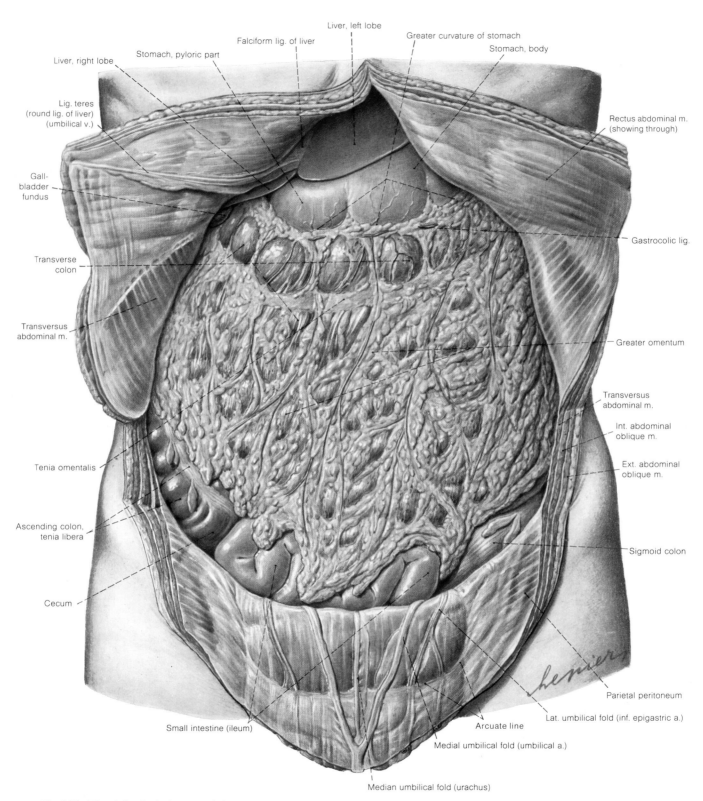

Liver, left lobe

Falciform lig. of liver

Greater curvature of stomach

Stomach, body

Liver, right lobe

Stomach, pyloric part

Lig. teres
(round lig. of liver)
(umbilical v.)

Rectus abdominal m.
(showing through)

Gall-
bladder
fundus

Gastrocolic lig.

Transverse
colon

Transversus
abdominal m.

Greater omentum

Transversus
abdominal m.

Int. abdominal
oblique m.

Ext. abdominal
oblique m.

Tenia omentalis

Ascending colon,
tenia libera

Sigmoid colon

Cecum

Parietal peritoneum

Lat. umbilical fold (inf. epigastric a.)

Small intestine (ileum)

Arcuate line

Medial umbilical fold (umbilical a.)

Median umbilical fold (urachus)

Fig. 206. The abdominal viscera and the greater omentum.

144

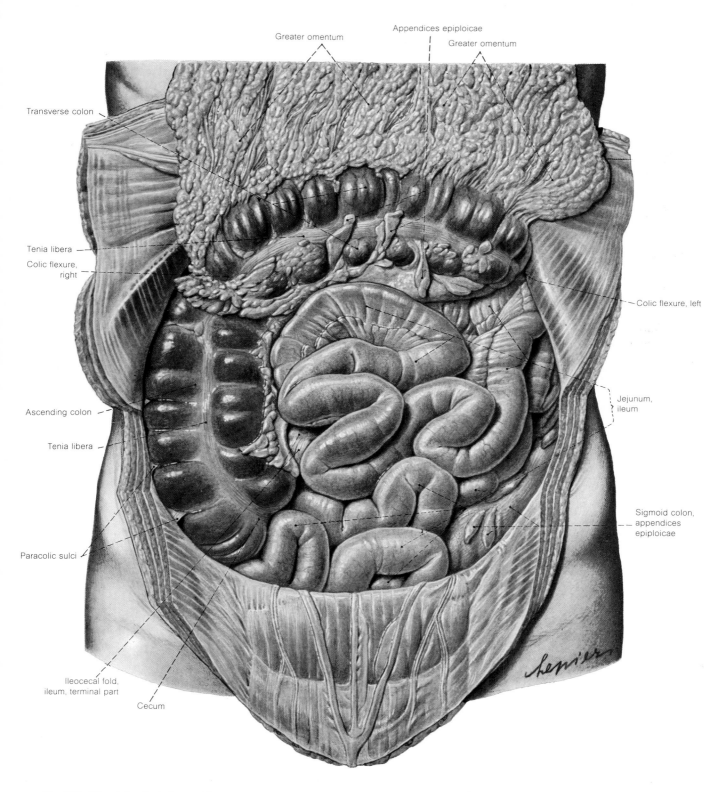

Greater omentum

Appendices epiploicae

Greater omentum

Transverse colon

Tenia libera

Colic flexure, right

Colic flexure, left

Ascending colon

Jejunum, ileum

Tenia libera

Paracolic sulci

Sigmoid colon, appendices epiploicae

Ileocecal fold, ileum, terminal part

Cecum

Fig. 207. The abdominal viscera. The greater omentum and transverse colon reflected cranially so that the intraperitoneal organs of the middle and lower abdominal cavity may be seen.

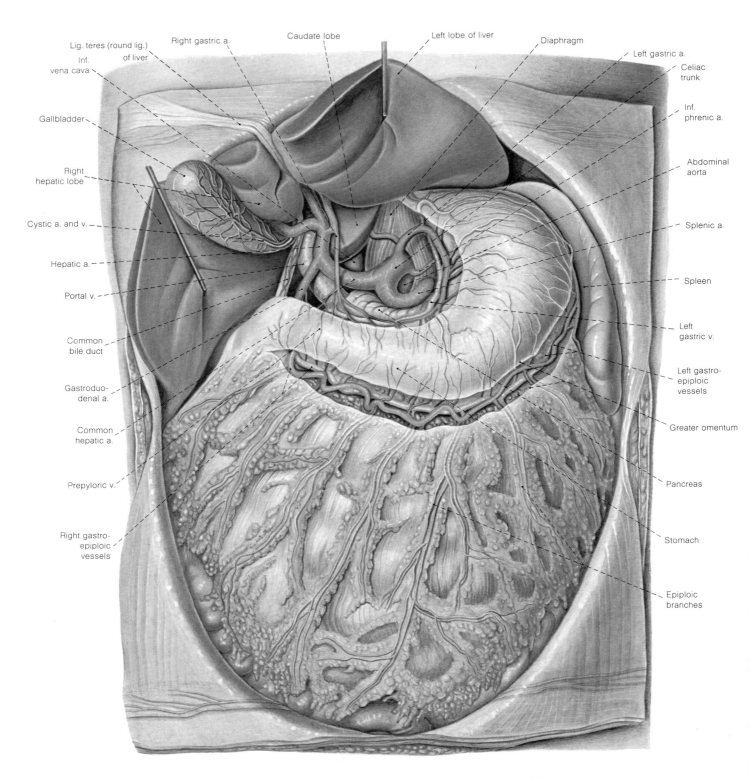

Lig. teres (round lig.) of liver
Inf. vena cava
Gallbladder
Right hepatic lobe
Cystic a. and v.
Hepatic a.
Portal v.
Common bile duct
Gastroduo- denal a.
Common hepatic a.
Prepyloric v.
Right gastro- epiploic vessels

Right gastric a.
Caudate lobe
Left lobe of liver
Diaphragm

Left gastric a.
Celiac trunk
Inf. phrenic a.
Abdominal aorta
Splenic a.
Spleen
Left gastric v.
Left gastro- epiploic vessels
Greater omentum
Pancreas
Stomach
Epiploic branches

Fig. 208. Blood vessels of stomach and liver. The celiac trunk has been exposed; the ventral plane of the greater omentum has been opened along the greater curvature of the stomach in order to expose the gastroepiploic vessels; the lesser omentum and peritoneal membrane in the region of the vestibule to the omental bursa have been removed.

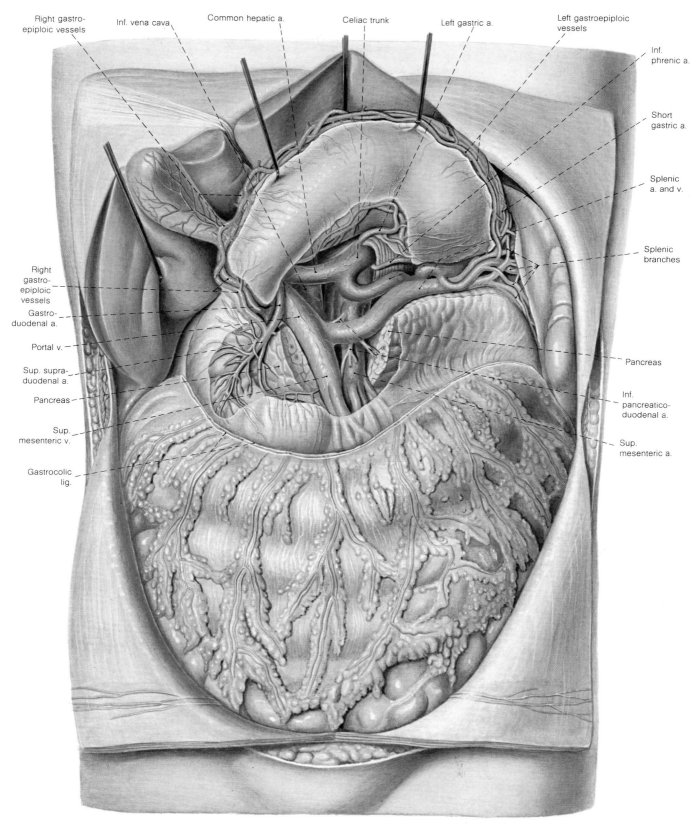

Fig. 209. Blood vessels of the stomach, tributaries to the portal vein, branches of the celiac trunk. The greater omentum has been sectioned and the stomach pulled upward so as to expose its posterior wall. A portion of the pancreas has been removed in order to expose the superior mesenteric artery and vein.

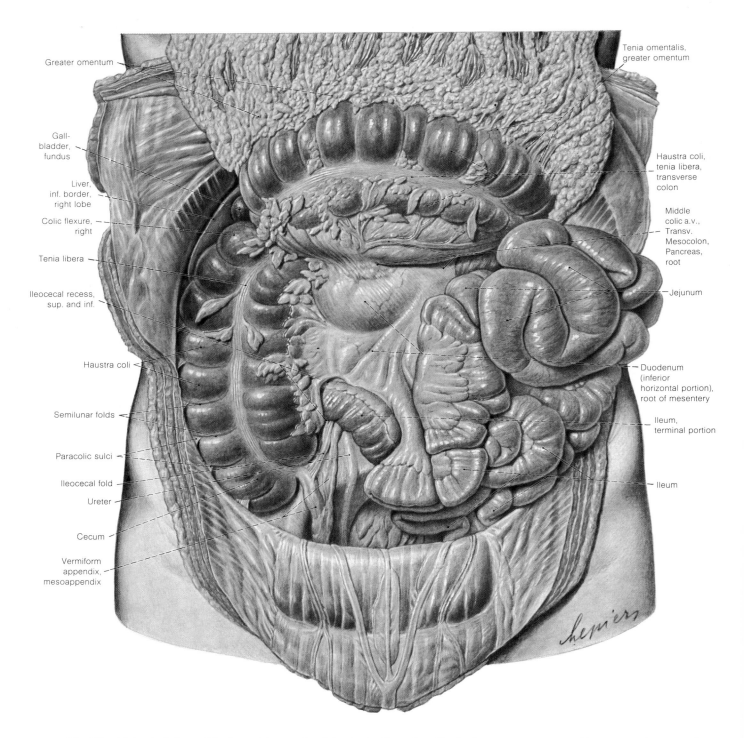

Greater omentum

Gall-
bladder,
fundus

Liver,
inf. border,
right lobe

Colic flexure,
right

Tenia libera

Ileocecal recess,
sup. and inf.

Haustra coli

Semilunar folds

Paracolic sulci

Ileocecal fold

Ureter

Cecum

Vermiform
appendix,
mesoappendix

Tenia omentalis,
greater omentum

Haustra coli,
tenia libera,
transverse
colon

Middle
colic a.v.,
Transv.
Mesocolon,
Pancreas,
root

Jejunum

Duodenum
(inferior
horizontal portion),
root of mesentery

Ileum,
terminal portion

Ileum

Fig. 210. Abdominal viscera. The flaps of the anterior abdominal wall are pinned back, the greater omentum and transverse colon upward, the small intestine toward the left. The vermiform appendix and the terminal part of the ileum are seen in the right iliac region. In the right hypochondrium, the sharp lower edge of the right liver lobe and the fundus of the gallbladder may be seen.

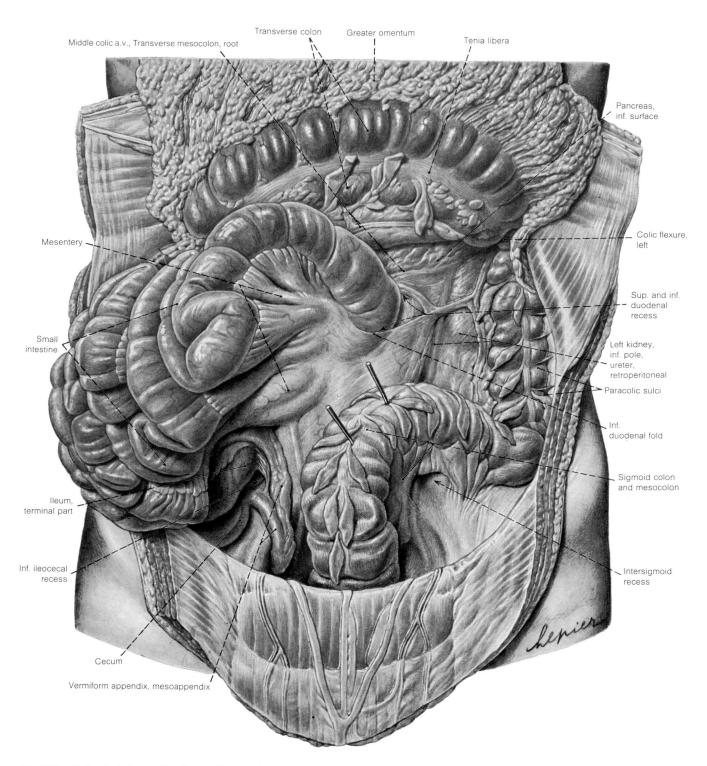

Middle colic a.v., Transverse mesocolon, root

Transverse colon

Greater omentum

Tenia libera

Pancreas, inf. surface

Mesentery

Colic flexure, left

Sup. and inf. duodenal recess

Small intestine

Left kidney, inf. pole, ureter, retroperitoneal

Paracolic sulci

Inf. duodenal fold

Sigmoid colon and mesocolon

Ileum, terminal part

Inf. ileocecal recess

Intersigmoid recess

Cecum

Vermiform appendix, mesoappendix

Fig. 211. Abdominal viscera. The flaps of the anterior abdominal wall, pushed laterally above and pulled down below. The greater omentum and transverse colon are pushed upward, the convolutions of the small intestine are laid toward the right, the sigmoid colon pulled forward and upward with hooks.

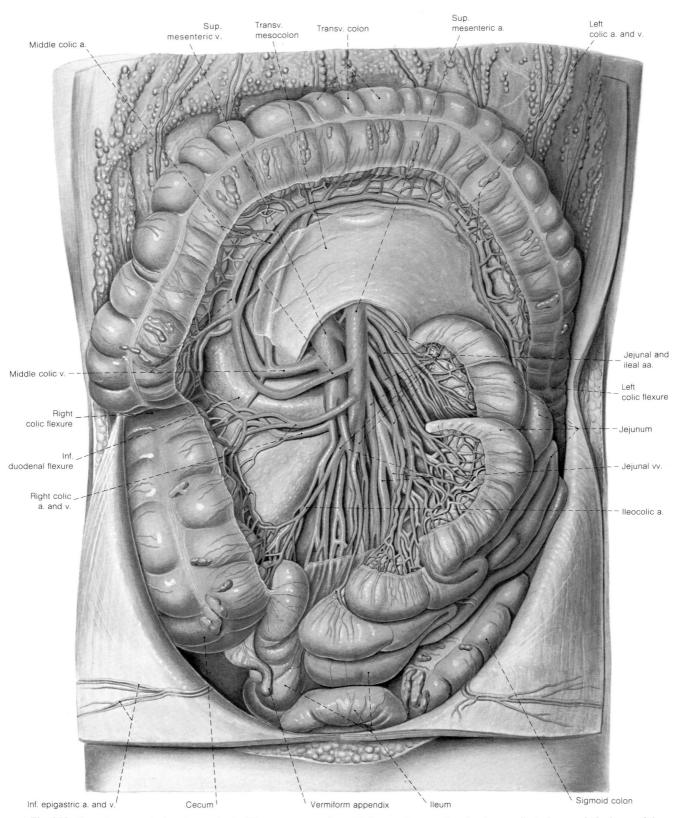

Middle colic a.

Sup. mesenteric v.

Transv. mesocolon

Transv. colon

Sup. mesenteric a.

Left colic a. and v.

Jejunal and ileal aa.

Middle colic v.

Left colic flexure

Right colic flexure

Jejunum

Inf. duodenal flexure

Jejunal vv.

Right colic a. and v.

Ileocolic a.

Inf. epigastric a. and v.

Cecum

Vermiform appendix

Ileum

Sigmoid colon

Fig. 212. Superior mesenteric artery and vein. The transverse colon with the greater omentum has been reflected upward, the loops of the small intestine have been moved toward the left. The parietal peritoneal membrane has been partially removed in order to expose the blood vessels.

150

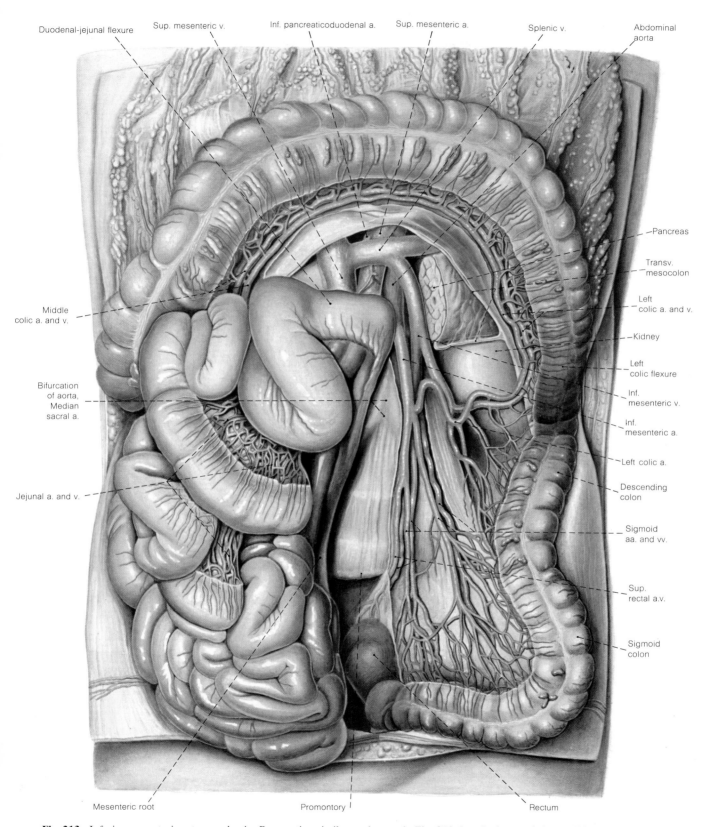

Duodenal-jejunal flexure

Sup. mesenteric v.

Inf. pancreaticoduodenal a.

Sup. mesenteric a.

Splenic v.

Abdominal aorta

Pancreas

Transv. mesocolon

Left colic a. and v.

Kidney

Left colic flexure

Inf. mesenteric v.

Inf. mesenteric a.

Left colic a.

Descending colon

Sigmoid aa. and vv.

Sup. rectal a.v.

Sigmoid colon

Middle colic a. and v.

Bifurcation of aorta, Median sacral a.

Jejunal a. and v.

Mesenteric root

Promontory

Rectum

Fig. 213. Inferior mesenteric artery and vein. Preparation similar to the one in Fig. 212, but the loops of the small intestine have been moved toward the right.

151

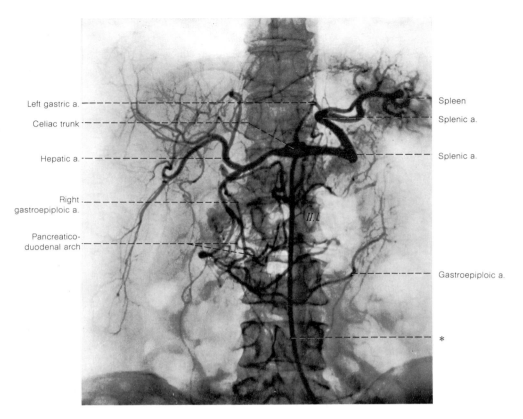

Left gastric a.

Celiac trunk

Hepatic a.

Right gastroepiploic a.

Pancreatico-duodenal arch

Spleen

Splenic a.

Splenic a.

Il. l.

Gastroepiploic a.

*

Fig. 214.

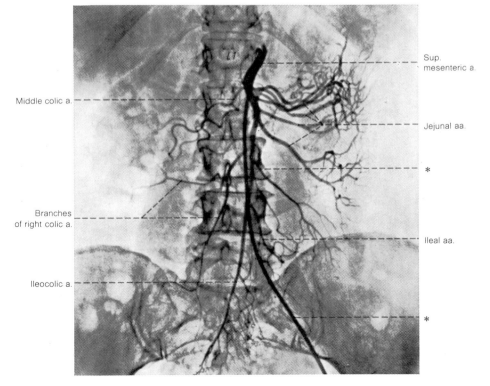

Middle colic a.

Branches of right colic a.

Ileocolic a.

Sup. mesenteric a.

Jejunal aa.

*

Ileal aa.

*

Fig. 215.

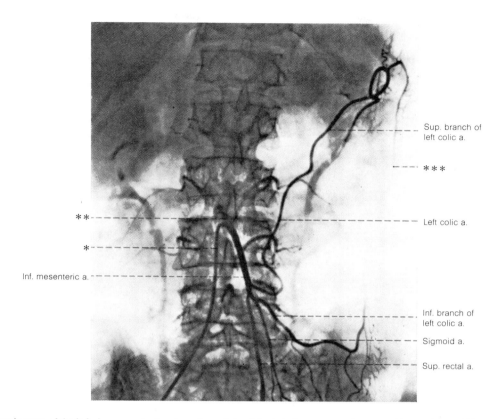

Sup. branch of
left colic a.

* * *

Left colic a.

Inf. branch of
left colic a.

Sigmoid a.

Sup. rectal a.

* *

*

Inf. mesenteric a.

Fig. 216. Arteriogram of the inferior mesenteric artery. * = origin of the inferior mesenteric artery; ** = catheter; *** = anastomosis along the descending colon.

◁ **Fig. 214.** Normal arteriogram of the branches of the celiac trunk. * = catheter in the aorta with its tip at the origin of the celiac trunk. (From BENNINGHOFF/GOERTTLER: Lehrbuch der Anatomie des Menschen, Vol. 2, 12th ed. [Eds. H. FERNER and J. STAUBESAND]. Urban & Schwarzenberg, Munich–Berlin–Vienna 1979.)

◁ **Fig. 215.** Arteriogram of the superior mesenteric artery. * = catheter in the abdominal aorta.

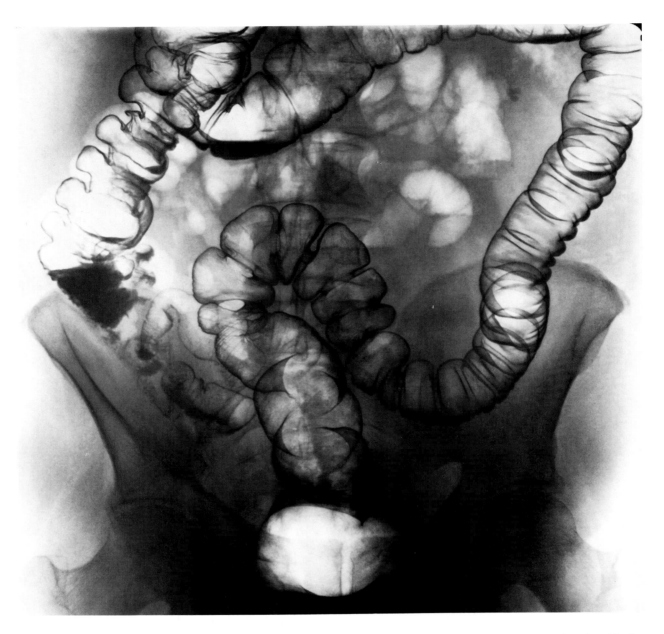

Fig. 217. Survey radiogram of the large intestine: right colic flexure, transverse colon, left colic flexure, descending colon, sigmoid colon and rectum. Double-contrast method. (Original: Prof. Dr. J. ALTARAS, Zentrum für Radiologie am Klinikum der Universität Giessen.)

The large intestine can be x-ray-examined optimally by means of the double-contrast method. After extended filling of all colonic portions with a positive contrast medium, subsequent emptying and insufflation with air the large intestine can be unfolded into a transparent tube. This transparency gives a spatial impression of the entire colon whose interior surface can be viewed at the same time en profil and en face. This makes it possible to evaluate organic changes not only as to their location but also as to their size and shape.

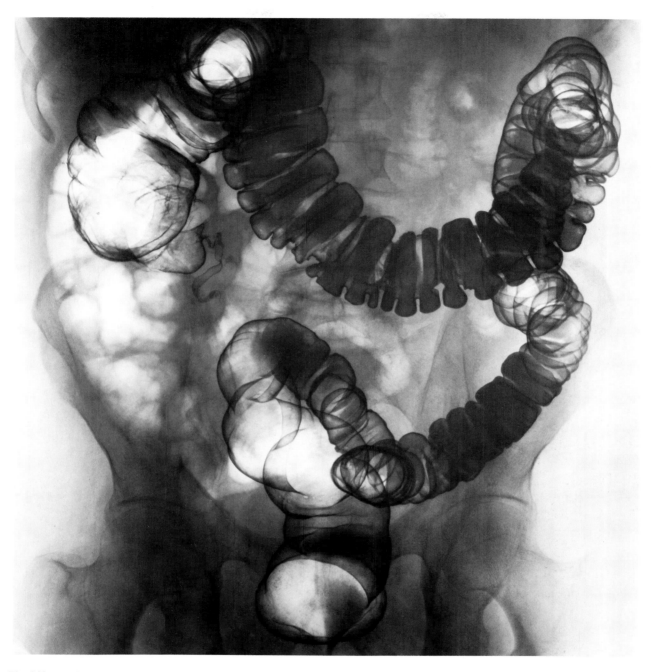

Fig. 218. Radiogram of rectum and sigmoid colon. (Original: Prof. Dr. J. ALTARAS, Zentrum für Radiologie am Klinikum der Universität Giessen.)

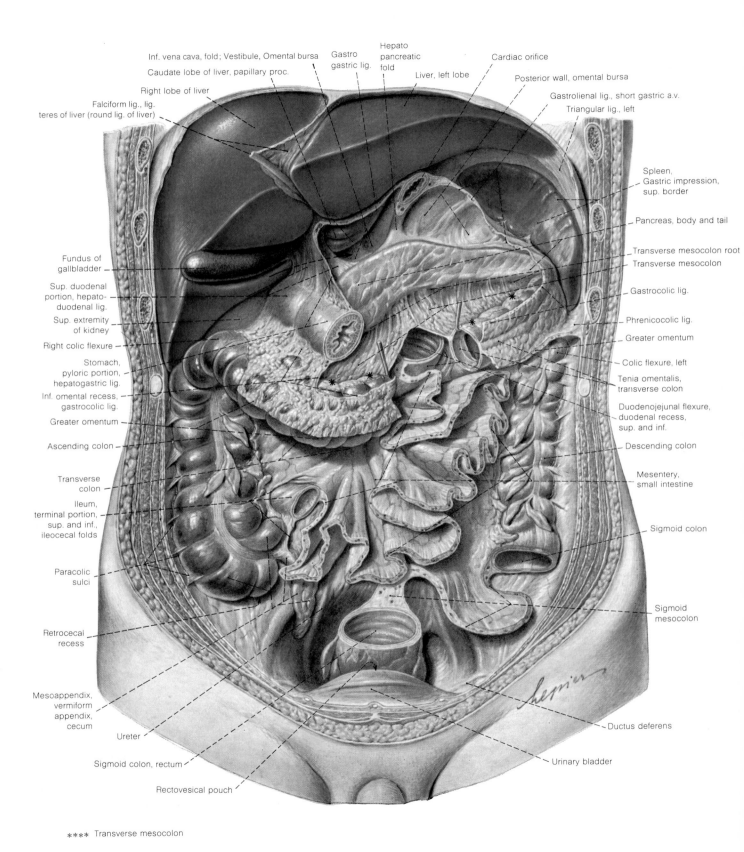

Inf. vena cava, fold; Vestibule, Omental bursa

Caudate lobe of liver, papillary proc.

Right lobe of liver

Falciform lig., lig.
teres of liver (round lig. of liver)

Gastro
gastric lig.

Hepato
pancreatic
fold

Liver, left lobe

Cardiac orifice

Posterior wall, omental bursa

Gastrolienal lig., short gastric a.v.

Triangular lig., left

Spleen,
Gastric impression,
sup. border

Pancreas, body and tail

Transverse mesocolon root

Transverse mesocolon

Gastrocolic lig.

Phrenicocolic lig.

Greater omentum

Colic flexure, left

Tenia omentalis,
transverse colon

Duodenojejunal flexure,
duodenal recess,
sup. and inf.

Descending colon

Mesentery,
small intestine

Sigmoid colon

Sigmoid
mesocolon

Ductus deferens

Urinary bladder

Fundus of
gallbladder

Sup. duodenal
portion, hepato-
duodenal lig.

Sup. extremity
of kidney

Right colic flexure

Stomach,
pyloric portion,
hepatogastric lig.

Inf. omental recess,
gastrocolic lig.

Greater omentum

Ascending colon

Transverse
colon

Ileum,
terminal portion,
sup. and inf.,
ileocecal folds

Paracolic
sulci

Retrocecal
recess

Mesoappendix,
vermiform
appendix,
cecum

Ureter

Sigmoid colon, rectum

Rectovesical pouch

✳✳✳✳ Transverse mesocolon

Fig. 219. Abdominal viscera. The stomach was removed from the cardiac portion to the pyloric portion, revealing the omental bursa and structures on the dorsal wall.

156

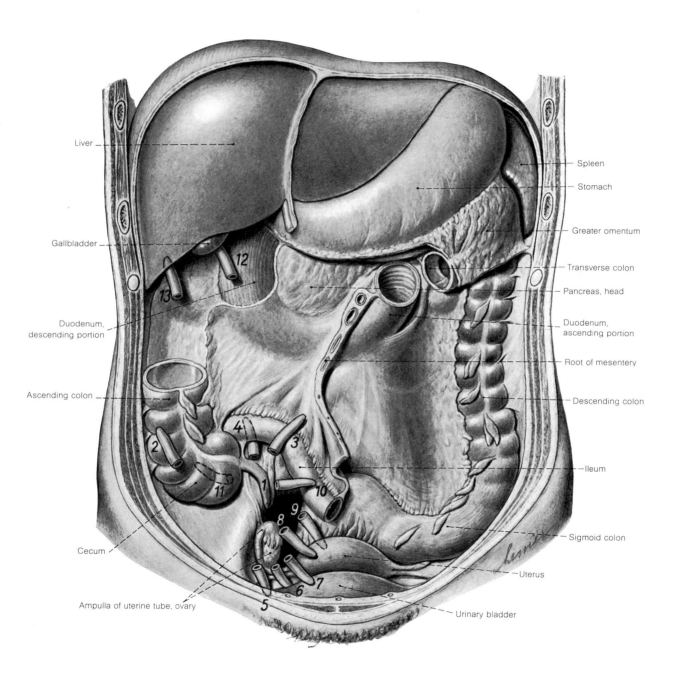

Liver

Gallbladder

Duodenum, descending portion

Ascending colon

Cecum

Ampulla of uterine tube, ovary

Spleen

Stomach

Greater omentum

Transverse colon

Pancreas, head

Duodenum, ascending portion

Root of mesentery

Descending colon

Ileum

Sigmoid colon

Uterus

Urinary bladder

1 Normal	6 In the uterovesical pouch	10 Toward the ileum and sigmoid colon
2 Lateral	7 On the urinary bladder	11 Rectocecal
3 Toward umbilicus and root of mesentery	8 On the uterus, uterine tube, or ovary	12 Toward the gallbladder
4 Dorsal to terminal part of ileum	9 In the rectouterine pouch (of DOUGLAS)	13 Toward the liver
5 In inguinal region		

Fig. 220. Variations in the location of the vermiform appendix: The deviations from the normal position are influenced by the length of the appendix and the mobility of the cecum.

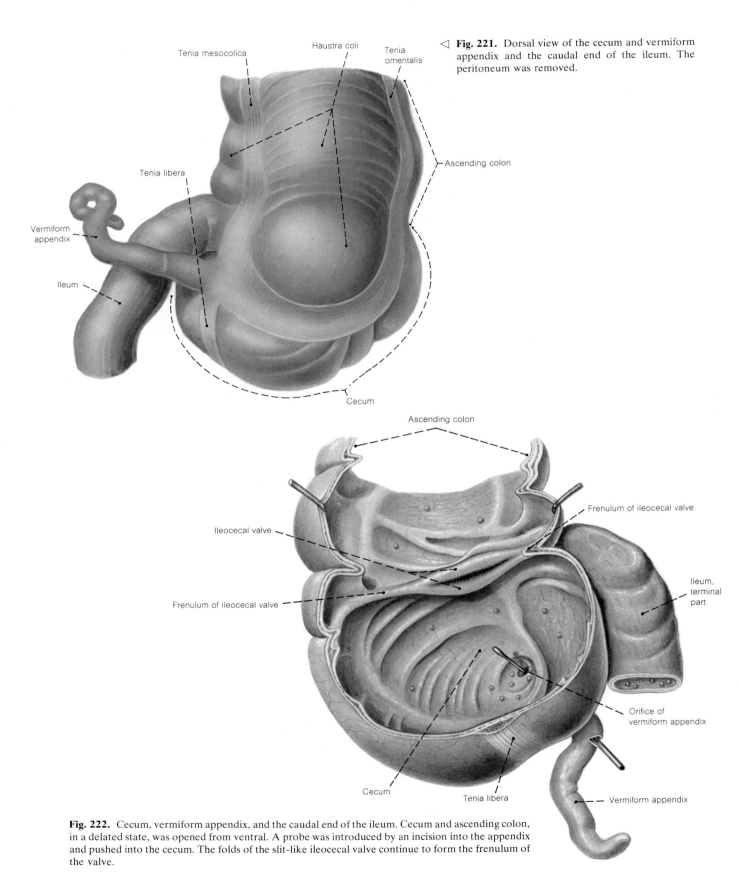

Tenia mesocolica

Haustra coli

Tenia omentalis

◁ **Fig. 221.** Dorsal view of the cecum and vermiform appendix and the caudal end of the ileum. The peritoneum was removed.

Tenia libera

Ascending colon

Vermiform appendix

Ileum

Cecum

Ascending colon

Ileocecal valve

Frenulum of ileocecal valve

Frenulum of ileocecal valve

Ileum, terminal part

Orifice of vermiform appendix

Cecum

Tenia libera

Vermiform appendix

Fig. 222. Cecum, vermiform appendix, and the caudal end of the ileum. Cecum and ascending colon, in a delated state, was opened from ventral. A probe was introduced by an incision into the appendix and pushed into the cecum. The folds of the slit-like ileocecal valve continue to form the frenulum of the valve.

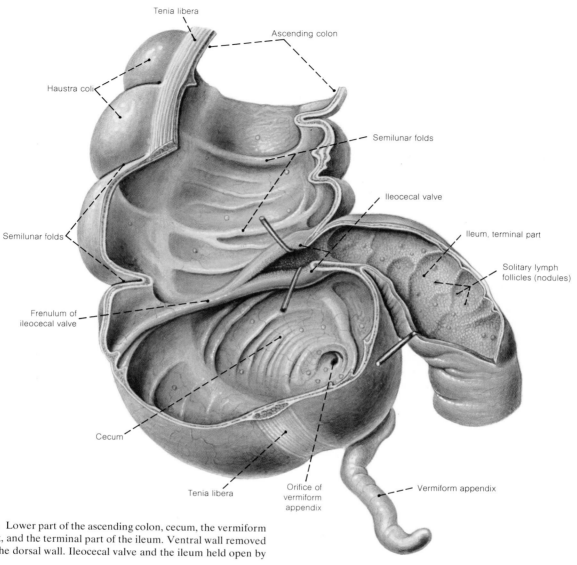

Tenia libera

Ascending colon

Haustra coli

Semilunar folds

Ileocecal valve

Ileum, terminal part

Semilunar folds

Solitary lymph
follicles (nodules)

Frenulum of
ileocecal valve

Cecum

Tenia libera

Orifice of
vermiform
appendix

Vermiform appendix

Fig. 223. Lower part of the ascending colon, cecum, the vermiform appendix, and the terminal part of the ileum. Ventral wall removed to view the dorsal wall. Ileocecal valve and the ileum held open by hooks.

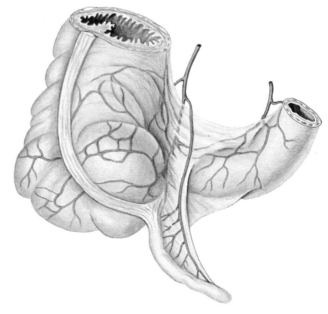

Fig. 224. Vascular supply of the vermiform appendix through the appendicular artery (having no arcades). The ostial segment is supplied by a branch from the ileocolic artery. After F. STELZNER and W. LIERSE, Langenbecks Arch. Chir. 330 (1972).

159

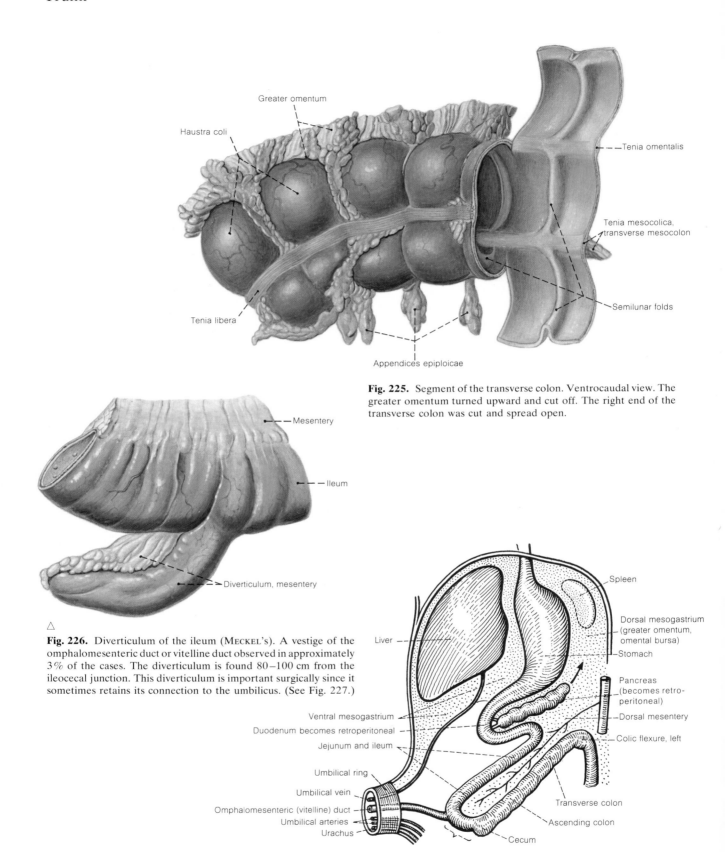

Greater omentum

Haustra coli

Tenia omentalis

Tenia mesocolica, transverse mesocolon

Semilunar folds

Tenia libera

Appendices epiploicae

Fig. 225. Segment of the transverse colon. Ventrocaudal view. The greater omentum turned upward and cut off. The right end of the transverse colon was cut and spread open.

Mesentery

Ileum

Diverticulum, mesentery

△

Fig. 226. Diverticulum of the ileum (MECKEL's). A vestige of the omphalomesenteric duct or vitelline duct observed in approximately 3% of the cases. The diverticulum is found 80–100 cm from the ileocecal junction. This diverticulum is important surgically since it sometimes retains its connection to the umbilicus. (See Fig. 227.)

Spleen

Liver

Dorsal mesogastrium (greater omentum, omental bursa)

Stomach

Pancreas (becomes retroperitoneal)

Dorsal mesentery

Colic flexure, left

Ventral mesogastrium

Duodenum becomes retroperitoneal

Jejunum and ileum

Umbilical ring

Umbilical vein

Omphalomesenteric (vitelline) duct

Umbilical arteries

Urachus

Transverse colon

Ascending colon

Cecum

Fig. 227. Development of the gastrointestinal tract in a 5-week old embryo. The stomach, liver, and spleen are in a sagittal plane and do not reach their definitive stage until the stomach rotates through 90°. MECKEL's diverticulum is a vestige of the omphalomesenteric duct. The course of the superior mesenteric artery is in the navel loop.

160

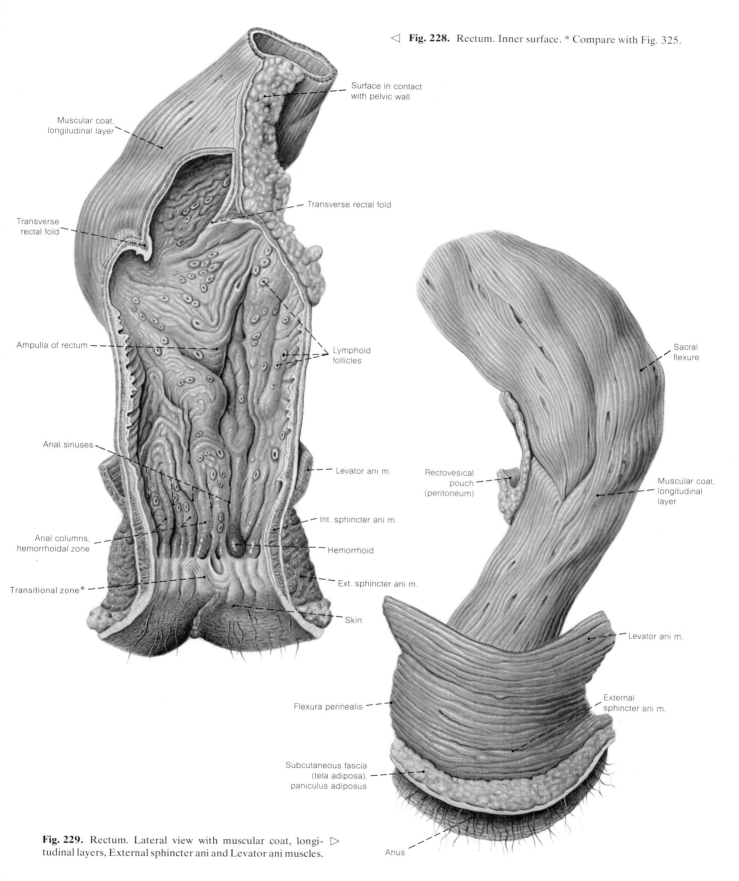

◁ **Fig. 228.** Rectum. Inner surface. * Compare with Fig. 325.

Surface in contact with pelvic wall

Muscular coat, longitudinal layer

Transverse rectal fold

Transverse rectal fold

Ampulla of rectum

Lymphoid follicles

Anal sinuses

Levator ani m.

Int. sphincter ani m.

Anal columns, hemorrhoidal zone

Hemorrhoid

Transitional zone*

Ext. sphincter ani m.

Skin

Flexura perinealis

Subcutaneous fascia (tela adiposa), paniculus adiposus

Sacral flexure

Rectovesical pouch (peritoneum)

Muscular coat, longitudinal layer

Levator ani m.

External sphincter ani m.

Anus

Fig. 229. Rectum. Lateral view with muscular coat, longitudinal layers, External sphincter ani and Levator ani muscles. ▷

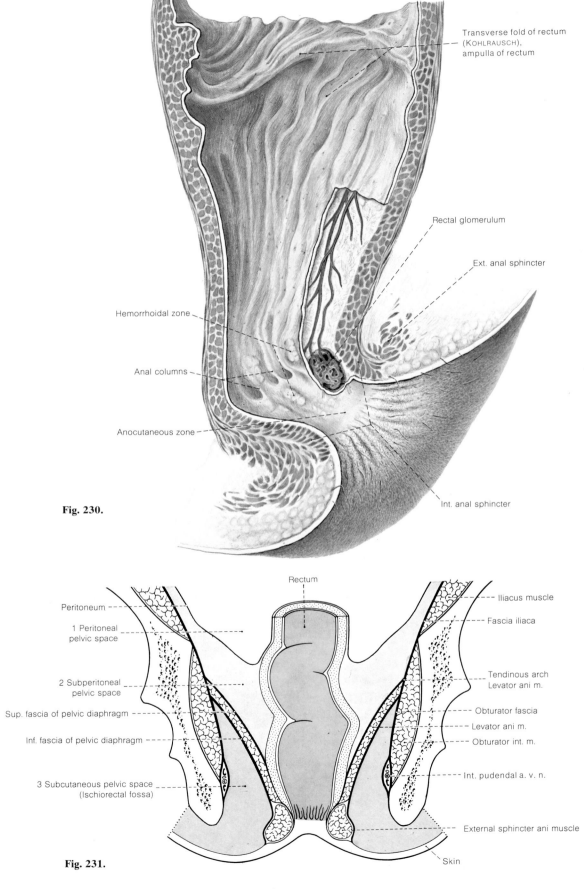

Transverse fold of rectum (KOHLRAUSCH), ampulla of rectum

Rectal glomerulum

Ext. anal sphincter

Hemorrhoidal zone

Anal columns

Anocutaneous zone

Int. anal sphincter

Fig. 230.

Rectum

Peritoneum

1 Peritoneal pelvic space

2 Subperitoneal pelvic space

Sup. fascia of pelvic diaphragm

Inf. fascia of pelvic diaphragm

3 Subcutaneous pelvic space (Ischiorectal fossa)

Iliacus muscle

Fascia iliaca

Tendinous arch Levator ani m.

Obturator fascia

Levator ani m.

Obturator int. m.

Int. pudendal a. v. n.

External sphincter ani muscle

Skin

Fig. 231.

◁ **Fig. 230.** Corpus cavernosum recti. Median section through the rectum. The mucous membrane has been partially removed in order to display the submucous afferent and efferent vessels of a rectal glomerulum. From J. STAUBESAND, Phlebol. u. Proctol. 1, 55–68 (1972).

Fig. 231. Diagrammatic frontal section through the pelvis in the region of the rectum (1, 2, 3): the three pelvic levels. Note the internal pudendal artery, the pudendal nerve, and the internal pudendal veins in the pudendal canal (ALCOCK's).

The corpus cavernosum recti is formed by the sum of all rectal glomerula (Fig. 230). It is essential for the muscular and mucous closure of the anus ("continence organ"). The arterio-venous rectal glomerula form the normal anatomical basis for the internal hemorrhoids and, therefore, should not be considered as pathologically extended veins or varicosities.

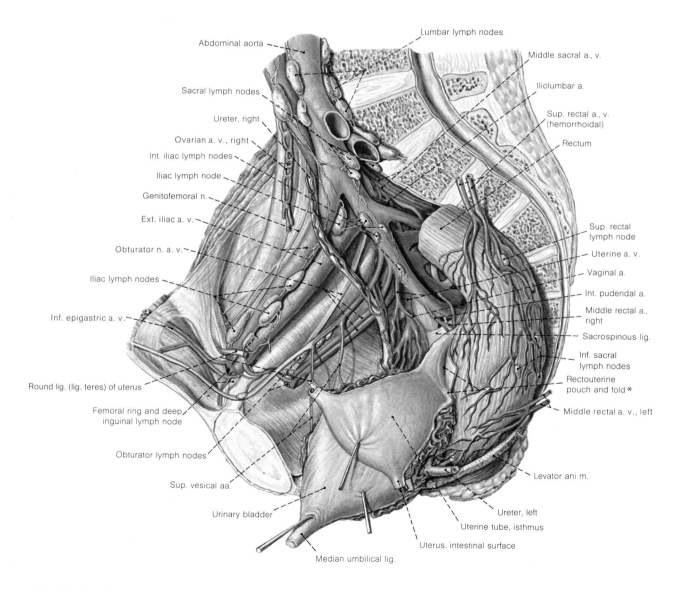

Fig. 232. Lymphatic vessels and nodes of the right lateral wall of the large and small pelvis. The pelvis was sectioned in the midline, but the urinary bladder, uterus, and rectum remain; the blood vessels, nerves, and lymphatics are displayed. Compare with Figs. 247 and 248. * DOUGLAS's pouch.

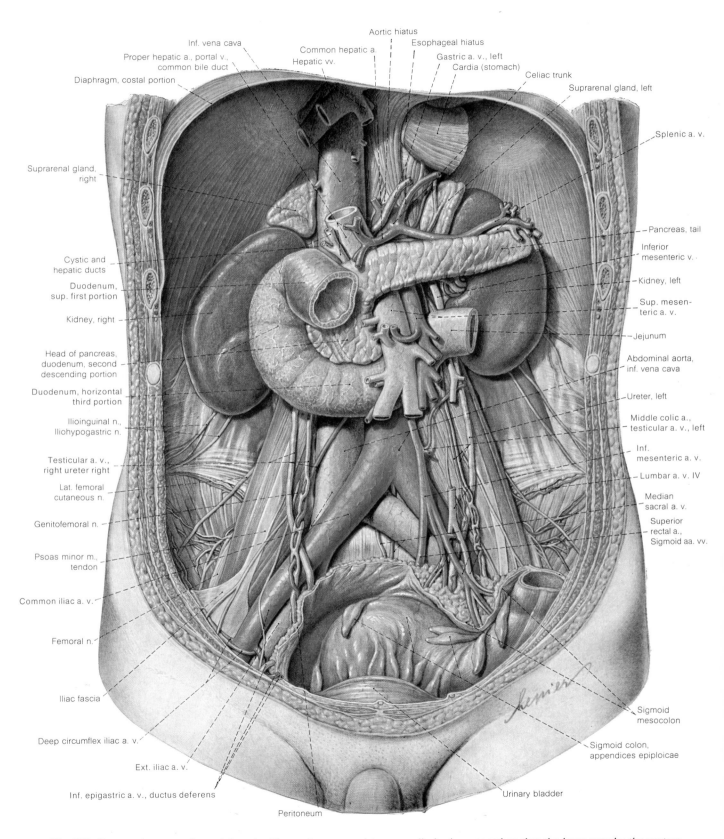

Inf. vena cava

Proper hepatic a., portal v., common bile duct

Diaphragm, costal portion

Aortic hiatus

Common hepatic a.
Hepatic vv.

Esophageal hiatus

Gastric a. v., left
Cardia (stomach)

Celiac trunk

Suprarenal gland, left

Splenic a. v.

Suprarenal gland, right

Pancreas, tail

Inferior mesenteric v.

Cystic and hepatic ducts

Kidney, left

Duodenum, sup. first portion

Sup. mesenteric a. v.

Kidney, right

Jejunum

Head of pancreas, duodenum, second descending portion

Abdominal aorta, inf. vena cava

Duodenum, horizontal third portion

Ureter, left

Ilioinguinal n., iliohypogastric n.

Middle colic a., testicular a. v., left

Testicular a. v., right ureter right

Inf. mesenteric a. v.

Lat. femoral cutaneous n.

Lumbar a. v. IV

Genitofemoral n.

Median sacral a. v.

Superior rectal a., Sigmoid aa. vv.

Psoas minor m., tendon

Common iliac a. v.

Femoral n.

Iliac fascia

Sigmoid mesocolon

Deep circumflex iliac a. v.

Sigmoid colon, appendices epiploicae

Ext. iliac a. v.

Inf. epigastric a. v., ductus deferens

Urinary bladder

Peritoneum

Fig. 233. Retroperitoneum of an adult male. The peritoneum and transversalis fascia removed so that the large vessels: the ureters, branches of the lumbar plexus, and a piece of the right ductus deferens, may be seen.

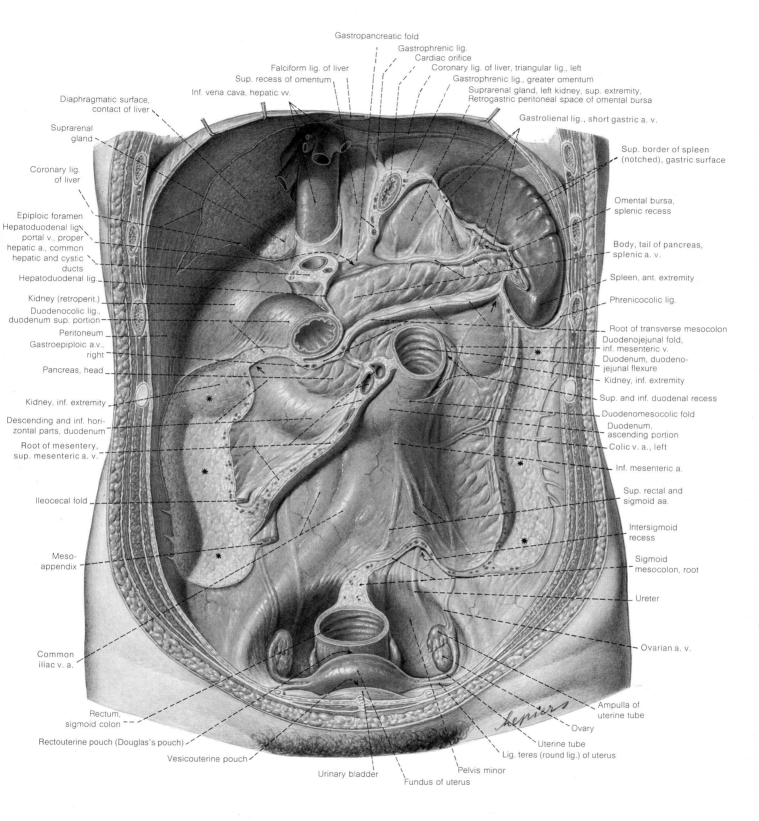

Fig. 234. Retroperitoneum of an adult woman. Posterior to the transverse cut of the hepatoduodenal ligament is an arrow in the epiploic foramen (WINSLOW's). The place of adhesion of ascending and descending colon with the dorsal body wall is marked with asterisks (*). Arrows on the right and left niche for the colic flexures.

165

Computerized tomography is a radiological procedure that utilizes a computer for image construction. A thinly focussed bundle of rays (layer thickness 1.5–10 mm) rotates around the body. An oppositely arranged detector measures the decrease in intensity of the x-rays behind the object at different angles. About 300,000 individual values per layer are transformed by the computer into graytones of a monitor image. The computerized tomographical picture is a topographically exact image of a section through the body. During the last few years, computerized tomography has played a leading role in the Roentgendiagnosis of the head and it gains increasing significance also for the examination of body cavities and internal organs. Special computer programs permit the creation, without additional exposure to x-rays, of so-called computer reformations, a "rearrangement" of computer data into sectional images in any plane and, thereby, an exact three-dimensional orientation. An essential prerequisite for the correct interpretation of computerized tomographic images and the optimal use of the reformation technique is, besides the familiarity with technical procedures, the detailed knowledge of the topography of various body regions.

Abdominal Computerized Tomograms
Topography of Internal Organs

Those abdominal and retroperitoneal organs that are surrounded by fat are sharply depicted.
By application of diluted gastrografin solutions and contrast media that clear through the Kidneys, the gastro-intestinal tract, Kidneys and urinary passages can be better visualized. Note the detailed demonstration of aorta, inferior vena cava, and splenic and renal vessels. Originals: Radiologische Abteilung Elisabeth-Krankenhaus Neuwied. Arrangement: Dr. R. UNSÖLD, Univ.-Augenklinik, Freiburg i. Brsg.

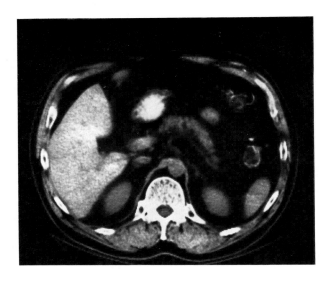

Fig. 235. Visualization of the upper margin of the pancreas and a loop of the splenic artery, further of liver, spleen, upper poles of the kidneys and suprarenal glands.

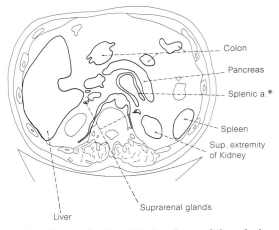

Fig. 236. Outline diagram for Fig. 235. * = Loop of the splenic artery.

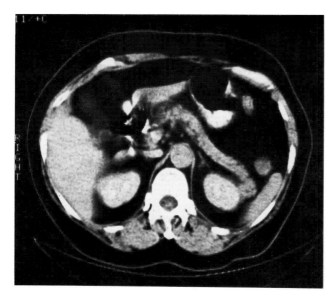

Fig. 237. Visualization of pancreas, splenic vein, liver, upper renal poles and left suprarenal gland.

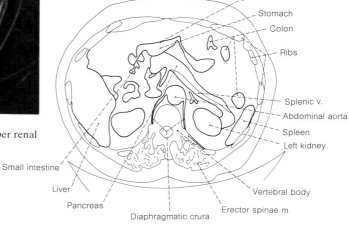

Fig. 238. Outline diagram for Fig. 237. * = Border between air and contrast medium.

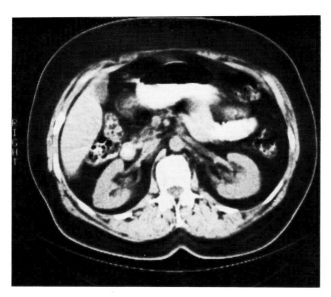

Fig. 239. Visualization of stomach, kidney and renal vessels.

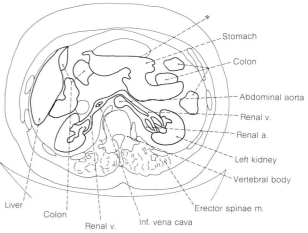

Fig. 240. Outline diagram for Fig. 239. * = Border between air and contrast medium.

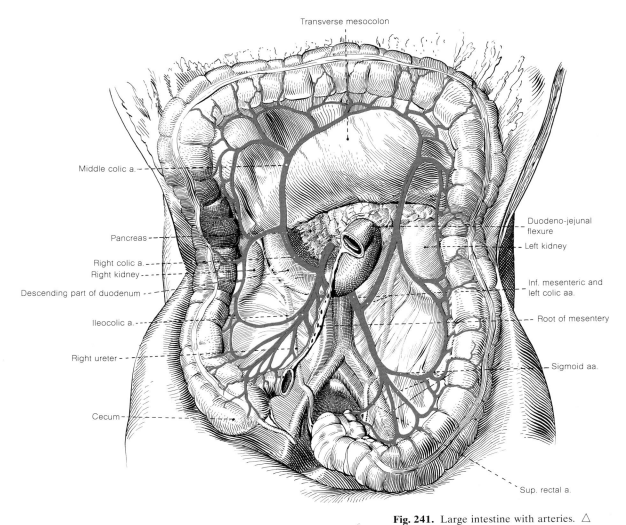

Transverse mesocolon

Middle colic a.

Pancreas

Right colic a.
Right kidney
Descending part of duodenum

Ileocolic a.

Right ureter

Cecum

Duodeno-jejunal flexure

Left kidney

Inf. mesenteric and left colic aa.

Root of mesentery

Sigmoid aa.

Sup. rectal a.

Fig. 241. Large intestine with arteries. △

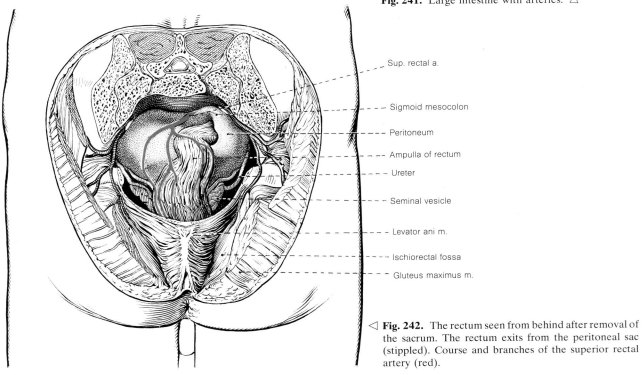

Sup. rectal a.

Sigmoid mesocolon

Peritoneum

Ampulla of rectum

Ureter

Seminal vesicle

Levator ani m.

Ischiorectal fossa

Gluteus maximus m.

◁ **Fig. 242.** The rectum seen from behind after removal of the sacrum. The rectum exits from the peritoneal sac (stippled). Course and branches of the superior rectal artery (red).

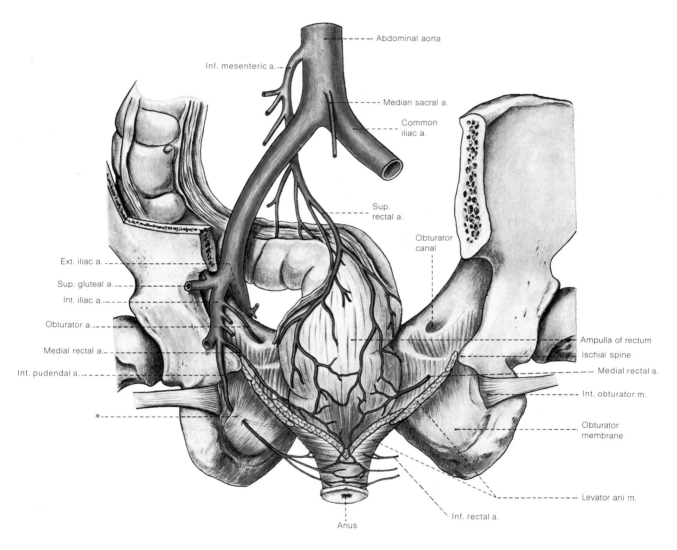

Abdominal aorta

Inf. mesenteric a.

Median sacral a.

Common
iliac a.

Sup.
rectal a.

Obturator
canal

Ext. iliac a.

Sup. gluteal a.

Int. iliac a.

Obturator a.

Medial rectal a.

Int. pudendal a.

Ampulla of rectum

Ischial spine

Medial rectal a.

Int. obturator m.

Obturator
membrane

*

Levator ani m.

Anus

Inf. rectal a.

Fig. 243. Schematic presentation of the blood supply of the rectum. Dorsal view of the ampulla of the rectum. Note the origin of the superior rectal artery from the inferior mesenteric artery, the branching of the middle rectal artery from the internal iliac artery and the origin of the inferior rectal artery from the internal pudendal artery. Based on an illustration by F. H. NETTER (1969). (From H. SCHMIDT and J. STAUBESAND, Fortschr. Röntgenstr. 116, 297–305, 1972.) * Origin of the inferior rectal artery within ALCOCK's canal.

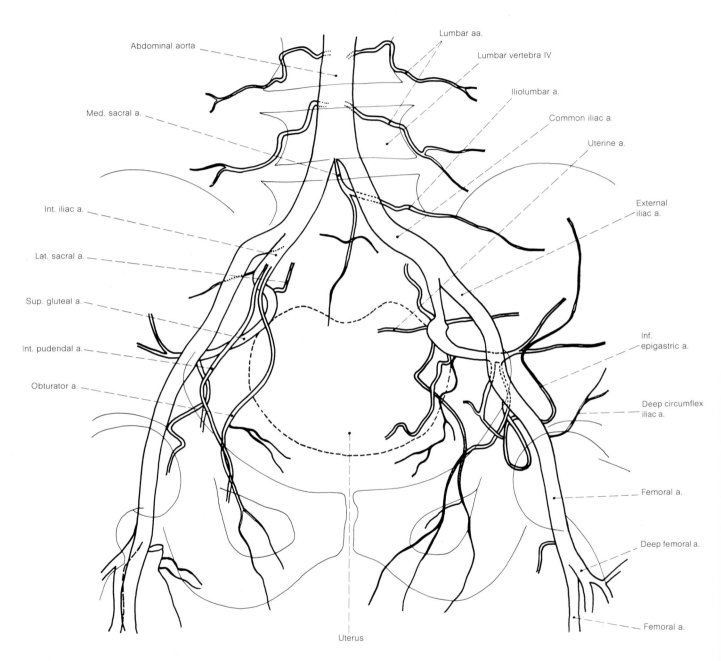

Abdominal aorta

Lumbar aa.

Lumbar vertebra IV

Med. sacral a.

Iliolumbar a.

Common iliac a.

Uterine a.

Int. iliac a.

External
iliac a.

Lat. sacral a.

Sup. gluteal a.

Inf.
epigastric a.

Int. pudendal a.

Deep circumflex
iliac a.

Obturator a.

Femoral a.

Deep femoral a.

Femoral a.

Uterus

Fig. 244. Outline diagram for Fig. 245.

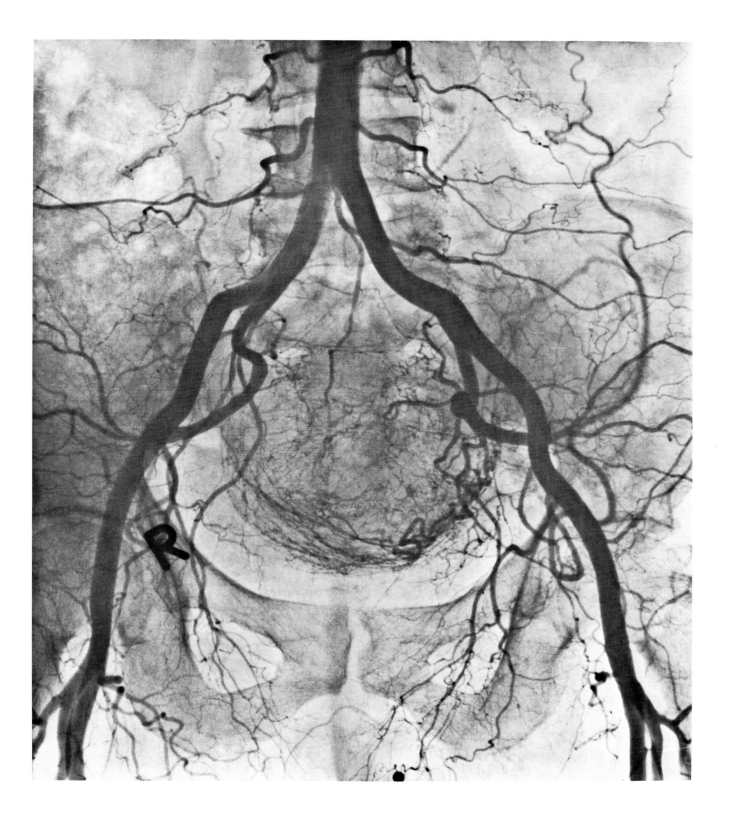

Fig. 245. Angiogram of the lower abdominal aorta, common iliac arteries, external and internal iliac arteries and their branches. A–P projection. (From L. WICKE: Atlas der Röntgenanatomie, 2nd ed. Urban & Schwarzenberg, Munich–Vienna–Baltimore 1980.)

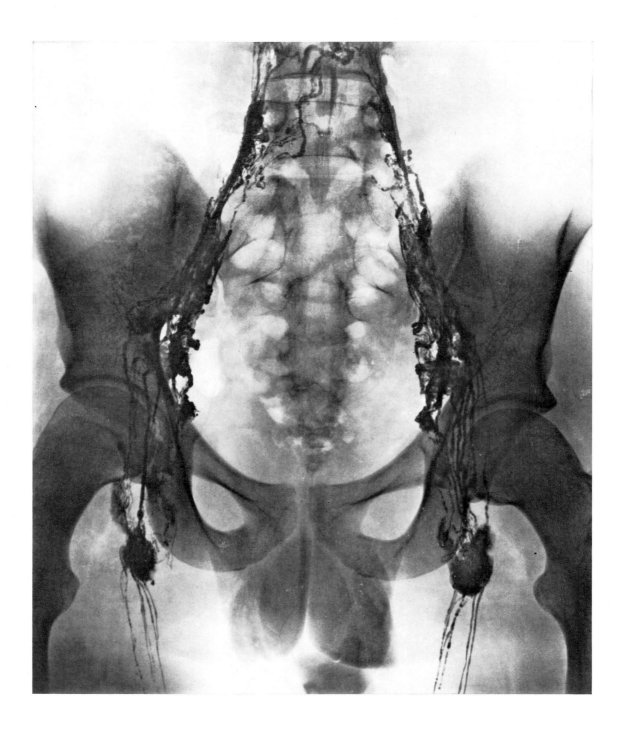

Fig. 246. Lymph angiogram of an 18-year old; sagittal exposure. Demonstration of the inguinal, ileocecal, and lumbar lymphatic vessels as well as the prevertebral anastomosis by means of an iodine-containing oil as contrast material (Lipiodol®). The beaded distentions of lymphatic vessels are brought about by one after another valve segments in succession. Initial storage of contrast medium in individual lymph nodes, especially in the inguinal region. (Photo: Dr. L. BAUMEISTER, Zentrum Radiologie am Klinikum der Universität Freiburg i. Brsg.).

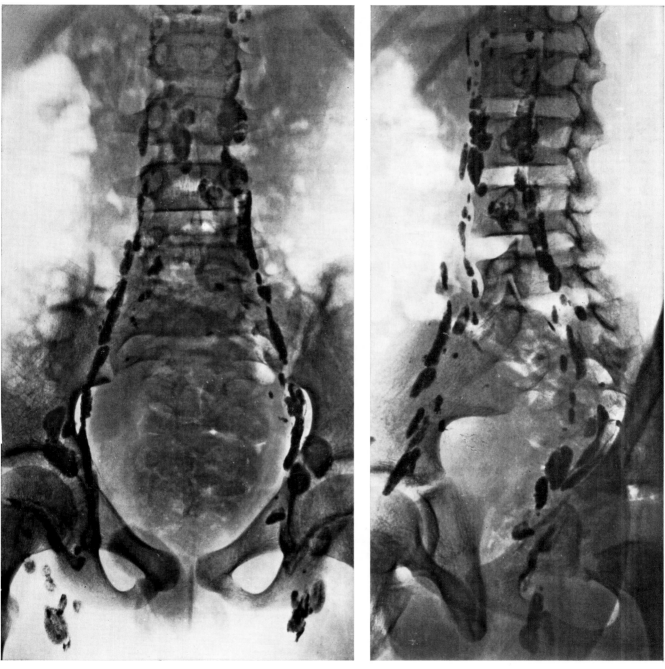

Fig. 247.   **Fig. 248.**

Figs. 247 and 248. Lymph angiogram of a 10-year old boy in supine (Fig. 247) and left anterior oblique position (Fig. 248). Storage of an iodine-containing oil contrast medium (Lipiodol®) in the inguinal, external iliac, common iliac, and lumbar lymph nodes. The combination of both photographic positions permits a more precise localization of individual lymph nodes. (Photo: Dr. L. BAUMEISTER, Zentrum Radiologie am Klinikum der Universität Freiburg i. Brsg.).

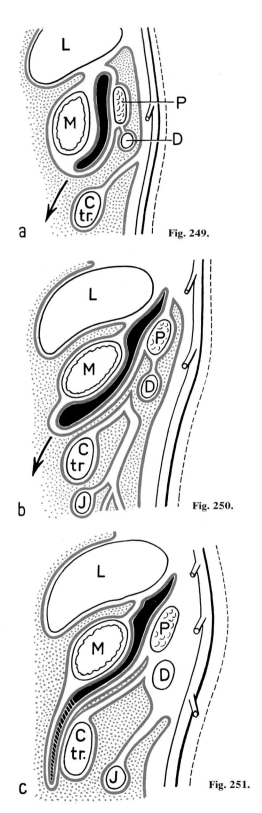

a   **Fig. 249.**

b   **Fig. 250.**

c   **Fig. 251.**

d   **Fig. 252.**

Figs. 249–252. Origin and development of the serous sacs of the abdominal cavity as well as the changes in the peritoneum. Schematic medial sagittal sections. Peritoneal membrane = red lines, peritoneal cavity = red dots. Figs. 249, 250, 251 embryonic stages. Fig. 252 Final condition (female situs) before fusion of the four layers (I–IV) of the greater omentum. Red broken line = original arrangement of the peritoneal membrane. Arrow in the epiploic foramen going into the omental bursa.

I–IV = 4 layers of the greater omentum	M = Stomach (ventriculus)	D = Duodenum	I = Ileum
L = Liver (hepar)	P = Pancreas	C tr = Transverse Colon	cs = Sigmoid colon
		J = Jejunum	S = Symphysis pubis

Urogenital System

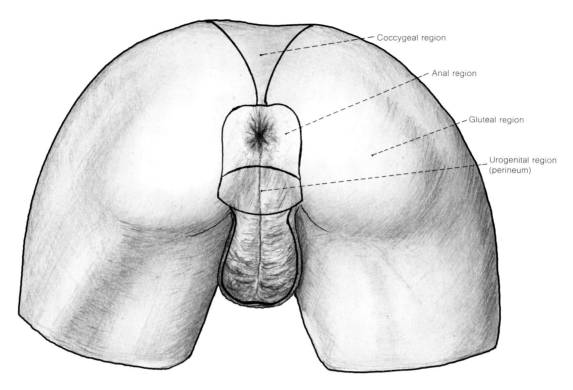

Coccygeal region

Anal region

Gluteal region

Urogenital region
(perineum)

Fig. 253. Regions of the male perineum.

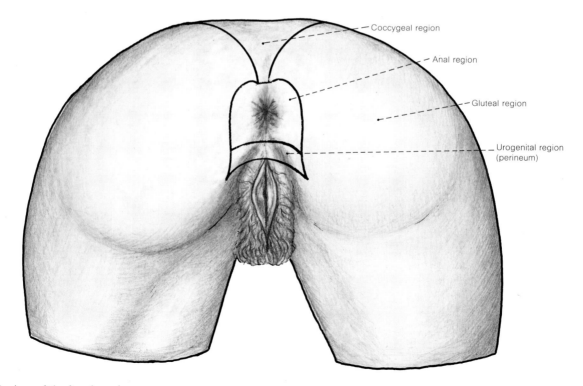

Coccygeal region

Anal region

Gluteal region

Urogenital region
(perineum)

Fig. 254. Regions of the female perineum.

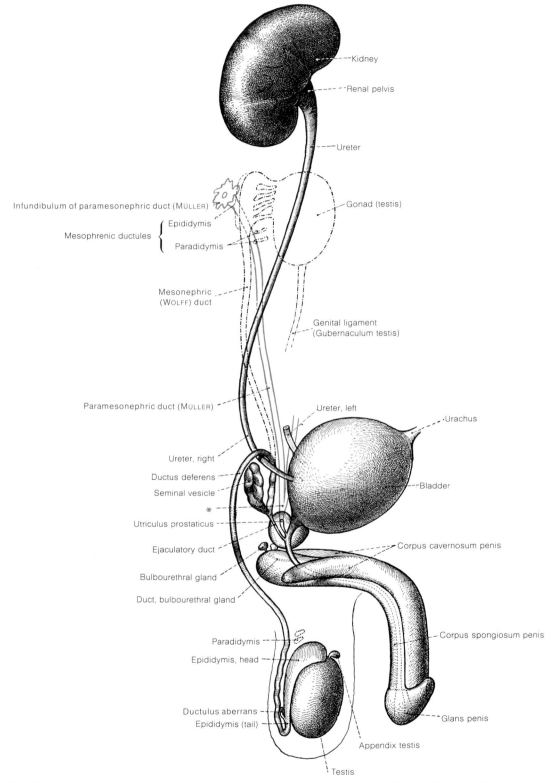

Kidney

Renal pelvis

Ureter

Infundibulum of paramesonephric duct (MÜLLER)

Gonad (testis)

Mesophrenic ductules { Epididymis

Paradidymis

Mesonephric (WOLFF) duct

Genital ligament (Gubernaculum testis)

Paramesonephric duct (MÜLLER)

Ureter, left

Urachus

Ureter, right

Ductus deferens

Seminal vesicle

Bladder

*

Utriculus prostaticus

Corpus cavernosum penis

Ejaculatory duct

Bulbourethral gland

Duct, bulbourethral gland

Corpus spongiosum penis

Paradidymis

Epididymis, head

Ductulus aberrans

Epididymis (tail)

Glans penis

Appendix testis

Testis

Fig. 255. Diagram of the male urogenital structure with regard to its development. Each diagram (255 and 256) shows the derivation from the undifferentiated bisexuell state. Red: Parts of the genital system wholly or partially lost in later stages of development. Interrupted black lines: Relative position of gonads and associated tracts before the caudal migration of gonads. * = Union of Müllerian ducts (paramesonephric duct).

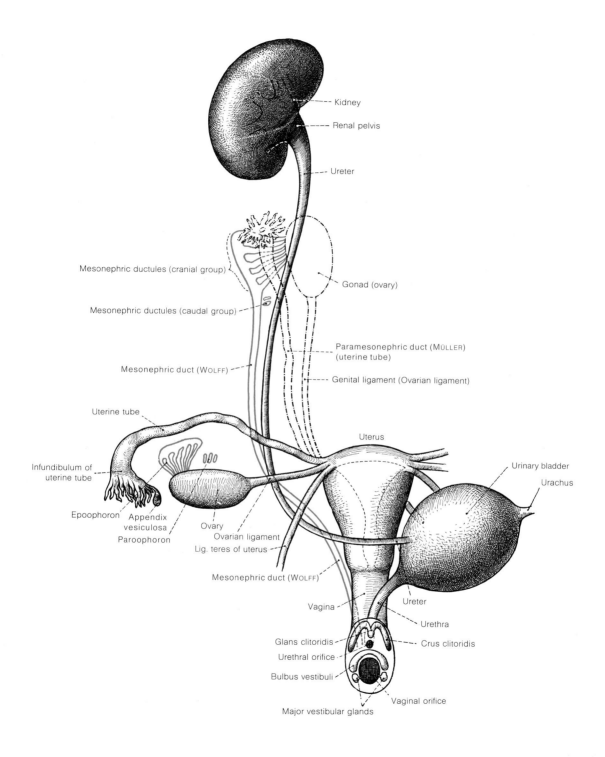

Kidney

Renal pelvis

Ureter

Mesonephric ductules (cranial group)

Gonad (ovary)

Mesonephric ductules (caudal group)

Paramesonephric duct (MÜLLER) (uterine tube)

Mesonephric duct (WOLFF)

Genital ligament (Ovarian ligament)

Uterine tube

Uterus

Urinary bladder

Urachus

Infundibulum of uterine tube

Epoophoron   Appendix vesiculosa
Paroophoron

Ovary

Ovarian ligament

Lig. teres of uterus

Mesonephric duct (WOLFF)

Vagina

Ureter

Urethra

Glans clitoridis

Crus clitoridis

Urethral orifice

Bulbus vestibuli

Vaginal orifice

Major vestibular glands

Fig. 256. Diagram of the female urogenital tract with regard to its development. Red: Parts of the genital system wholly or partially lost in later stages of development. Interrupted black lines: Relative position of gonads and associated tracts before the caudal migration of the gonads.

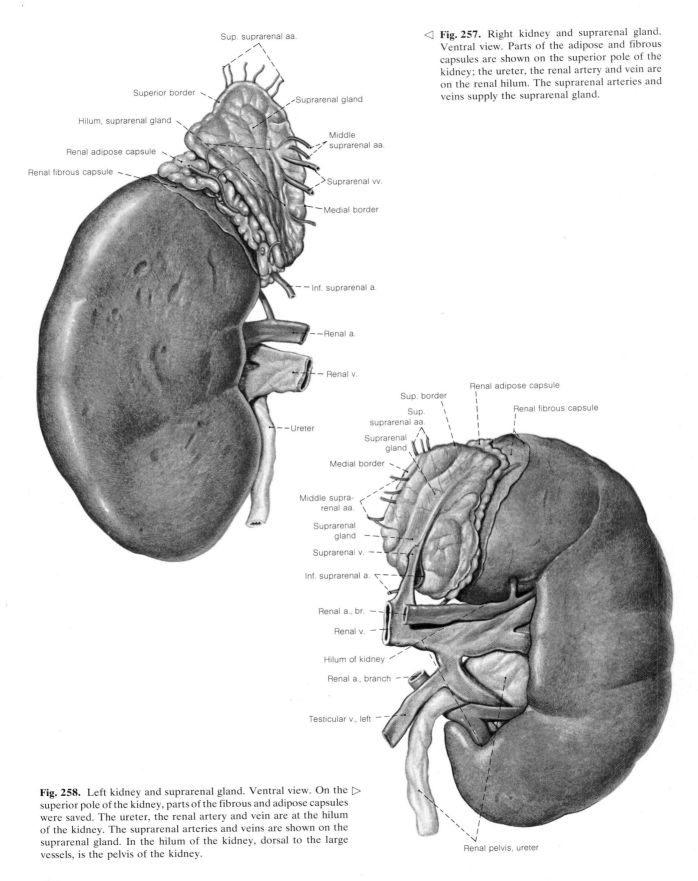

Sup. suprarenal aa.

Superior border

Hilum, suprarenal gland

Renal adipose capsule

Renal fibrous capsule

Suprarenal gland

Middle
suprarenal aa.

Suprarenal vv.

Medial border

Inf. suprarenal a.

Renal a.

Renal v.

Ureter

Fig. 257. Right kidney and suprarenal gland. Ventral view. Parts of the adipose and fibrous capsules are shown on the superior pole of the kidney; the ureter, the renal artery and vein are on the renal hilum. The suprarenal arteries and veins supply the suprarenal gland.

Sup. border

Sup.
suprarenal aa.

Suprarenal
gland

Medial border

Middle supra-
renal aa.

Suprarenal
gland

Suprarenal v.

Inf. suprarenal a.

Renal a., br.

Renal v.

Hilum of kidney

Renal a., branch

Testicular v., left

Renal adipose capsule

Renal fibrous capsule

Renal pelvis, ureter

Fig. 258. Left kidney and suprarenal gland. Ventral view. On the ▷ superior pole of the kidney, parts of the fibrous and adipose capsules were saved. The ureter, the renal artery and vein are at the hilum of the kidney. The suprarenal arteries and veins are shown on the suprarenal gland. In the hilum of the kidney, dorsal to the large vessels, is the pelvis of the kidney.

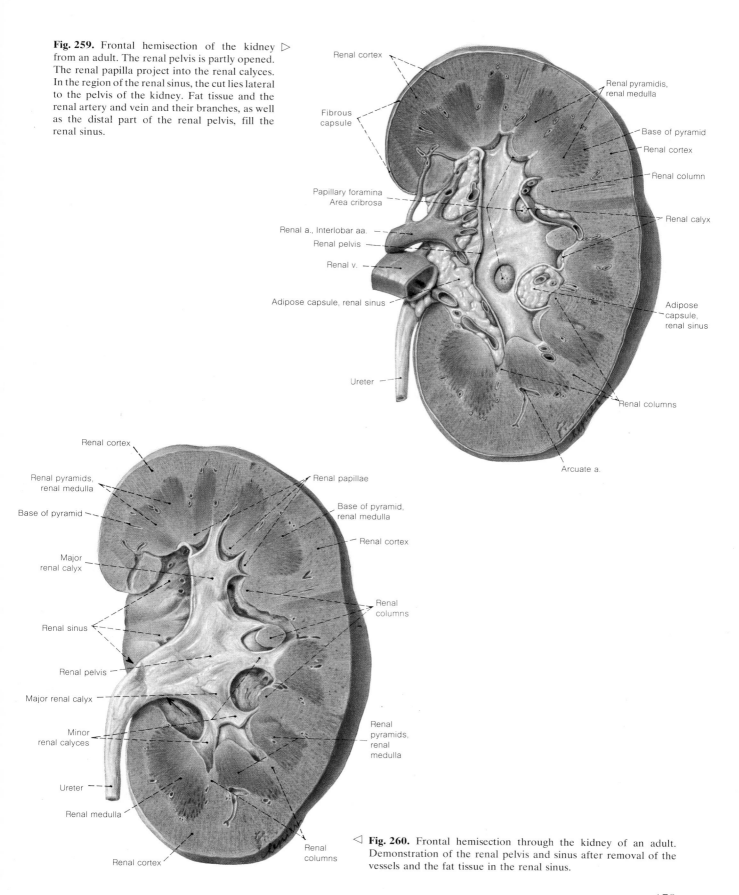

Fig. 259. Frontal hemisection of the kidney ▷ from an adult. The renal pelvis is partly opened. The renal papilla project into the renal calyces. In the region of the renal sinus, the cut lies lateral to the pelvis of the kidney. Fat tissue and the renal artery and vein and their branches, as well as the distal part of the renal pelvis, fill the renal sinus.

Renal cortex

Fibrous capsule

Papillary foramina
Area cribrosa

Renal a., Interlobar aa.

Renal pelvis

Renal v.

Adipose capsule, renal sinus

Ureter

Renal pyramidis, renal medulla

Base of pyramid

Renal cortex

Renal column

Renal calyx

Adipose capsule, renal sinus

Renal columns

Arcuate a.

Renal cortex

Renal pyramids, renal medulla

Base of pyramid

Major renal calyx

Renal sinus

Renal pelvis

Major renal calyx

Minor renal calyces

Ureter

Renal medulla

Renal cortex

Renal papillae

Base of pyramid, renal medulla

Renal cortex

Renal columns

Renal pyramids, renal medulla

Renal columns

◁ **Fig. 260.** Frontal hemisection through the kidney of an adult. Demonstration of the renal pelvis and sinus after removal of the vessels and the fat tissue in the renal sinus.

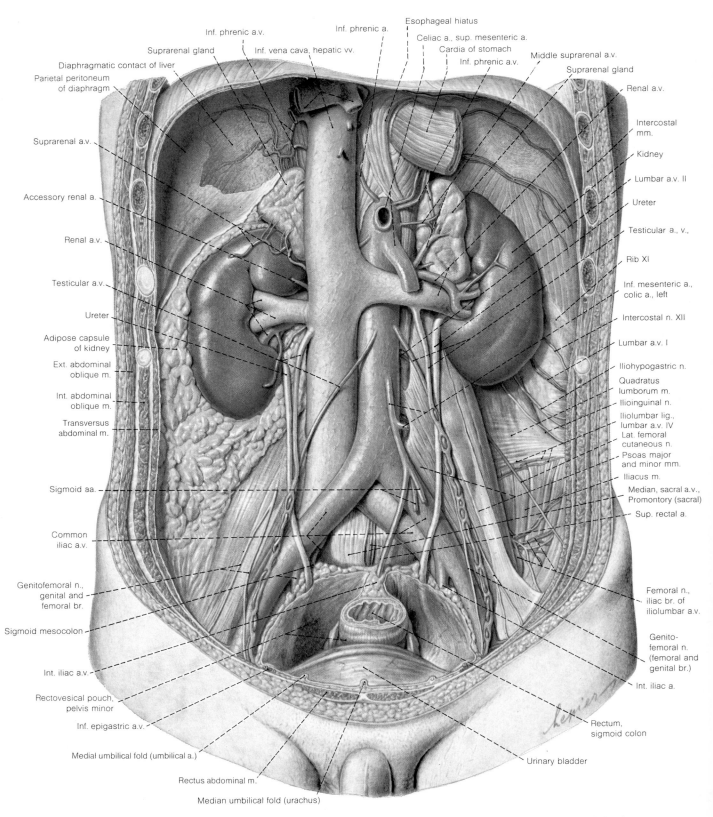

Inf. phrenic a.v.

Suprarenal gland

Diaphragmatic contact of liver

Parietal peritoneum of diaphragm

Suprarenal a.v.

Accessory renal a.

Renal a.v.

Testicular a.v.

Ureter

Adipose capsule of kidney

Ext. abdominal oblique m.

Int. abdominal oblique m.

Transversus abdominal m.

Sigmoid aa.

Common iliac a.v.

Genitofemoral n., genital and femoral br.

Sigmoid mesocolon

Int. iliac a.v.

Rectovesical pouch, pelvis minor

Inf. epigastric a.v.

Medial umbilical fold (umbilical a.)

Rectus abdominal m.

Median umbilical fold (urachus)

Inf. phrenic a.

Esophageal hiatus

Inf. vena cava, hepatic vv.

Celiac a., sup. mesenteric a.

Cardia of stomach

Inf. phrenic a.v.

Middle suprarenal a.v.

Suprarenal gland

Renal a.v.

Intercostal mm.

Kidney

Lumbar a.v. II

Ureter

Testicular a., v.,

Rib XI

Inf. mesenteric a., colic a., left

Intercostal n. XII

Lumbar a.v. I

Iliohypogastric n.

Quadratus lumborum m.

Ilioinguinal n.

Iliolumbar lig., lumbar a.v. IV

Lat. femoral cutaneous n.

Psoas major and minor mm.

Iliacus m.

Median, sacral a.v., Promontory (sacral)

Sup. rectal a.

Femoral n., iliac br. of iliolumbar a.v.

Genito-femoral n. (femoral and genital br.)

Int. iliac a.

Rectum, sigmoid colon

Urinary bladder

Fig. 261. Abdominal viscera on the dorsal body wall. The retroperitoneal space. Note the positions of kidneys, suprarenal glands, ureters, and great vessels.

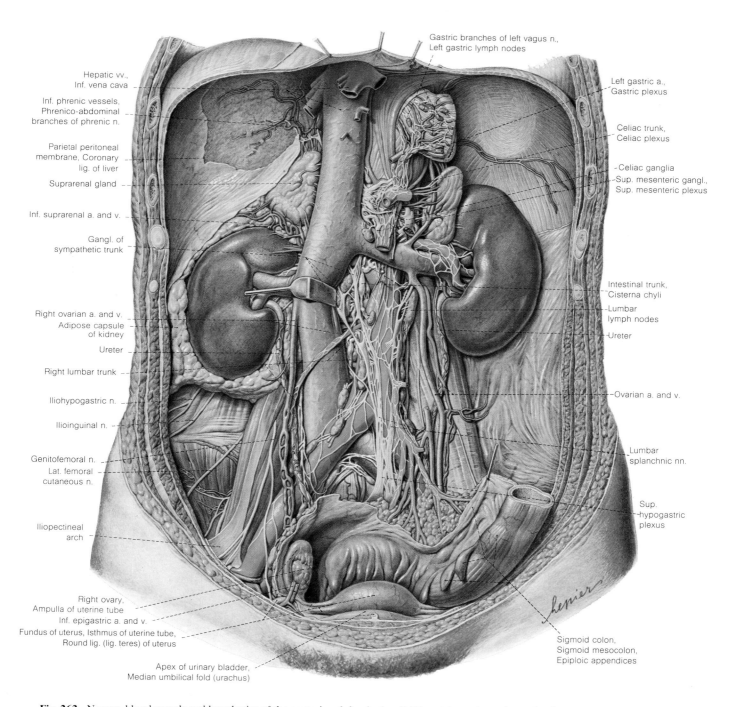

Fig. 262. Nerves, blood vessels and lymphatics of the posterior abdominal wall. The peritoneal membrane has been mostly removed and is retained only in the lesser pelvis, in the left iliac fossa and in the area of the coronary ligament of the liver. The adipose capsule of the left kidney is removed entirely, that of the right partially.

181

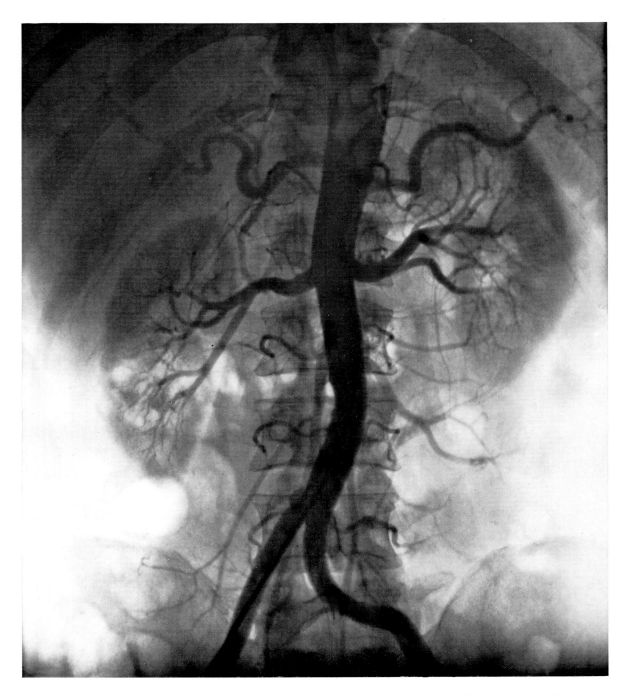

Fig. 263. Arteriogram of the abdominal aorta and of both renal arteries. Injection of the contrast medium was performed via a SELDINGER-catheter which was introduced through the femoral artery and the tip of which had come to rest immediately above the origin of the renal arteries. (Sagittal film by Prof. Dr. H. SCHMIDT, Pforzheim.)

1 Descending colon
2 Ascending colon
3 Psoas major muscle,
  lateral border
4 Renal pelvis
5 Renal papilla
6 Ureter
7 Left kidney, inferior extremity

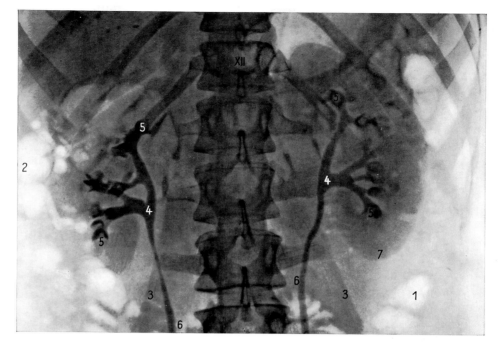

Fig. 264. Bilateral retrograde pylogram. The minor renal calyces are cup-shaped and unite to form the major calyces, which in turn form the renal pelvis. The renal papilla, light; their investment, dark, owing to the calyx filled with the contrast medium.

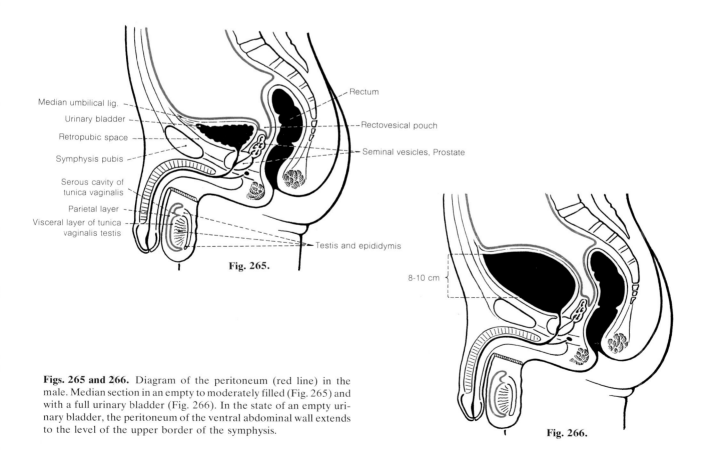

Median umbilical lig.
Urinary bladder
Retropubic space
Symphysis pubis
Serous cavity of
tunica vaginalis
Parietal layer
Visceral layer of tunica
vaginalis testis

Rectum
Rectovesical pouch
Seminal vesicles, Prostate
Testis and epididymis

Fig. 265.

8-10 cm

Fig. 266.

Figs. 265 and 266. Diagram of the peritoneum (red line) in the male. Median section in an empty to moderately filled (Fig. 265) and with a full urinary bladder (Fig. 266). In the state of an empty urinary bladder, the peritoneum of the ventral abdominal wall extends to the level of the upper border of the symphysis.

183

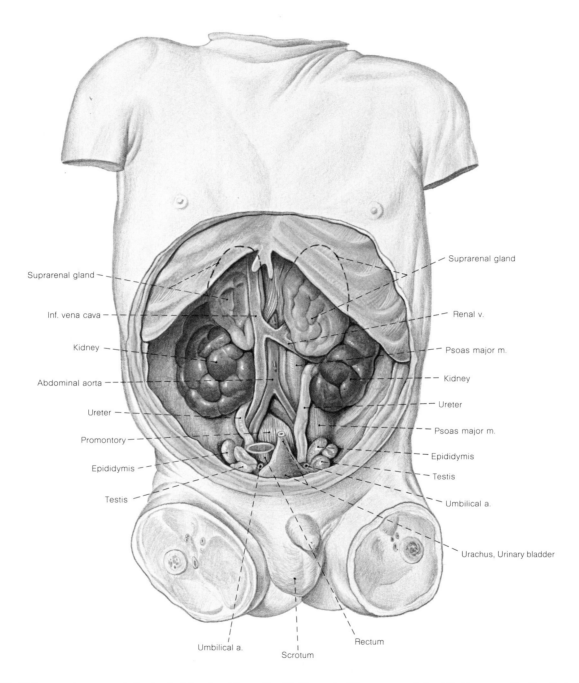

Suprarenal gland

Inf. vena cava

Kidney

Abdominal aorta

Ureter

Promontory

Epididymis

Testis

Suprarenal gland

Renal v.

Psoas major m.

Kidney

Ureter

Psoas major m.

Epididymis

Testis

Umbilical a.

Urachus, Urinary bladder

Umbilical a.

Scrotum

Rectum

Fig. 267. Kidneys and suprarenal glands of a fetus about 5 months old. The part of the suprarenal gland that is covered by the ribs is shown by the dotted line. The kidneys are definitely lobed, the suprarenals conspicuously large and folded on the surface. The ureter is wide and tortuous; the testes and epididymis lie in the true pelvis at the beginning of the inguinal canal. The urinary bladder tapers itself conically into the urachus, which is still open. The large organs of the abdomen are removed, such as the large and small intestine. The colon has been cut off the rectum so that is barely visible.

Fig. 268. Right kidney of an adult with retention of fetal lobulation. ▷

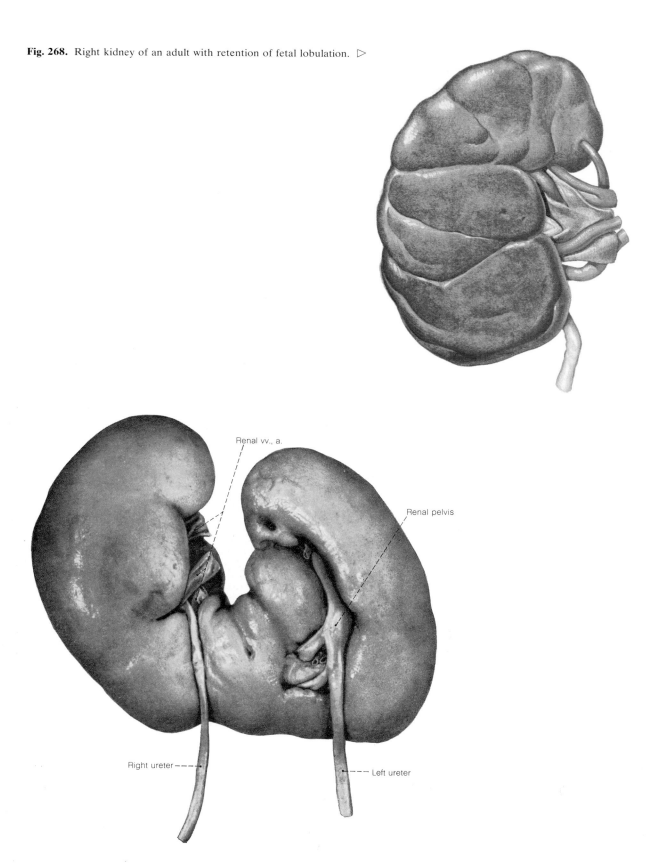

Renal vv., a.

Renal pelvis

Right ureter – – – –

– – – Left ureter

Fig. 269. Horseshoe-shaped kidney. Ventral view. Broad bridge of renal tissue between the lower poles of the kidneys.

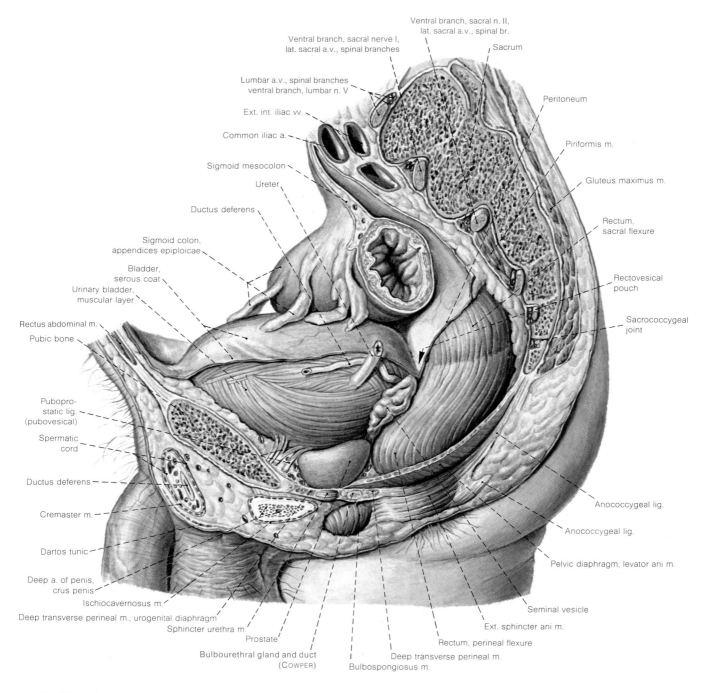

Ventral branch, sacral n. II,
lat. sacral a.v., spinal br.

Ventral branch, sacral nerve I,
lat. sacral a.v., spinal branches

Sacrum

Lumbar a.v., spinal branches
ventral branch, lumbar n. V

Ext. int. iliac vv.

Peritoneum

Common iliac a.

Piriformis m.

Sigmoid mesocolon

Gluteus maximus m.

Ureter

Ductus deferens

Rectum,
sacral flexure

Sigmoid colon,
appendices epiploicae

Rectovesical
pouch

Bladder,
serous coat

Urinary bladder,
muscular layer

Sacrococcygeal
joint

Rectus abdominal m.

Pubic bone

Pubopro-
static lig.
(pubovesical)

Spermatic
cord

Ductus deferens

Anococcygeal lig.

Cremaster m.

Anococcygeal lig.

Dartos tunic

Pelvic diaphragm, levator ani m.

Deep a. of penis,
crus penis

Seminal vesicle

Ischiocavernosus m.

Ext. sphincter ani m.

Deep transverse perineal m., urogenital diaphragm

Rectum, perineal flexure

Sphincter urethra m.

Deep transverse perineal m.

Prostate

Bulbospongiosus m.

Bulbourethral gland and duct
(COWPER)

Fig. 270. Right half of a paramedian section of the pelvis of an adult male. Viewed from the medial side. The peritoneum is removed from the side of the urinary bladder.

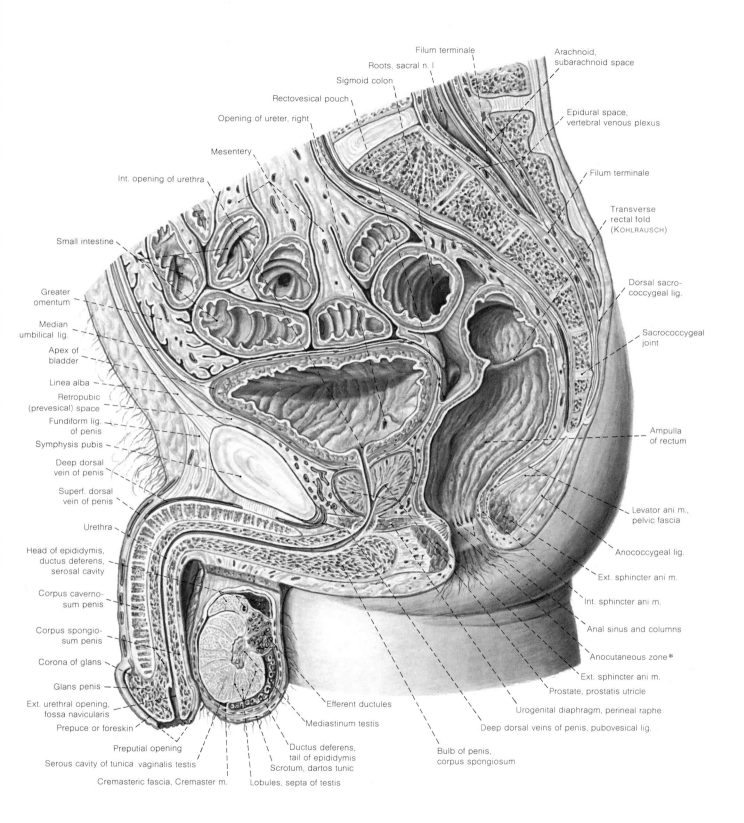

Filum terminale

Roots, sacral n. l

Sigmoid colon

Rectovesical pouch

Opening of ureter, right

Mesentery

Int. opening of urethra

Small intestine

Greater omentum

Median umbilical lig.

Apex of bladder

Linea alba

Retropubic (prevesical) space

Fundiform lig. of penis

Symphysis pubis

Deep dorsal vein of penis

Superf. dorsal vein of penis

Urethra

Head of epididymis, ductus deferens, serosal cavity

Corpus cavernosum penis

Corpus spongiosum penis

Corona of glans

Glans penis

Ext. urethral opening, fossa navicularis

Prepuce or foreskin

Preputial opening

Serous cavity of tunica vaginalis testis

Cremasteric fascia, Cremaster m.

Efferent ductules

Mediastinum testis

Ductus deferens, tail of epididymis

Scrotum, dartos tunic

Lobules, septa of testis

Bulb of penis, corpus spongiosum

Deep dorsal veins of penis, pubovesical lig.

Urogenital diaphragm, perineal raphe

Prostate, prostatis utricle

Ext. sphincter ani m.

Anocutaneous zone *

Anal sinus and columns

Int. sphincter ani m.

Ext. sphincter ani m.

Anococcygeal lig.

Levator ani m., pelvic fascia

Ampulla of rectum

Sacrococcygeal joint

Dorsal sacro-coccygeal lig.

Transverse rectal fold (KOHLRAUSCH)

Filum terminale

Epidural space, vertebral venous plexus

Arachnoid, subarachnoid space

Fig. 271. Right half of a median section through the pelvis of an adult male. Paramedian section of the scrotum. * The anocutaneous zone is the parchment-colored region between the deeply pigmented area (cutaneous zone) and the reddish mucous membrane of the rectum. The anocutaneous zone is also designated as zona alba, hemorrhoidal zone, or HILTON's line.

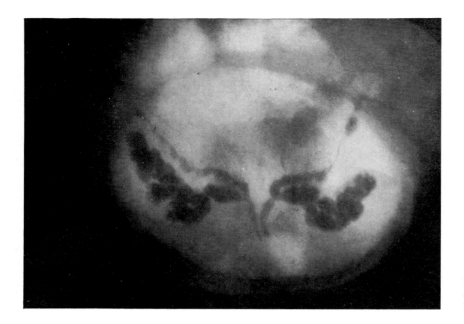

Fig. 272. X-ray film of seminal vesicles, ductus deferens, and ejaculatory ducts behind the air-inflated bladder.

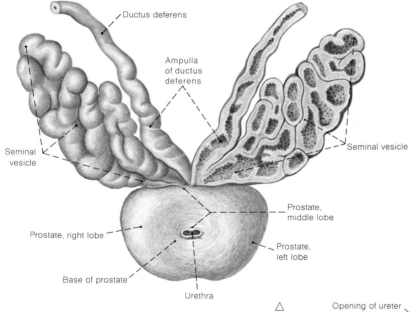

Ductus deferens

Ampulla of ductus deferens

Seminal vesicle

Seminal vesicle

Prostate, middle lobe

Prostate, right lobe

Prostate, left lobe

Base of prostate

Urethra

△

Fig. 273. Prostate with seminal vesicles. Ventrocranial view. On one side, the seminal versicles and the ampulla of the ductus deferens have been cut in half frontally. The male urethra has been cut off near the urinary bladder. Note the concave base of the prostate.

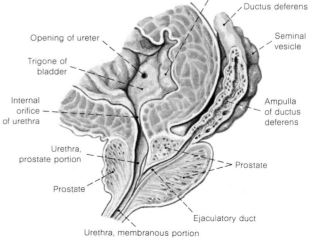

Urinary bladder, fundus

Ductus deferens

Opening of ureter

Seminal vesicle

Trigone of bladder

Internal orifice of urethra

Ampulla of ductus deferens

Urethra, prostate portion

Prostate

Prostate

Ejaculatory duct

Urethra, membranous portion

Fig. 274. Median section of the fundus of the bladder, the prostate ▷ gland, and ductus deferens.

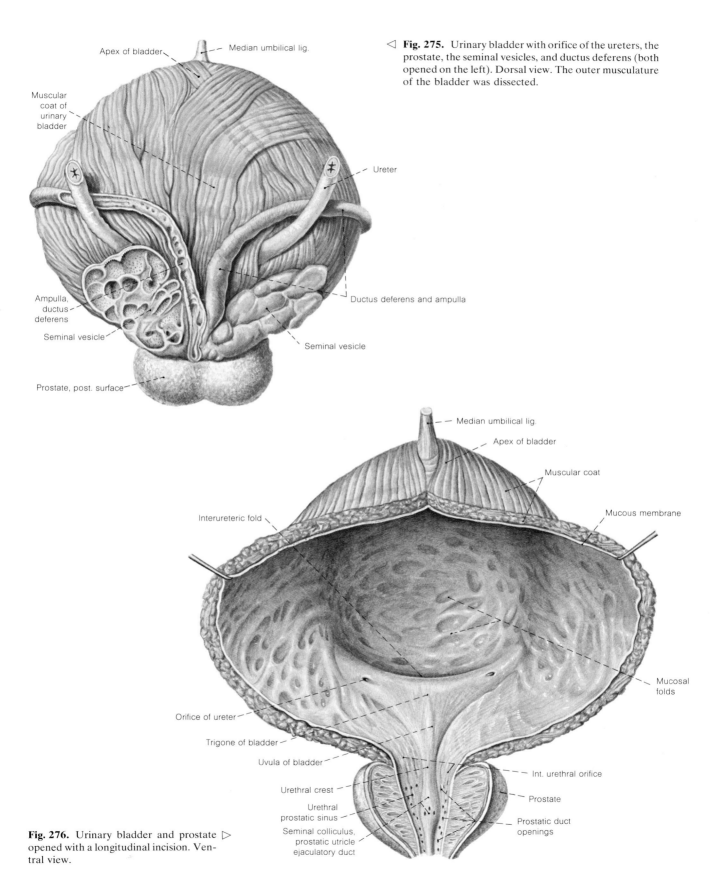

Apex of bladder

Median umbilical lig.

Muscular coat of urinary bladder

Ureter

Ampulla, ductus deferens

Seminal vesicle

Ductus deferens and ampulla

Seminal vesicle

Prostate, post. surface

◁ **Fig. 275.** Urinary bladder with orifice of the ureters, the prostate, the seminal vesicles, and ductus deferens (both opened on the left). Dorsal view. The outer musculature of the bladder was dissected.

Median umbilical lig.

Apex of bladder

Muscular coat

Mucous membrane

Interureteric fold

Mucosal folds

Orifice of ureter

Trigone of bladder

Uvula of bladder

Int. urethral orifice

Urethral crest

Prostate

Urethral prostatic sinus

Seminal colliculus, prostatic utricle ejaculatory duct

Prostatic duct openings

Fig. 276. Urinary bladder and prostate ▷ opened with a longitudinal incision. Ventral view.

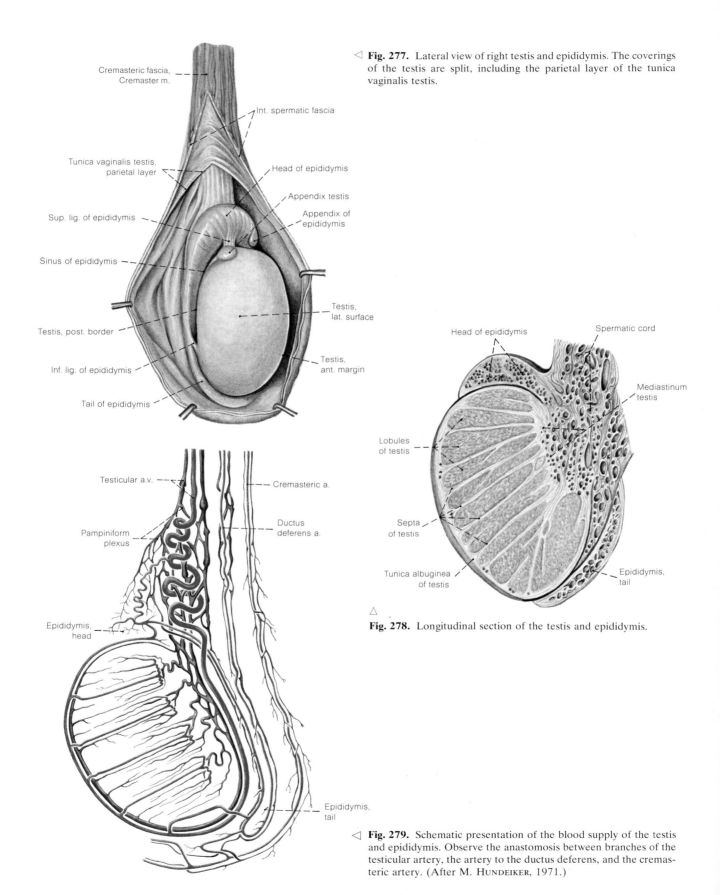

Cremasteric fascia,
Cremaster m.

Int. spermatic fascia

Tunica vaginalis testis,
parietal layer

Head of epididymis

Appendix testis

Appendix of
epididymis

Sup. lig. of epididymis

Sinus of epididymis

Testis,
lat. surface

Testis, post. border

Inf. lig. of epididymis

Tail of epididymis

Testis,
ant. margin

◁ **Fig. 277.** Lateral view of right testis and epididymis. The coverings of the testis are split, including the parietal layer of the tunica vaginalis testis.

Head of epididymis

Spermatic cord

Mediastinum
testis

Lobules
of testis

Septa
of testis

Tunica albuginea
of testis

Epididymis,
tail

△
Fig. 278. Longitudinal section of the testis and epididymis.

Testicular a.v.

Cremasteric a.

Pampiniform
plexus

Ductus
deferens a.

Epididymis,
head

Epididymis,
tail

◁ **Fig. 279.** Schematic presentation of the blood supply of the testis and epididymis. Observe the anastomosis between branches of the testicular artery, the artery to the ductus deferens, and the cremasteric artery. (After M. HUNDEIKER, 1971.)

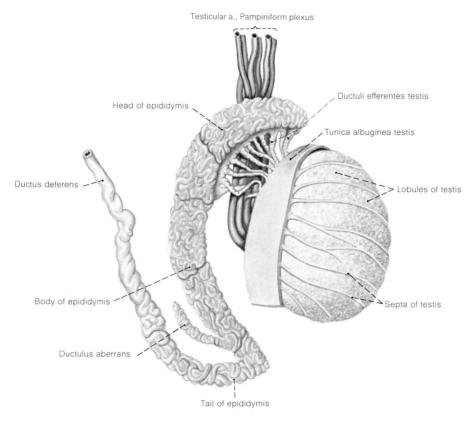

Testicular a., Pampiniform plexus

Head of epididymis

Ductuli efferentes testis

Tunica albuginea testis

Ductus deferens

Lobules of testis

Body of epididymis

Septa of testis

Ductulus aberrans

Tail of epididymis

Fig. 280. Testis, epididymis, and the beginning of the ductus deferens. Nearly all of the tunica albuginea of the testis was removed. The duct of the epididymis stretches 5–6 meters in length. The spermatozoa mature within the long duct system.

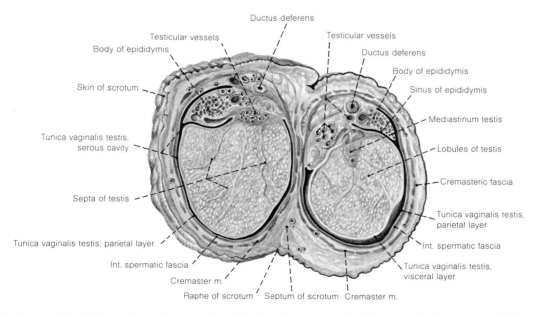

Ductus deferens

Testicular vessels

Testicular vessels

Body of epididymis

Ductus deferens

Skin of scrotum

Body of epididymis

Sinus of epididymis

Mediastinum testis

Tunica vaginalis testis, serous cavity

Lobules of testis

Cremasteric fascia

Septa of testis

Tunica vaginalis testis, parietal layer

Tunica vaginalis testis, parietal layer

Int. spermatic fascia

Int. spermatic fascia

Cremaster m.

Tunica vaginalis testis, visceral layer

Raphe of scrotum   Septum of scrotum   Cremaster m.

Fig. 281. Cross section of the scrotum with testes of an adult. Since the testes are in different levels of the scrotum (left usually lower than the right), they appear to be different sizes in this section.

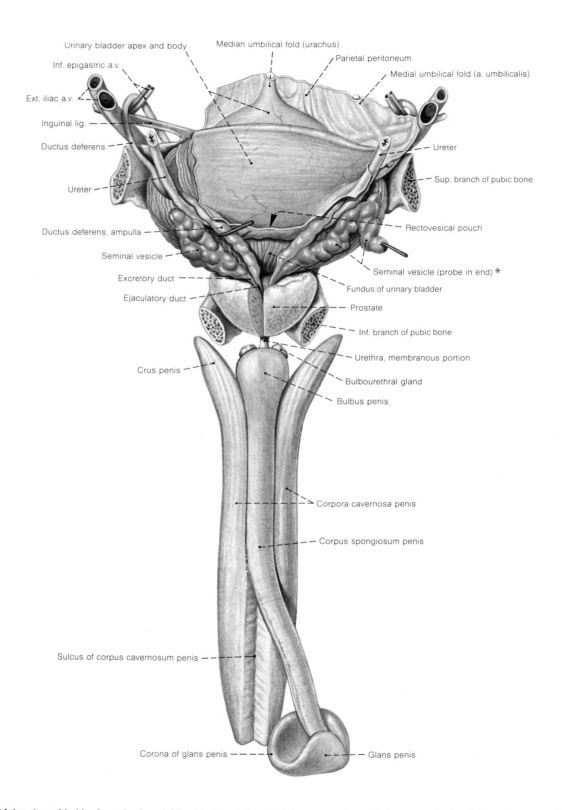

Fig. 282. Male urinary bladder from the dorsal side with the pelvic part of the ureters, ductus deferens, seminal vesicles, and prostate. Note: The membranous and the spongy portions of the urethra and the glans penis as well as the corpora cavernosa penis. The tortuous duct system of the seminal vesicles is pulled out on the right and untwisted (* a sound in the end). A wedge-shaped piece ist cut from the isthmus of the prostate in order to show the ejaculatory ducts.

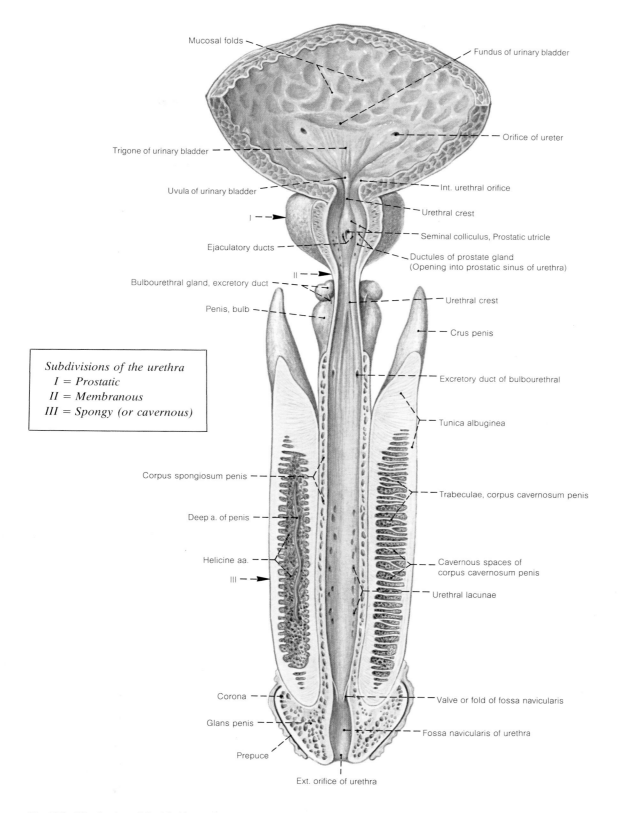

Mucosal folds

Fundus of urinary bladder

Orifice of ureter

Trigone of urinary bladder

Int. urethral orifice

Uvula of urinary bladder

Urethral crest

I

Seminal colliculus, Prostatic utricle

Ejaculatory ducts

Ductules of prostate gland
(Opening into prostatic sinus of urethra)

II

Bulbourethral gland, excretory duct

Urethral crest

Penis, bulb

Crus penis

Subdivisions of the urethra
I = Prostatic
II = Membranous
III = Spongy (or cavernous)

Excretory duct of bulbourethral

Tunica albuginea

Corpus spongiosum penis

Trabeculae, corpus cavernosum penis

Deep a. of penis

Helicine aa.

Cavernous spaces of
corpus cavernosum penis

III

Urethral lacunae

Corona

Valve or fold of fossa navicularis

Glans penis

Fossa navicularis of urethra

Prepuce

Ext. orifice of urethra

Fig. 283. The fundus of the bladder and male urethra opened lengthwise. Note: The prostate and bulbourethral glands. The skin of the penis is removed up to the prepuce over the glans penis.

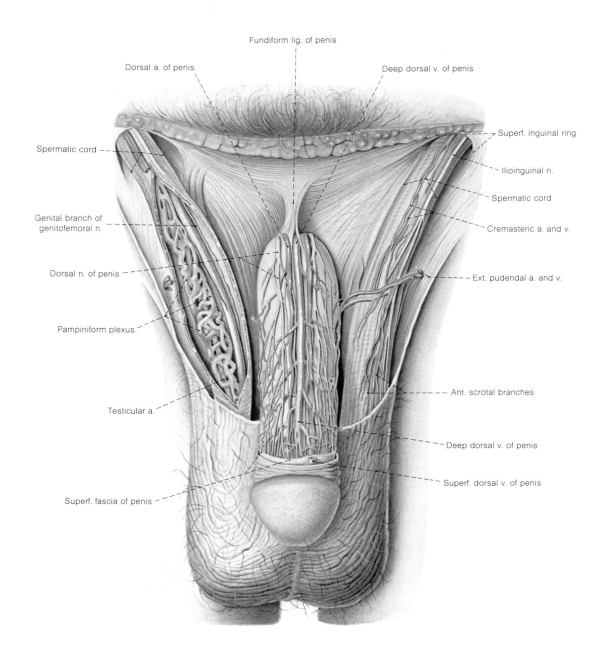

Fundiform lig. of penis

Dorsal a. of penis

Deep dorsal v. of penis

Superf. inguinal ring

Spermatic cord

Ilioinguinal n.

Spermatic cord

Genital branch of genitofemoral n.

Cremasteric a. and v.

Dorsal n. of penis

Ext. pudendal a. and v.

Pampiniform plexus

Ant. scrotal branches

Testicular a.

Deep dorsal v. of penis

Superf. dorsal v. of penis

Superf. fascia of penis

Fig. 284. Nerves and vessels of the external male genitalia. Skin and fascia of the penis have been removed. The right spermatic cord has been openend in order to expose the testicular artery and the pampiniform plexus.

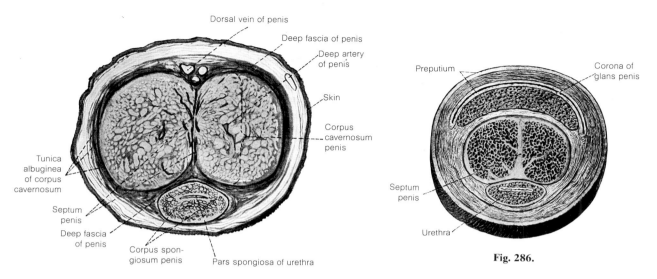

Fig. 285.

Dorsal vein of penis
Deep fascia of penis
Deep artery of penis
Skin
Corpus cavernosum penis
Tunica albuginea of corpus cavernosum
Septum penis
Deep fascia of penis
Corpus spongiosum penis
Pars spongiosa of urethra

Preputium
Corona of glans penis
Septum penis
Urethra

Fig. 286.

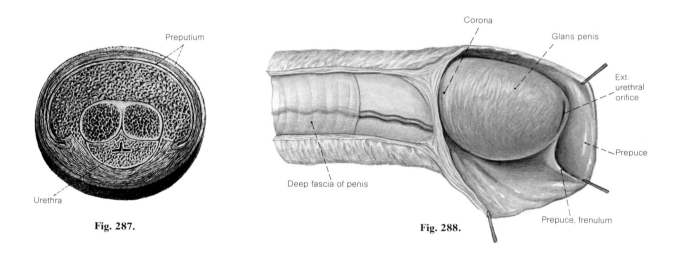

Preputium
Urethra

Fig. 287.

Corona
Glans penis
Ext. urethral orifice
Prepuce
Deep fascia of penis
Prepuce, frenulum

Fig. 288.

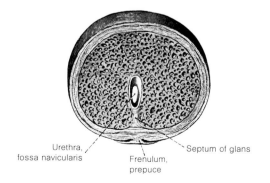

Urethra, fossa navicularis
Frenulum, prepuce
Septum of glans

Fig. 289.

Figs. 285–287, 289. Cross sections of the penis. The enlarged cross section of the penis. Fig. 285 (cut at midlength) shows the cavernous spaces filled; that of Fig. 286 goes through the neck of the glans with the tapered ends of the corpus cavernosum; that of Fig. 287 at the level of the corona of the glans penis; while that of Fig. 289 goes through the glans penis.

Fig. 288. The free distal end of the penis with preputial sac. The skin and deep penile fascia were partially removed.

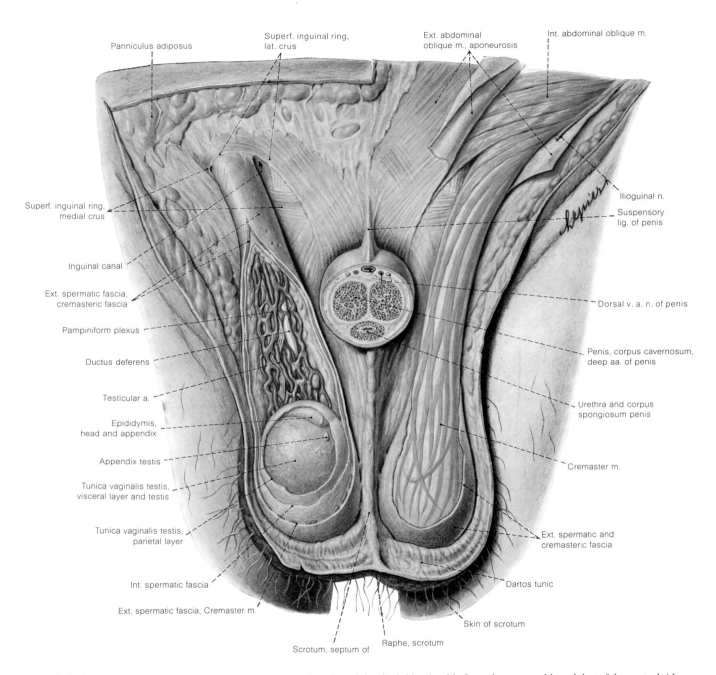

Panniculus adiposus

Superf. inguinal ring, lat. crus

Ext. abdominal oblique m., aponeurosis

Int. abdominal oblique m.

Superf. inguinal ring, medial crus

Inguinal canal

Ext. spermatic fascia, cremasteric fascia

Pampiniform plexus

Ductus deferens

Testicular a.

Epididymis, head and appendix

Appendix testis

Tunica vaginalis testis, visceral layer and testis

Tunica vaginalis testis, parietal layer

Int. spermatic fascia

Ext. spermatic fascia, Cremaster m.

Scrotum, septum of

Raphe, scrotum

Ilioguinal n.

Suspensory lig. of penis

Dorsal v. a. n. of penis

Penis, corpus cavernosum, deep aa. of penis

Urethra and corpus spongiosum penis

Cremaster m.

Ext. spermatic and cremasteric fascia

Dartos tunic

Skin of scrotum

Fig. 290. The male pubic and inguinal regions. Ventral view. The abdominal skin, the skin from the mons pubis and that of the ventral side of the scrotum were removed, partially reflected. The body of the penis was sectioned transversely. At the left is the inguinal canal opened, displaying the aponeurosis of the External abdominal oblique muscle and the Cremaster muscle after dissecting the external spermatic fascia. On the right, coverings of the spermatic cord were opened and, in the parietal lamina, an oval window was cut in the tunica vaginalis testis.

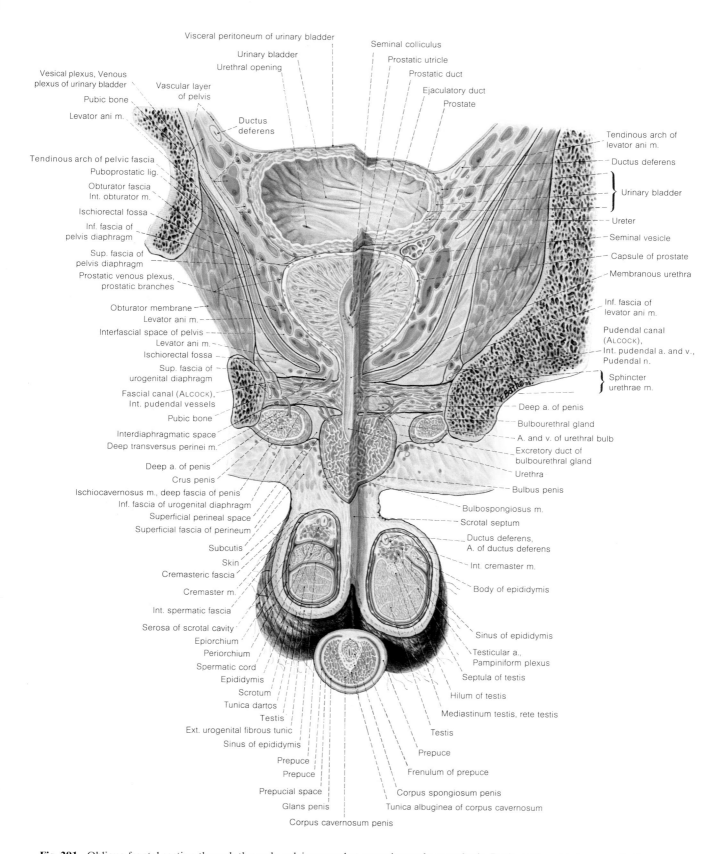

Visceral peritoneum of urinary bladder
Urinary bladder
Urethral opening
Seminal colliculus
Prostatic utricle
Prostatic duct
Ejaculatory duct
Prostate

Vesical plexus, Venous plexus of urinary bladder
Pubic bone
Levator ani m.
Vascular layer of pelvis
Ductus deferens

Tendinous arch of levator ani m.
Ductus deferens
Urinary bladder
Ureter
Seminal vesicle
Capsule of prostate
Membranous urethra

Tendinous arch of pelvic fascia
Puboprostatic lig.
Obturator fascia
Int. obturator m.
Ischiorectal fossa
Inf. fascia of pelvis diaphragm
Sup. fascia of pelvis diaphragm
Prostatic venous plexus, prostatic branches
Obturator membrane
Levator ani m.
Interfascial space of pelvis
Levator ani m.
Ischiorectal fossa
Sup. fascia of urogenital diaphragm
Fascial canal (ALCOCK), Int. pudendal vessels
Pubic bone
Interdiaphragmatic space
Deep transversus perinei m.
Deep a. of penis
Crus penis
Ischiocavernosus m., deep fascia of penis
Inf. fascia of urogenital diaphragm
Superficial perineal space
Superficial fascia of perineum
Subcutis
Skin
Cremasteric fascia
Cremaster m.
Int. spermatic fascia
Serosa of scrotal cavity
Epiorchium
Periorchium
Spermatic cord
Epididymis
Scrotum
Tunica dartos
Testis
Ext. urogenital fibrous tunic
Sinus of epididymis
Prepuce
Prepuce
Prepucial space
Glans penis
Corpus cavernosum penis

Inf. fascia of levator ani m.
Pudendal canal (ALCOCK),
Int. pudendal a. and v., Pudendal n.
Sphincter urethrae m.
Deep a. of penis
Bulbourethral gland
A. and v. of urethral bulb
Excretory duct of bulbourethral gland
Urethra
Bulbus penis
Bulbospongiosus m.
Scrotal septum
Ductus deferens, A. of ductus deferens
Int. cremaster m.
Body of epididymis
Sinus of epididymis
Testicular a., Pampiniform plexus
Septula of testis
Hilum of testis
Mediastinum testis, rete testis
Testis
Prepuce
Frenulum of prepuce
Corpus spongiosum penis
Tunica albuginea of corpus cavernosum

Fig. 291. Oblique frontal section through the male pelvis somewhat posterior to the symphysis. Penis sectioned twice: once in the area of the root, once in the area of the glans. (From PERNKOPF: Atlas der topographischen und angewandten Anatomie des Menschen, Vol. 2, 2nd ed. [Ed. H. FERNER]. Urban & Schwarzenberg, Munich–Vienna–Baltimore 1980.)

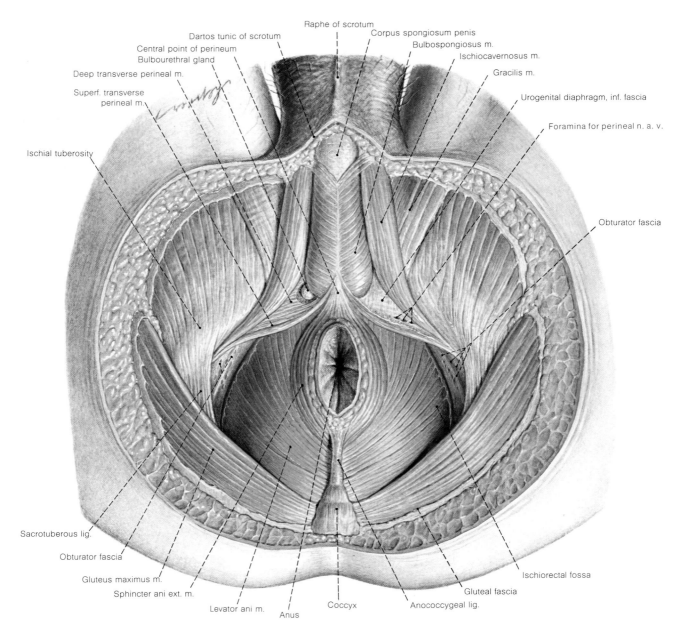

Raphe of scrotum

Dartos tunic of scrotum

Corpus spongiosum penis

Central point of perineum

Bulbospongiosus m.

Bulbourethral gland

Ischiocavernosus m.

Deep transverse perineal m.

Gracilis m.

Superf. transverse perineal m.

Urogenital diaphragm, inf. fascia

Foramina for perineal n. a. v.

Ischial tuberosity

Obturator fascia

Sacrotuberous lig.

Obturator fascia

Gluteus maximus m.

Ischiorectal fossa

Sphincter ani ext. m.

Gluteal fascia

Levator ani m.

Anus

Coccyx

Anococcygeal lig.

Fig. 292. The superficial layer of the muscles of the male perineum. Skin and subcutaneous fat tissues of the anal and perineal regions were removed, as well as the fat from the ischiorectal fossa. On the right, the bulbourethral gland was dissected from the deep transverse perineal muscles, after removal of the inferior urogenital diaphragmatic fascia. (Compare with Fig. 329.)

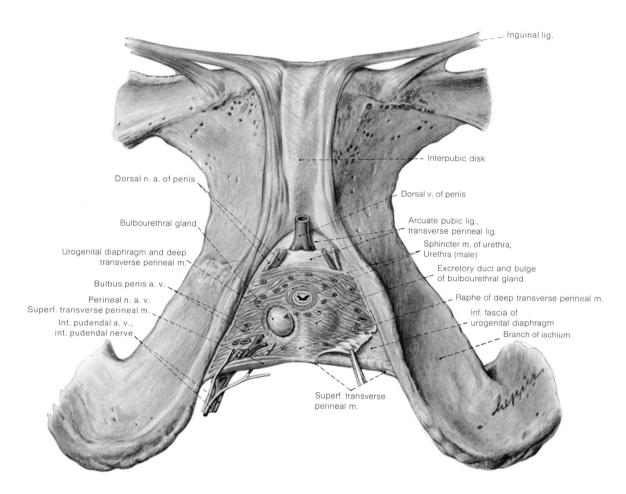

Inguinal lig.

Interpubic disk

Dorsal n. a. of penis

Dorsal v. of penis

Bulbourethral gland

Arcuate pubic lig., transverse perineal lig.

Urogenital diaphragm and deep transverse perineal m.

Sphincter m. of urethra, Urethra (male)

Excretory duct and bulge of bulbourethral gland

Bulbus penis a. v.

Raphe of deep transverse perineal m.

Perineal n. a. v.
Superf. transverse perineal m.

Inf. fascia of urogenital diaphragm

Int. pudendal a. v., int. pudendal nerve

Branch of ischium

Superf. transverse perineal m.

Fig. 293. Urogenital diaphragm of the male. The skin and the subcutaneous adipose tissue of the anal and perineal region as well as of the ischiorectal fossa have been removed. On the right side the inferior fascia of the urogenital diaphragm has been removed in order to display the bulbourethral gland within the transversus perinei muscle. (Compare with Fig. 322.)

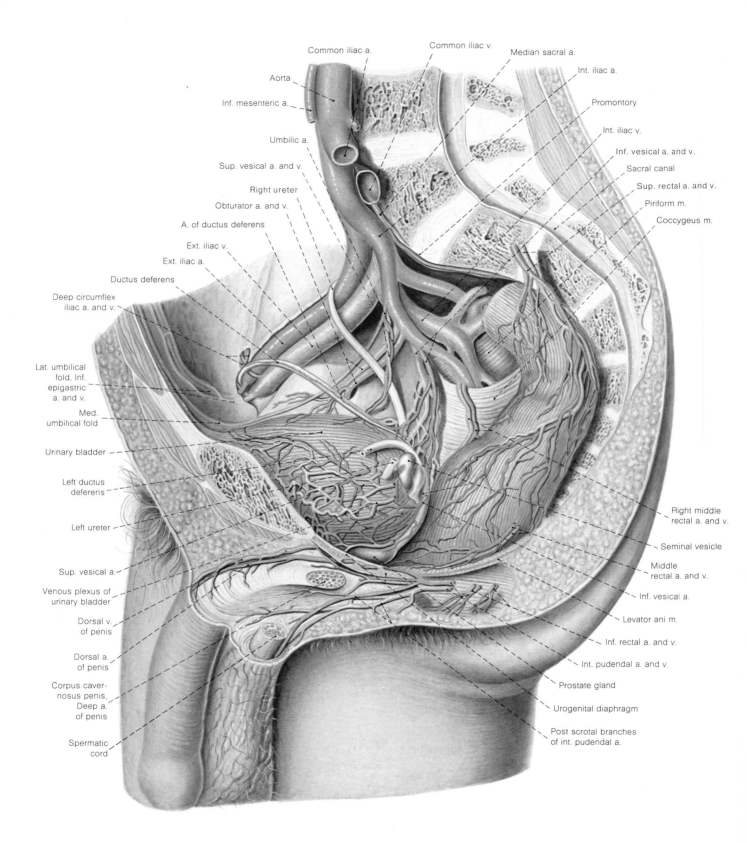

Common iliac a.

Common iliac v.

Median sacral a.

Aorta

Int. iliac a.

Inf. mesenteric a.

Promontory

Int. iliac v.

Umbilic a.

Inf. vesical a. and v.

Sup. vesical a. and v.

Sacral canal

Right ureter

Sup. rectal a. and v.

Obturator a. and v.

Piriform m.

A. of ductus deferens

Coccygeus m.

Ext. iliac v.

Ext. iliac a.

Ductus deferens

Deep circumflex iliac a. and v.

Lat. umbilical fold, Inf. epigastric a. and v.

Med. umbilical fold

Urinary bladder

Right middle rectal a. and v.

Left ductus deferens

Seminal vesicle

Left ureter

Middle rectal a. and v.

Sup. vesical a.

Inf. vesical a.

Venous plexus of urinary bladder

Levator ani m.

Dorsal v. of penis

Inf. rectal a. and v.

Dorsal a. of penis

Int. pudendal a. and v.

Corpus cavernosus penis, Deep a. of penis

Prostate gland

Urogenital diaphragm

Spermatic cord

Post scrotal branches of int. pudendal a.

Fig. 294. Blood vessels of the pelvic viscera in the male. The left half of the pelvis has been removed by a parasagittal section.

200

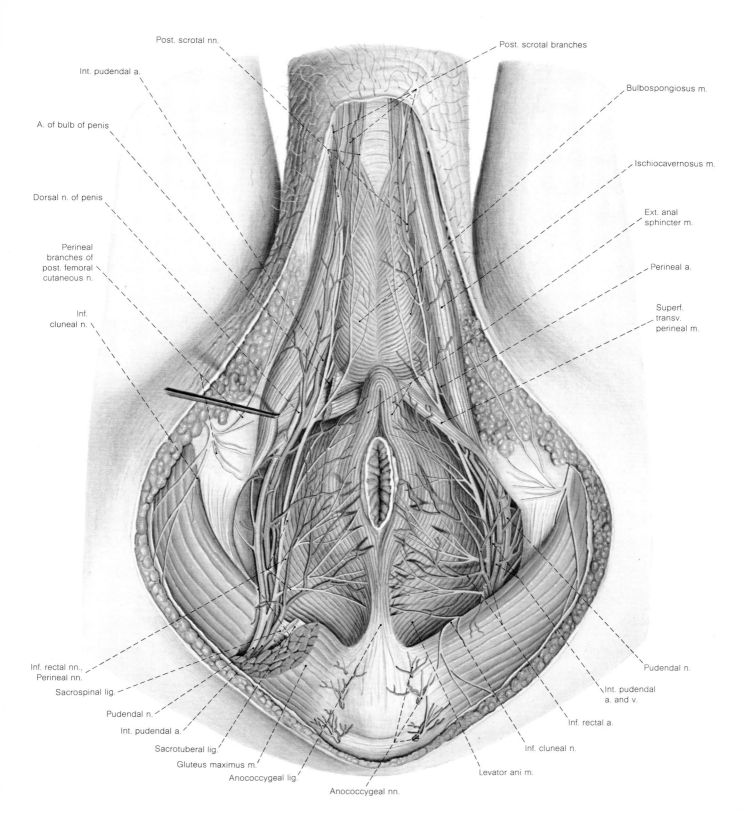

Post. scrotal nn.

Int. pudendal a.

A. of bulb of penis

Dorsal n. of penis

Perineal
branches of
post. femoral
cutaneous n.

Inf.
cluneal n.

Post. scrotal branches

Bulbospongiosus m.

Ischiocavernosus m.

Ext. anal
sphincter m.

Perineal a.

Superf.
transv.
perineal m.

Inf. rectal nn.,
Perineal nn.

Sacrospinal lig.

Pudendal n.

Int. pudendal a.

Sacrotuberal lig.

Gluteus maximus m.

Anococcygeal lig.

Anococcygeal nn.

Pudendal n.

Int. pudendal
a. and v.

Inf. rectal a.

Inf. cluneal n.

Levator ani m.

Fig. 295. Nerves and vessels of the male perineum. Superficial perineal muscles are shown on the left side, fat of the ischiorectal fossa has been removed, nerves and vessels are exposed by incisions into the musculature on the right side.

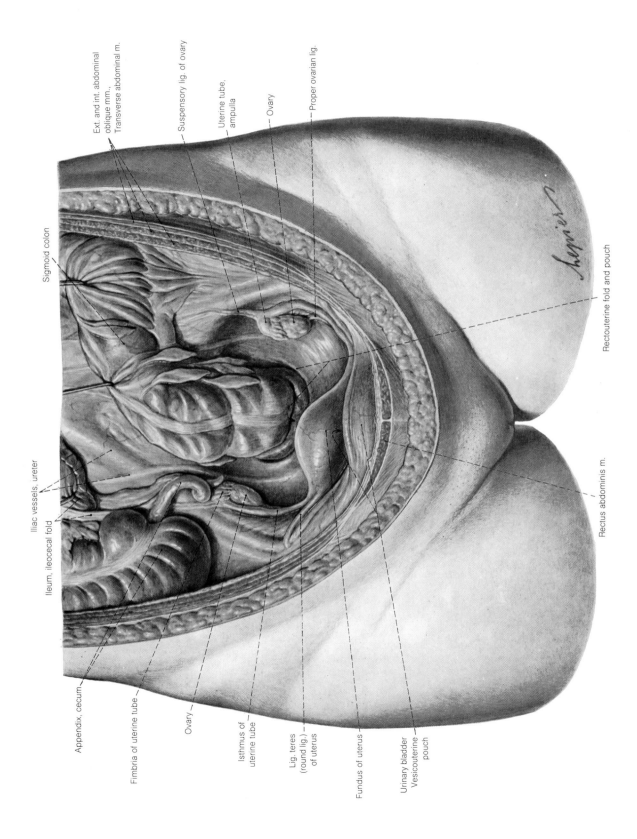

Ext. and int. abdominal
oblique mm.,
Transverse abdominal m.

Suspensory lig. of ovary

Uterine tube,
ampulla

Ovary

Proper ovarian lig.

Sigmoid colon

Rectouterine fold and pouch

Iliac vessels, ureter

Ileum, ileocecal fold

Rectus abdominis m.

Appendix, cecum

Fimbria of uterine tube

Ovary

Isthmus of
uterine tube

Lig. teres
(round lig.)
of uterus

Fundus of uterus

Urinary bladder
Vesicouterine
pouch

Fig. 296. Pelvic viscera of an adult female. The pelvis minor (or true pelvis) from above. The uterus lies, in this case, not in the exact midplane, but is lying to the right. (Dextro position frequently seen.) Observe the nearness of the appendix vermiformis to the right ovary and uterine tube. (Difficult differential diagnose in diseases of this organ complex!)

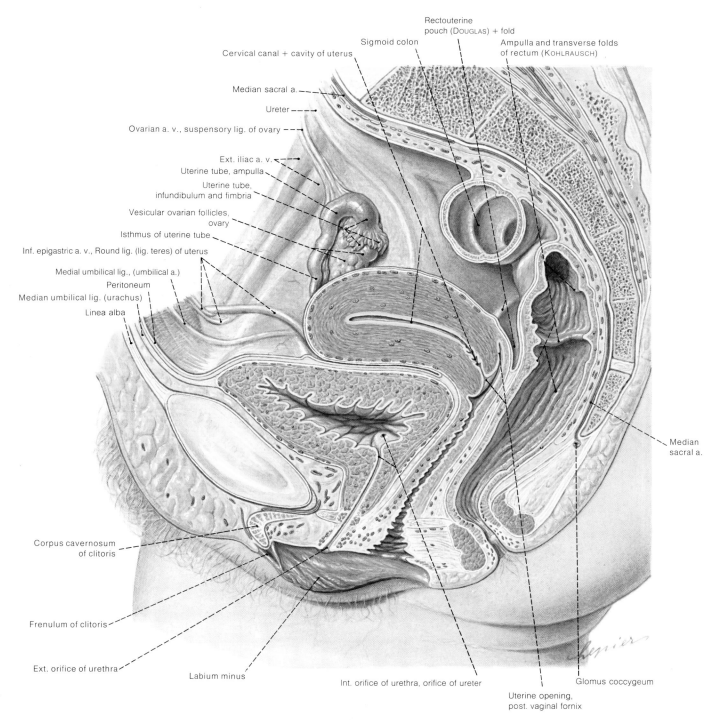

Rectouterine pouch (DOUGLAS) + fold

Sigmoid colon

Ampulla and transverse folds of rectum (KOHLRAUSCH)

Cervical canal + cavity of uterus

Median sacral a.

Ureter

Ovarian a. v., suspensory lig. of ovary

Ext. iliac a. v.

Uterine tube, ampulla

Uterine tube, infundibulum and fimbria

Vesicular ovarian follicles, ovary

Isthmus of uterine tube

Inf. epigastric a. v., Round lig. (lig. teres) of uterus

Medial umbilical lig., (umbilical a.)

Peritoneum

Median umbilical lig. (urachus)

Linea alba

Median sacral a.

Corpus cavernosum of clitoris

Frenulum of clitoris

Ext. orifice of urethra

Labium minus

Int. orifice of urethra, orifice of ureter

Glomus coccygeum

Uterine opening, post. vaginal fornix

Fig. 297. Pelvis of an adult female showing the relationship of the uterine tube to the ovary. Median sagittal section, right half. Following ovulation, the fimbria of the uterine tube and the cilia guide the ovum (still surrounded by the corona radiata) to the opening of the uterine tube.

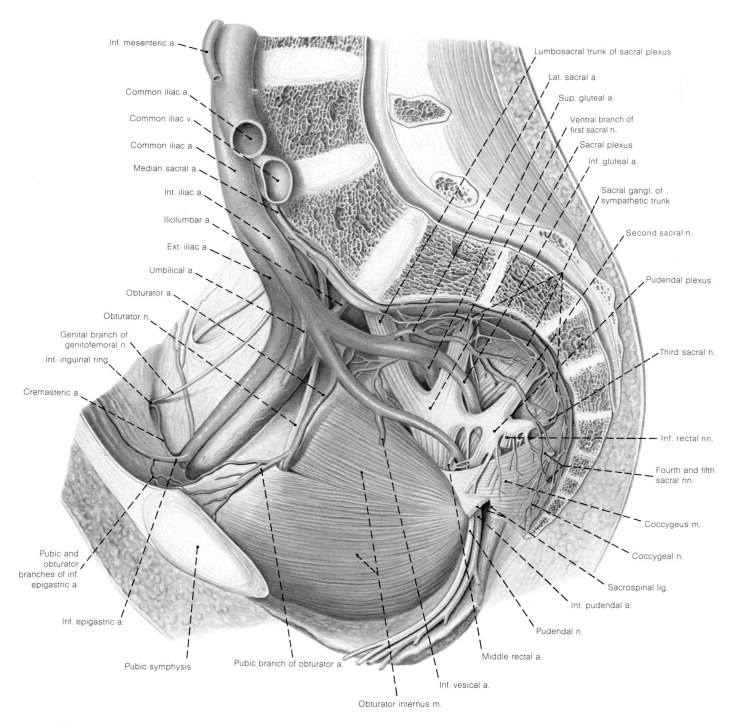

Inf. mesenteric a.

Common iliac a.

Common iliac v.

Common iliac a.

Median sacral a.

Int. iliac a.

Iliolumbar a.

Ext. iliac a.

Umbilical a.

Obturator a.

Obturator n.

Genital branch of
genitofemoral n.

Int. inguinal ring

Cremasteric a.

Pubic and
obturator
branches of inf.
epigastric a.

Inf. epigastric a.

Pubic symphysis

Pubic branch of obturator a.

Obturator internus m.

Inf. vesical a.

Middle rectal a.

Pudendal n.

Int. pudendal a.

Coccygeal n.

Sacrospinal lig.

Coccygeus m.

Fourth and fifth
sacral nn.

Inf. rectal nn.

Third sacral n.

Pudendal plexus

Second sacral n.

Sacral gangl. of
sympathetic trunk

Inf. gluteal a.

Sacral plexus

Ventral branch of
first sacral n.

Sup. gluteal a.

Lat. sacral a.

Lumbosacral trunk of sacral plexus

Fig. 298. Blood vessels and nerves of the right pelvic wall. Pelvis has been divided in the sagittal plane and pelvic viscera have been removed.

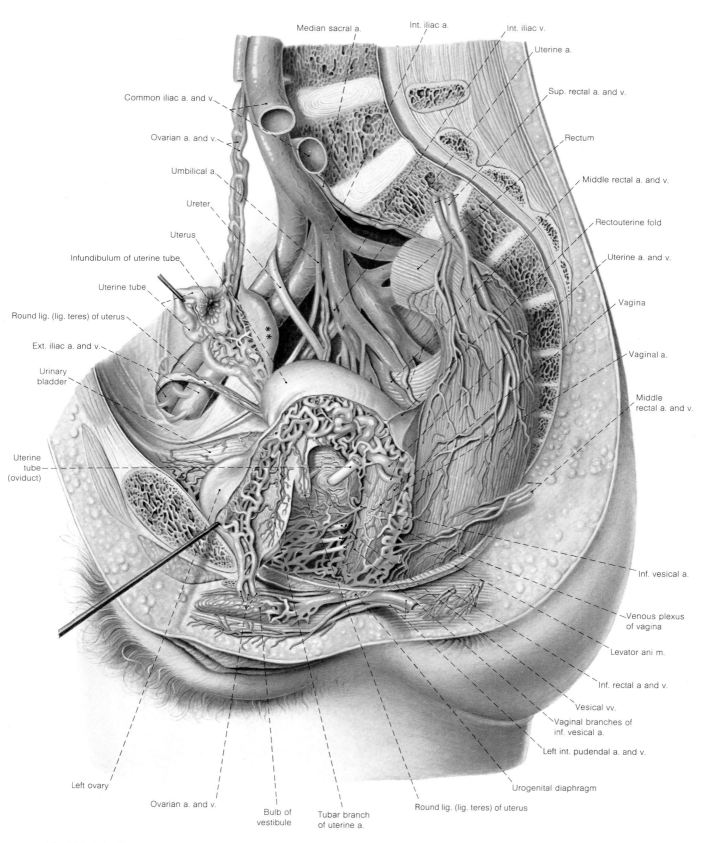

Fig. 299. Blood vessels of the pelvic viscera in the female. Preparation as in Fig. 294. Ovary and oviduct are pulled forward and downward on the left side, upward on the right side. ⁑ = Right ovary.

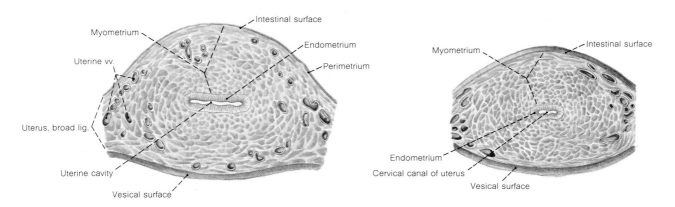

Fig. 300.

Myometrium

Uterine vv.

Uterus, broad lig.

Uterine cavity

Vesical surface

Intestinal surface

Endometrium

Perimetrium

Fig. 301.

Myometrium

Intestinal surface

Endometrium

Cervical canal of uterus

Vesical surface

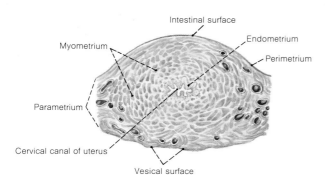

Myometrium

Parametrium

Cervical canal of uterus

Intestinal surface

Endometrium

Perimetrium

Vesical surface

Fig. 302.

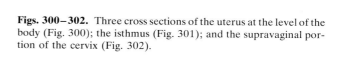

Figs. 300–302. Three cross sections of the uterus at the level of the body (Fig. 300); the isthmus (Fig. 301); and the supravaginal portion of the cervix (Fig. 302).

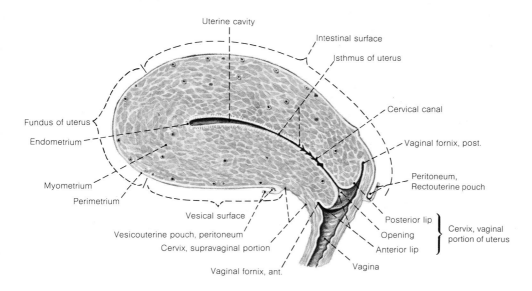

Uterine cavity

Intestinal surface

Isthmus of uterus

Cervical canal

Vaginal fornix, post.

Peritoneum, Rectouterine pouch

Fundus of uterus

Endometrium

Myometrium

Perimetrium

Vesical surface

Vesicouterine pouch, peritoneum

Cervix, supravaginal portion

Vaginal fornix, ant.

Posterior lip

Opening

Anterior lip

Cervix, vaginal portion of uterus

Vagina

Fig. 303. Sagittal section of the uterus and the cranial part of the vagina of an adult female.

206

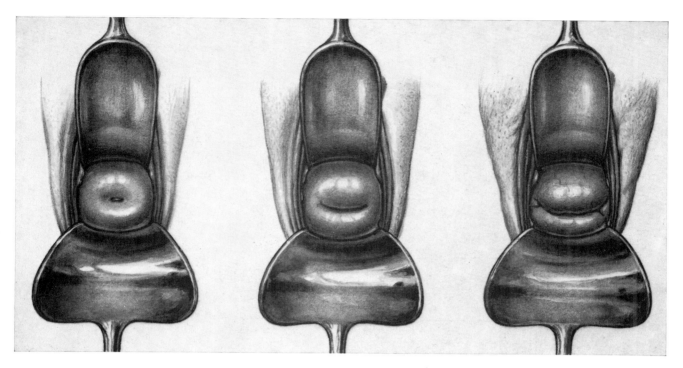

Fig. 304. Views of the vaginal portion of the cervix of the uterus (under gynecological examination, viewed through vaginal specula). 1. From a nullipara, one who has not given birth. Ostium of uterus (external os) is a round dimple, lip of ostium is a swollen ring. 2. The middle, from either a nullipara or one who has had only one birth. 3. On the right, the opening is slit-shaped, wider, and more irregular, which is evidence of having given birth to several children (multipara). See the definite lips of the external os.

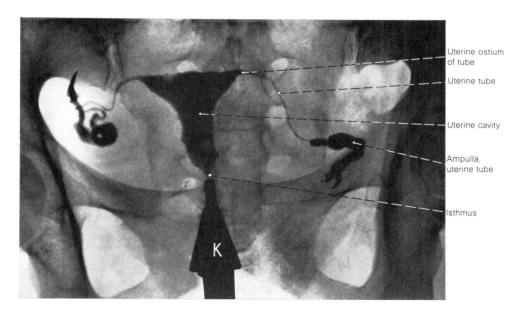

Uterine ostium of tube

Uterine tube

Uterine cavity

Ampulla, uterine tube

Isthmus

K

Fig. 305. X-ray of the lumen of the uterine cavity and tubes. The point of injection (K) lies in the canal at the cervix of the uterus. The injection medium is penetrated from the body of the uterus to the lumen of the tubes and fills them to the tube of the infundibulum. On the left side of the picture, a part of the injection material was forced into the free pelvic cavity. The left oviduct is tortuous. The uterine cavity shows the form of an isosceles triangle. On the cranial ends, lie the junction of the oviducts. The injection medium shows the vary narrow lumen of the isthmus of the uterine tube, while the ampulla and the infundibulum of the uterine tube also shows in the contrast medium as a wider lumen.

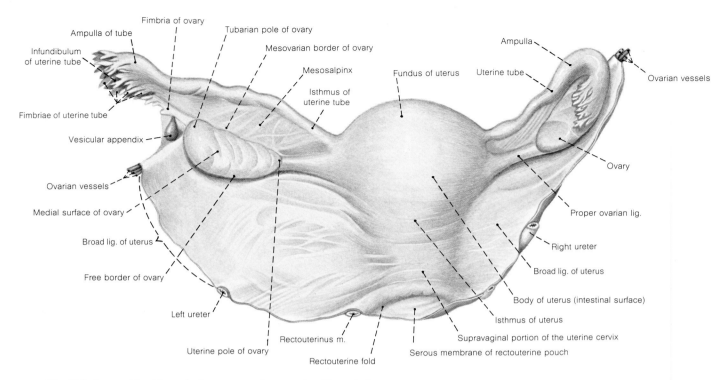

Fig. 306. Internal female genitalia, uterus, tubes, ovaries. Ventral view.

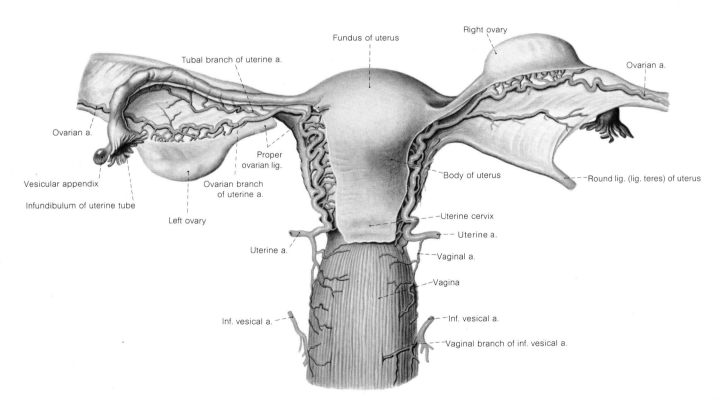

Fig. 307. Arteries of the internal female genitalia, dorsal view. The caudal portion of the broad ligament has been removed, the left proper ovarian ligament has been cut, the peritoneal covering of the mesosalpinx has been removed along the vessels.

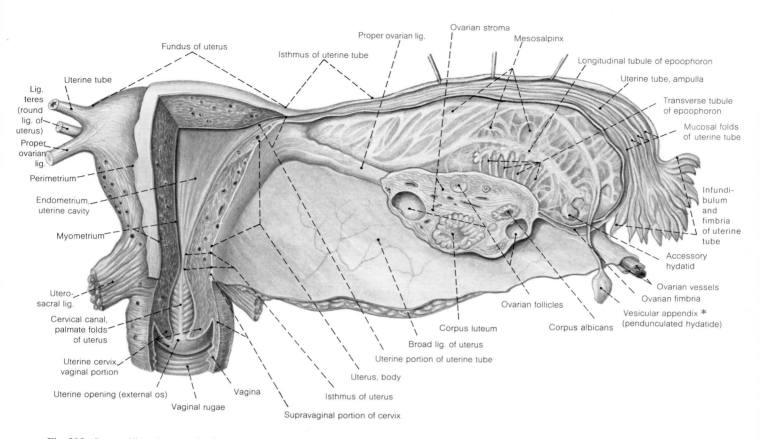

Fig. 308. Internal female reproductive organs on the right side with the uterine tube, ovary, and the broad ligament of the uterus. The right half of the uterus is opened from the front as well as cranial part of the vagina and the right oviduct. The ovary is cut frontally. The ventral layers of the peritoneal covering of the mesosalpinx, the suspensory ligament of the tube are removed so that these vessels and rudimentary structure are seen. Note: The smooth condition of the endometrium in the body of the uterus and the palmleaflike folds (plicae palmatae) of the mucous membrane of the cervical canal. * pedunculated hydatid.

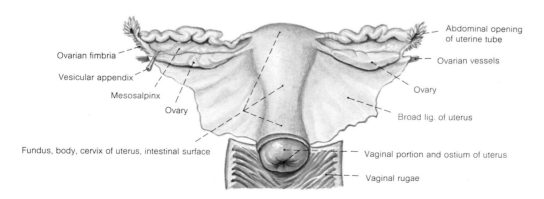

Fig. 309. Internal genital tract of a newborn female infant. The dorsal surface of the uterine tube is very convoluted, the ovaries are small and long. Note: The slender constricted shape of the uterus, the rounded vaginal part of the cervix, and the wrinkled, folded, pulled-in round aspect of the ostium of uterus.

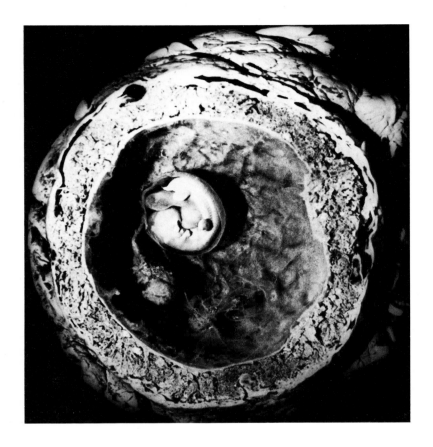

Fig. 310. Human embryo, 9 mm maximal length. Uterine and amniotic cavities are opened. Note the primordia of the paired segments and of the paddle-shaped extremital buds. (Collection of v. Hochstetter, Anatomical Institute, University of Vienna.)

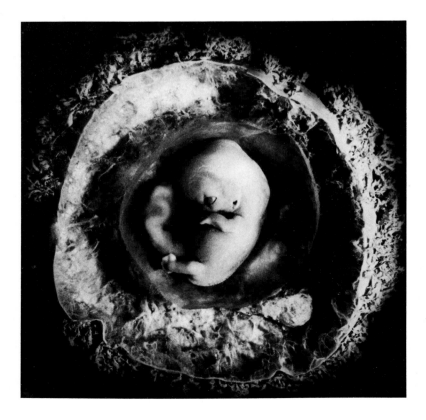

Fig. 311. Human fetus, CRL (Crown-Rump-Length) = 17.8 mm. Uterine and amniotic cavities opened. Formation of the face in progress; wide open eyes because eye lids have not yet developed. External auditory meatus prominent. Beginning development of finger and toe rays. (Collection of v. Hochstetter, Anatomical Institute, University of Vienna.)

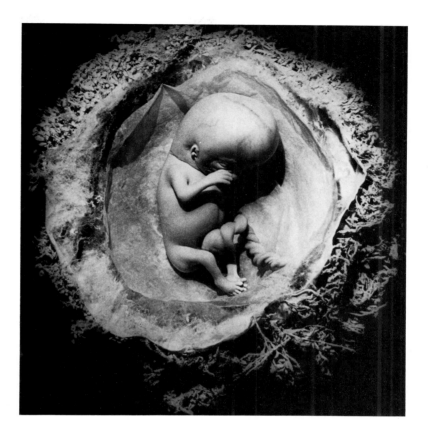

Fig. 312. Human fetus, CRL 31 mm. Uterine and amniotic cavities opened. Primordia of the eye lids. Further development of the extremities. (Collection of v. HOCHSTETTER, Anatomical Institute, University of Vienna.)

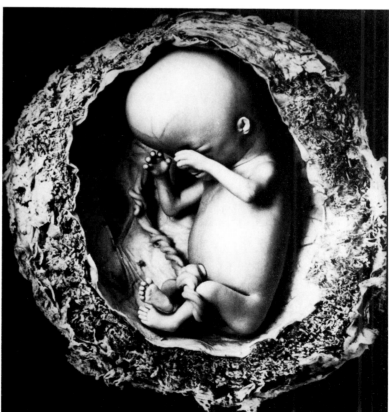

Fig. 313. Human fetus, CRL 54 mm. Uterine and amniotic cavities opened. Fusion of the eye lids. Note the prominent touch pads on the palmar and plantar surfaces of the extremities as well as the supination of the feet which is characteristic during the further total period. (Collection of v. HOCHSTETTER, Anatomical Institute, University of Vienna.)

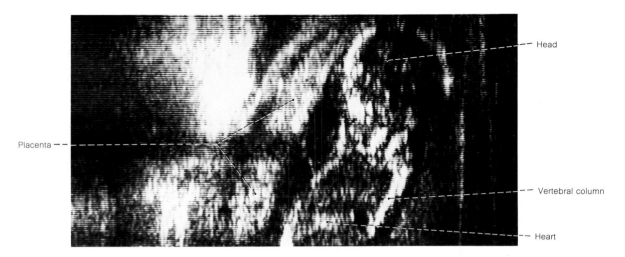

Fig. 314. Sonogram taken during the 16th week of pregnancy. (Original: Prof. Dr. G. KAUFFMANN, Zentrum Radiologie im Klinikum der Universität Freiburg i. Brsg.)

Principles of Sonography (= ultrasound examination):

Emission and reflexion of high frequency (1−5 MHz) sound waves: They penetrate through the skin into the tissues and are reflected at physical interfaces. Their registered signals from various depths can be transformed into sectional images. It is possible to visualize organs of the lesser pelvis (e.g. uterus, urinary bladder, ovaries, etc.) without the use of ionizing rays and to demonstrate physiological and pathological changes including motions (fetal movements).

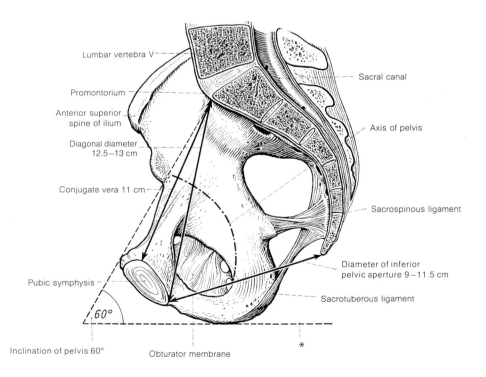

Fig. 315. Median sagittal section of the pelvis of an adult female, Angle of the pelvic inclination with the pelvic axis and pelvic diameter indicated. * = Horizontal line.

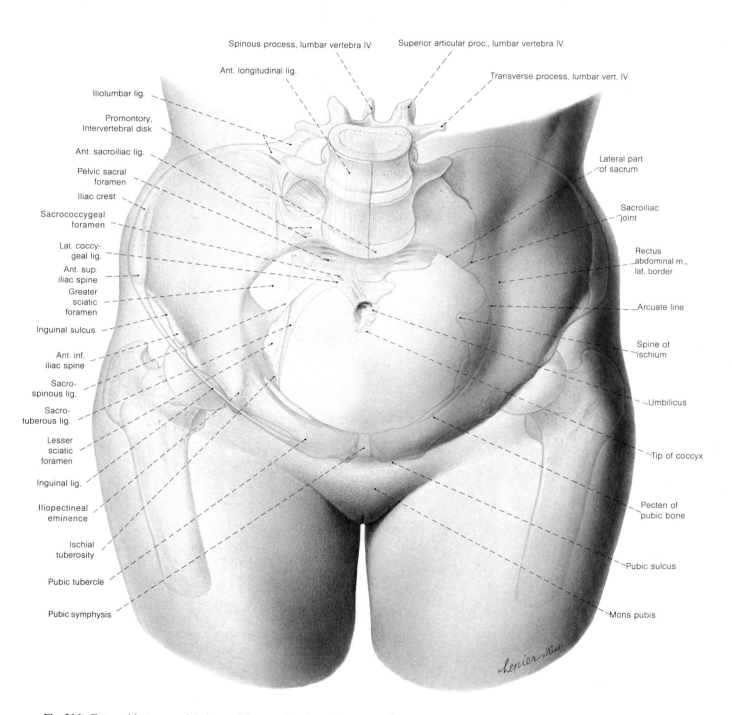

Fig. 316. External features and skeleton of the erect female pelvis. Antero-superior view. (From PERNKOPF: Atlas der topographischen und angewandten Anatomie des Menschen, Vol. 2, 2nd ed. [Ed. H. FERNER]. Urban & Schwarzenberg, Munich–Vienna–Baltimore 1980.)

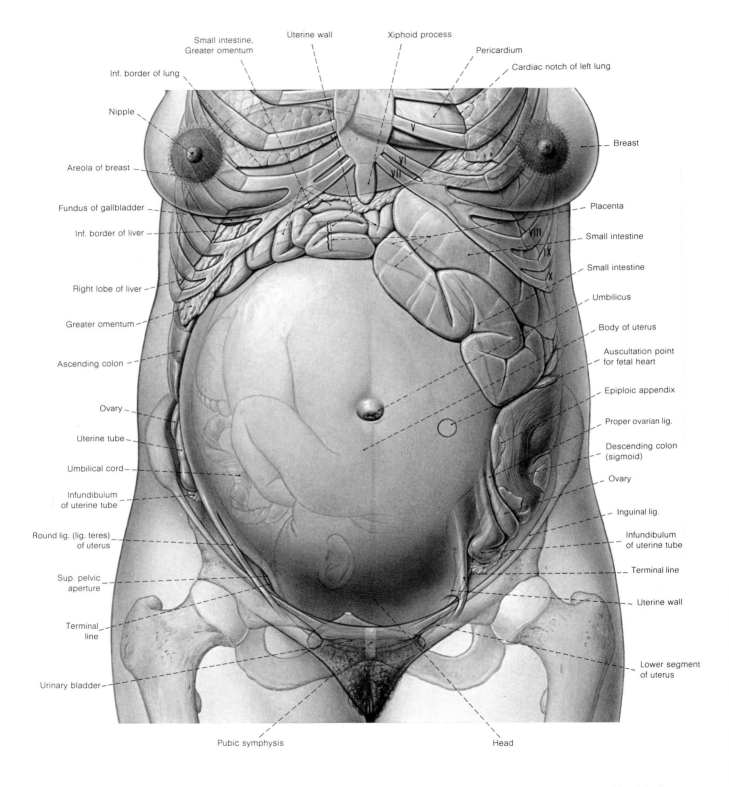

Inf. border of lung

Nipple

Areola of breast

Fundus of gallbladder

Inf. border of liver

Right lobe of liver

Greater omentum

Ascending colon

Ovary

Uterine tube

Umbilical cord

Infundibulum of uterine tube

Round lig. (lig. teres) of uterus

Sup. pelvic aperture

Terminal line

Urinary bladder

Small intestine, Greater omentum

Uterine wall

Xiphoid process

Pericardium

Cardiac notch of left lung

Breast

Placenta

Small intestine

Small intestine

Umbilicus

Body of uterus

Auscultation point for fetal heart

Epiploic appendix

Proper ovarian lig.

Descending colon (sigmoid)

Ovary

Inguinal lig.

Infundibulum of uterine tube

Terminal line

Uterine wall

Lower segment of uterus

Pubic symphysis

Head

Fig. 317. Abdominal viscera of a multipara shortly before the end of pregnancy. Sagittal projection, ventral view. Fetal head in dorso-anterior position. (From PERNKOPF: Atlas der topographischen und angewandten Anatomie des Menschen, Vol. 2, 2nd ed. [Ed. H. FERNER]. Urban & Schwarzenberg, Munich–Vienna–Baltimore 1980.)

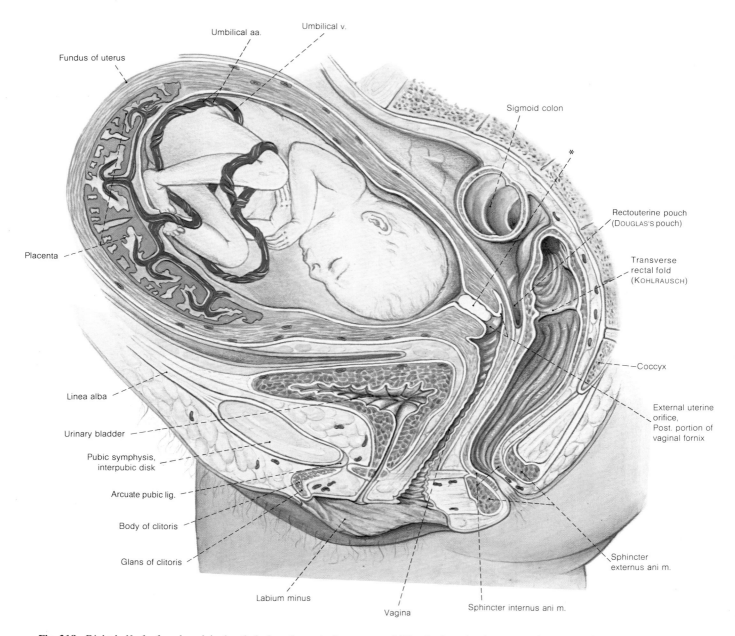

Fundus of uterus

Umbilical aa.

Umbilical v.

Sigmoid colon

*

Placenta

Rectouterine pouch
(DOUGLAS'S pouch)

Transverse
rectal fold
(KOHLRAUSCH)

Linea alba

Coccyx

Urinary bladder

External uterine
orifice,
Post. portion of
vaginal fornix

Pubic symphysis,
interpubic disk

Arcuate pubic lig.

Body of clitoris

Glans of clitoris

Sphincter
externus ani m.

Labium minus

Vagina

Sphincter internus ani m.

Fig. 318. Right half of a female pelvis shortly before the end of pregnancy. Midsagittal section (compare with Fig. 317). * Mucous plug
(KRISTELLER'S) in the cervical canal.

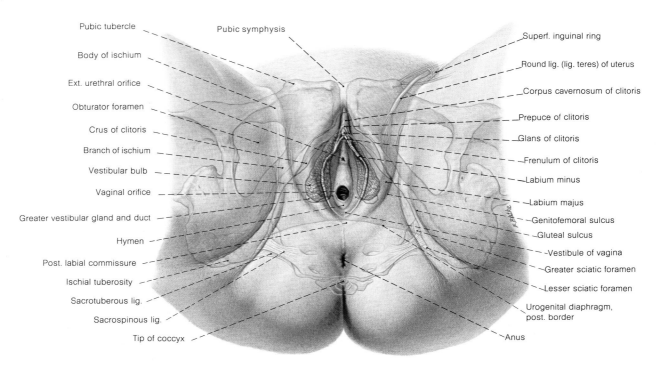

Fig. 319. Projection of external female genitalia on bony structures of the pelvis. Caudal view. (From PERNKOPF: Atlas der topographischen und angewandten Anatomie des Menschen, Vol. 2, 2nd ed. [Ed. H. FERNER]. Urban & Schwarzenberg, Munich–Vienna–Baltimore 1980.)

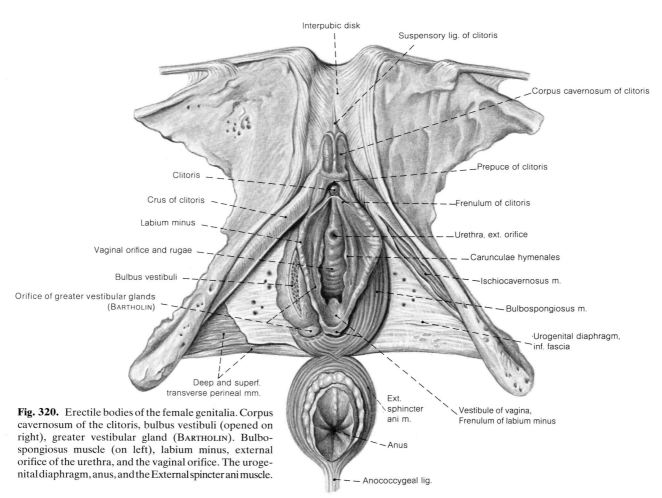

Fig. 320. Erectile bodies of the female genitalia. Corpus cavernosum of the clitoris, bulbus vestibuli (opened on right), greater vestibular gland (BARTHOLIN). Bulbo-spongiosus muscle (on left), labium minus, external orifice of the urethra, and the vaginal orifice. The urogenital diaphragm, anus, and the External spincter ani muscle.

Fig. 321. Uterus, vagina, and external genitalia of a multiparous woman. The vagina cut lengthwise and spread open. Transverse slit-like opening of the external os of the uterus with anterior and posterior lips and mucous plug (KRISTELLER's).

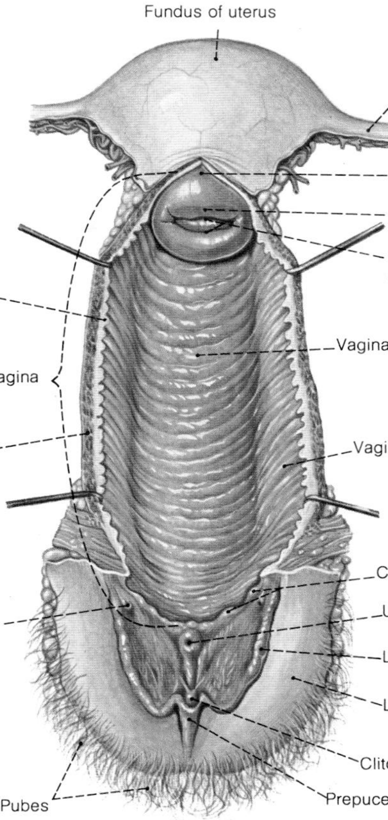

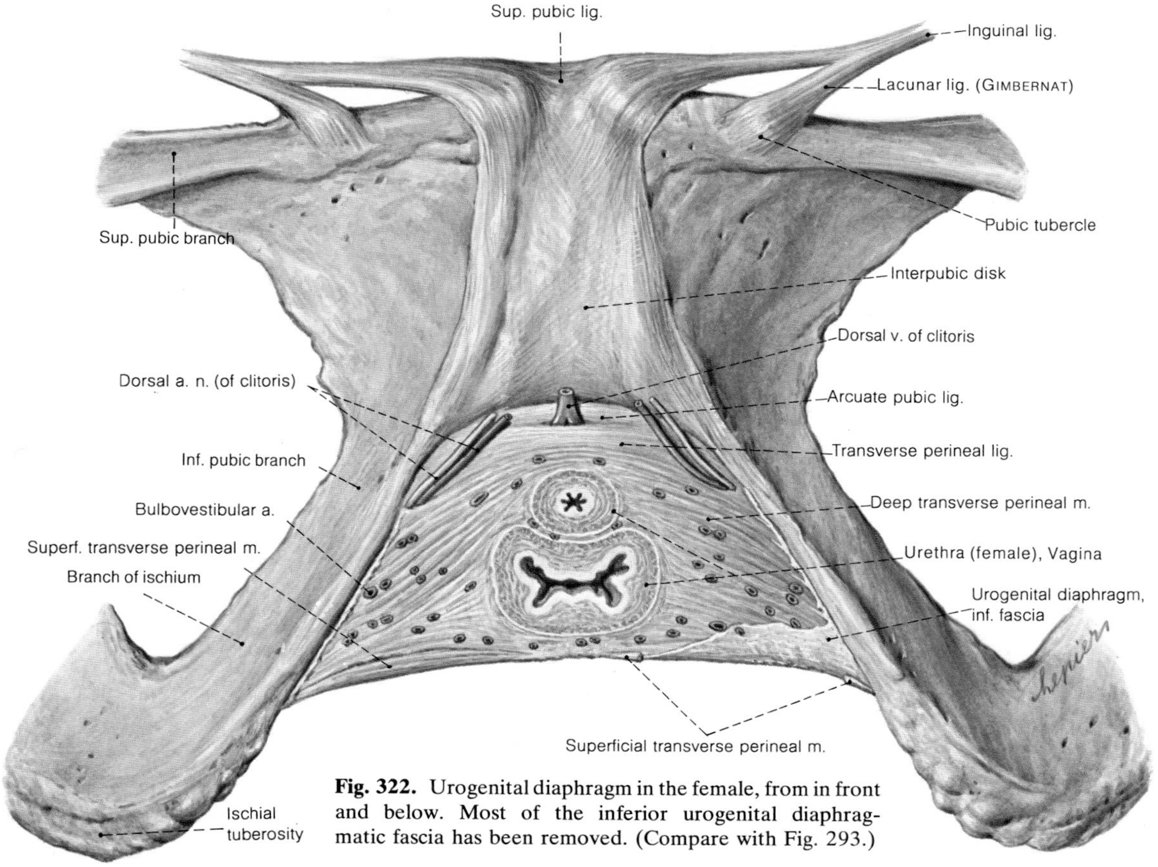

Fundus of uterus

Uterine tube, isthmus

Vaginal fornix, post.

Cervix, vaginal portion, post. lip

Uterine orifice (mucous plug)

Vaginal rugae, ant.

Vagina, mucous membrane

Vagina

Vaginal muscular coat

Vaginal rugae, post.

Carunculae hymenales

Urethral opening, ext.

Greater vestibular gland, excretory duct

Labium minus

Labium majus

Clitoris

Prepuce of clitoris

Pubes

Sup. pubic lig.

Inguinal lig.

Lacunar lig. (GIMBERNAT)

Pubic tubercle

Sup. pubic branch

Interpubic disk

Dorsal v. of clitoris

Dorsal a. n. (of clitoris)

Arcuate pubic lig.

Inf. pubic branch

Transverse perineal lig.

Bulbovestibular a.

Deep transverse perineal m.

Superf. transverse perineal m.

Urethra (female), Vagina

Branch of ischium

Urogenital diaphragm, inf. fascia

Superficial transverse perineal m.

Ischial tuberosity

Fig. 322. Urogenital diaphragm in the female, from in front and below. Most of the inferior urogenital diaphragmatic fascia has been removed. (Compare with Fig. 293.)

217

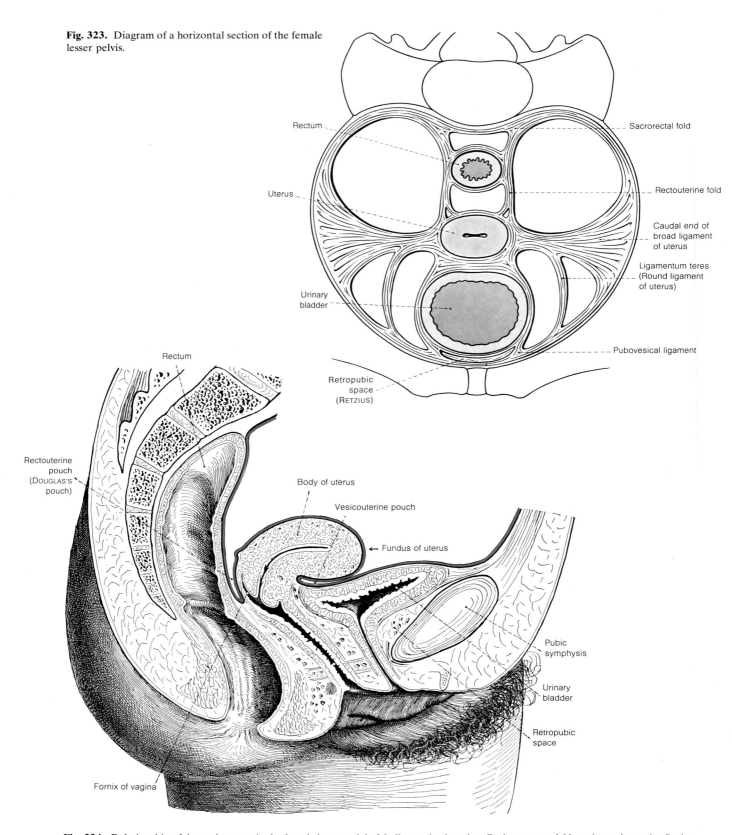

Fig. 323. Diagram of a horizontal section of the female lesser pelvis.

Rectum

Uterus

Urinary bladder

Retropubic space (Retzius)

Sacrorectal fold

Rectouterine fold

Caudal end of broad ligament of uterus

Ligamentum teres (Round ligament of uterus)

Pubovesical ligament

Rectum

Rectouterine pouch (Douglas's pouch)

Body of uterus

Vesicouterine pouch

Fundus of uterus

Pubic symphysis

Urinary bladder

Retropubic space

Fornix of vagina

Fig. 324. Relationship of the peritoneum in the female lesser pelvis. Median sagittal section. Peritoneum red. Note the peritoneal reflexion near the posterior fornix of the vagina.

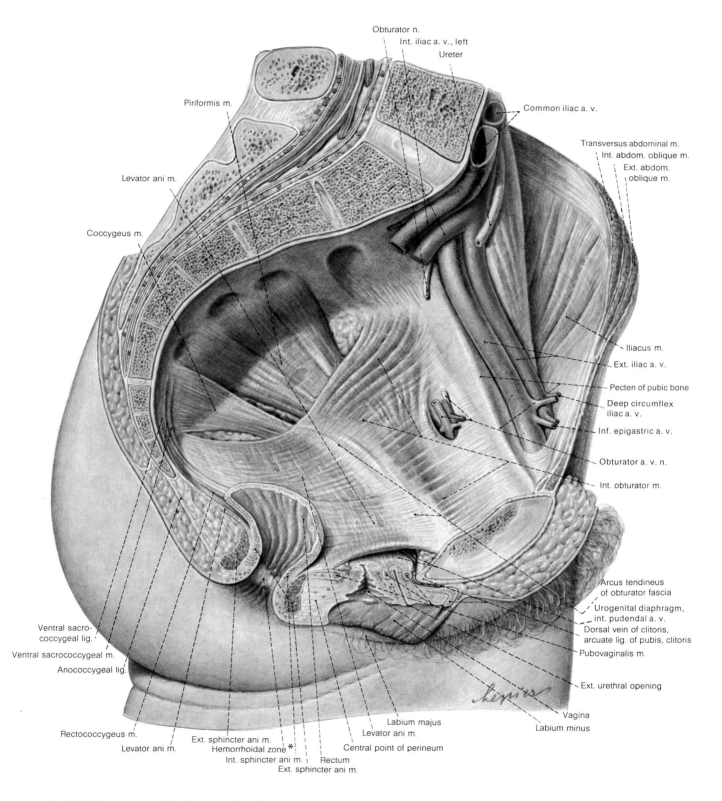

Fig. 325. Musculature of the lateral wall and floor of the pelvis (Pelvic muscles). Median section of the female pelvis, left half.
Note: * The zona alba or white line which is the parchment-colored region between the deeply pigmented area (cutaneous zone) and the reddish mucous membrane of the rectum. The hemorrhoidal zone is part of the anal canal which contains the important rectal venous plexus. The veins of this plexus are prone to become varicose and are then called hemorrhoids.

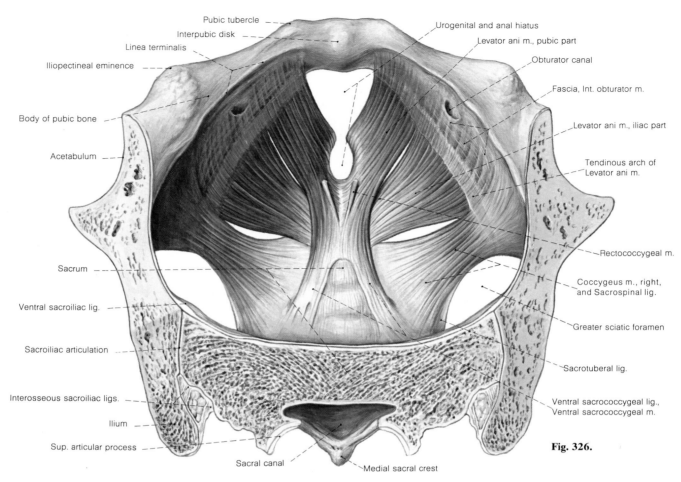

Fig. 326.

Perineal Muscles

Name		Origin	Insertion
Ischicavernosus muscle (paired)		Ischial ramus, together with the crus of penis (or clitoris)	Corpus cavernosum penis and deep fascia of penis (or clitoris)
Bulbospongiosus muscle	a) male	Perineal surface of bulb of penis	The superficial fibers transmit into the corpus cavernosum penis
	b) female	Sphincter-like surrounds entry into vagina	
Sphincter urethrae muscle (only in the male) (not paired)		Transverse ligament of perineum (part of the muscle substance of the urogenital diaphragm)	Surrounds the membranous part of the urethra with ring-shaped fibers

Innervation: Levator ani m. and coccygeus m. are innervated by the sacral plexus (3rd or 4th sacral nerve), all other perineal muscles by branches of the pudendal n.

Muscles of the Pelvic Floor

Name	Origin	Insertion
I. Pelvic diaphragm **1. Levator ani muscle,** funnel-shaped, made up of several muscle parts: Pubococcygeus, Puborectalis, Iliococcygeus, Levator prostatae mm.	Tendinous arch of Levator ani muscle (spans the Obturator internus muscle from the symphysis to the ischial spine)	Sacrum, coccyx, and External sphincter muscle

Nerve: Pudendal plexus, sacral nerves (S 3−5)

Function: Supports and slightly raises the pelvic floor

continued →

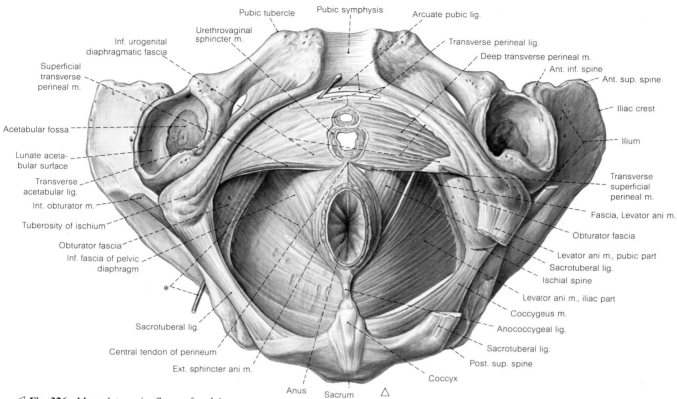

Fig. 326. Musculature in floor of pelvis of an adult female. Seen from above.

Fig. 327. Musculature in floor of pelvis of an adult female. Perineal view. * Probe in pudendal canal.

Muscles of the Pelvic Floor (continued)

Name	Origin	Insertion
2. Coccygeus muscle its fibers are embedded in the sacro-spinal ligament	Ischial spine	Sacrum, coccyx

Function: Enforces pelvic floor in conjunction with the sacrospinal ligament

II. External sphincter ani muscle Subcutaneous portion Superficial portion Deep portion	Radiates into the corium anterior and posterior to the anus; between centrum tendineum and anococcygeal ligament; more ring shaped, 3–4 cm anterior position	

Innervation: Pudendal n.

Function: Closes anus

III. Urogenital diaphragm **1. Transverse perinei profundus muscle**	Stretches between the ischial rami, completed by the transverse ligament of the perineum and the arcuate ligament of the pubis. The male urethra or the urethra and vagina pass through this	
2. Transverse perinei superf. muscle (variable)	Superficial portion of the previous, radiates into the centrum tendineum	

Innervation: Pudendal n.

Function: Closes the urogenital hiatus except for the openings for urethra and vagina

Central tendon of perineum (centrum tendineum): A knotty-like tendinous tissue for all muscles of the pelvic floor. It is interlaced anteriorly with the Sphincter ani externus muscle, with the dorsal border of the Transversus perinei profundus muscle, involving in addition, the Levator ani and the Bulbospongiosus muscles.

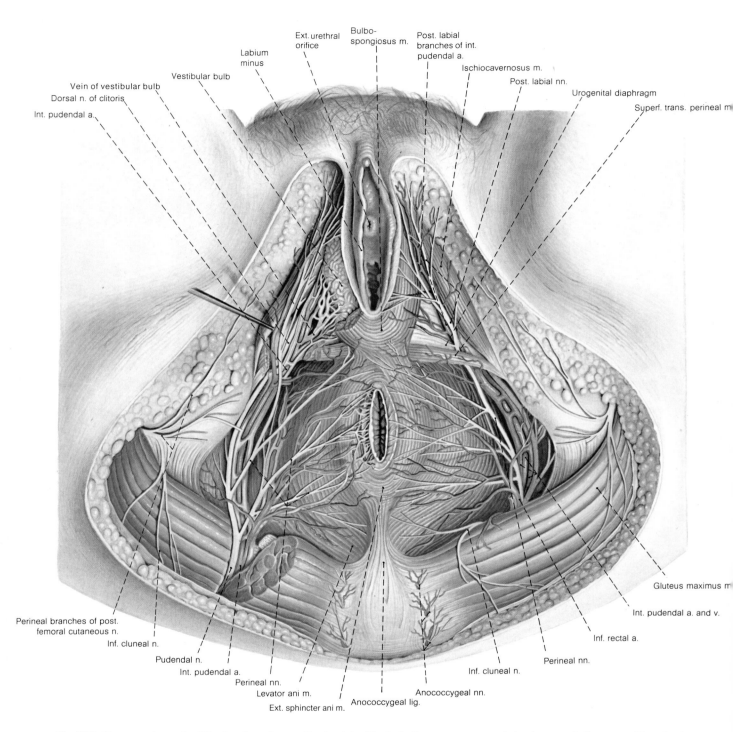

Fig. 328. Nerves and vessels of the female perineum. On the right side the bulbocavernosus muscle has been partially removed in order to expose the vestibular bulb. Nerves and vessels have been exposed by incisions into the musculature.

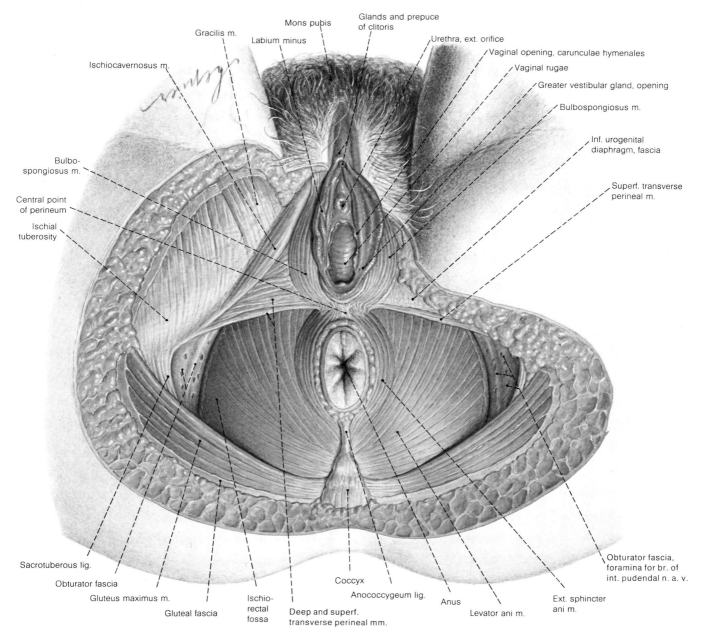

Ischiocavernosus m.
Gracilis m.
Mons pubis
Labium minus
Glands and prepuce of clitoris
Urethra, ext. orifice
Vaginal opening, carunculae hymenales
Vaginal rugae
Greater vestibular gland, opening
Bulbospongiosus m.
Inf. urogenital diaphragm, fascia
Superf. transverse perineal m.
Bulbo-spongiosus m.
Central point of perineum
Ischial tuberosity
Sacrotuberous lig.
Obturator fascia
Gluteus maximus m.
Gluteal fascia
Ischio-rectal fossa
Deep and superf. transverse perineal mm.
Coccyx
Anococcygeum lig.
Anus
Levator ani m.
Ext. sphincter ani m.
Obturator fascia, foramina for br. of int. pudendal n. a. v.

Fig. 329. Superficial perineal muscles of the female. On the right, the urogenital diaphragmatic fascia was removed, as well as a wide area of skin from the perineum, the labium major, and thigh. Deep transverse perineal, Bulbospongiosus, and Ischiocavernosus muscles are displayed. (Compare with Fig. 292, musculature of the male perineum.)

Perineal lacerations

During delivery, the soft tissue bridge (perineum) between vagina and rectum may be lacerated if it is stressed beyond capacity. Such lacerations may occur for various reasons: e.g. because of inadequate perineal protection by the obstetrician, because of constitutional conditions (infantilism, asthenia) or because of extensive strain. One distinguishes 3 degrees of perineal lacerations: 1st degree, vaginal wall and skin of the perineum rupture for a maximal distance of 2 cm; 2nd degree, the musculature of the perineum is involved, however, the external anal sphincter muscle remains fully intact; 3rd degree (= total perineal rupture), the laceration includes the external and internal sphincter muscle and may continue to the anterior wall of the rectum.

Back

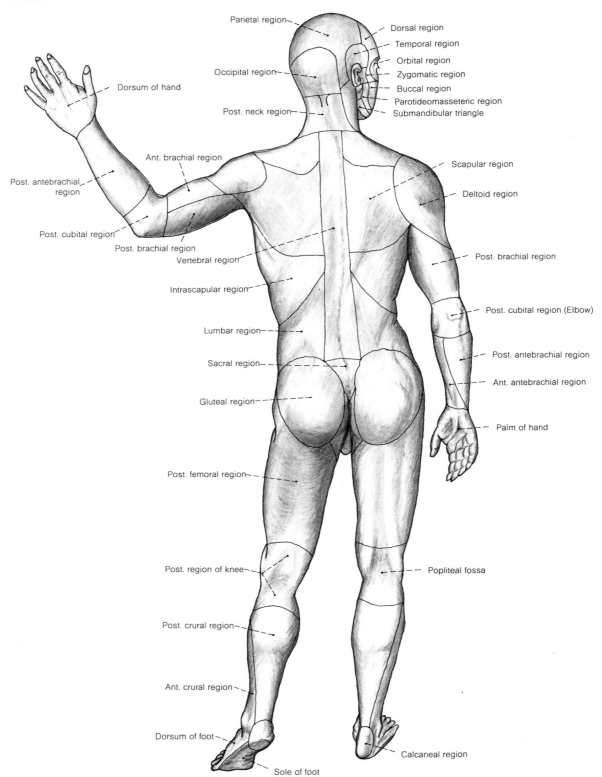

Parietal region

Dorsal region

Temporal region

Occipital region

Orbital region

Zygomatic region

Buccal region

Parotideomasseteric region

Post. neck region

Submandibular triangle

Dorsum of hand

Scapular region

Ant. brachial region

Deltoid region

Post. antebrachial region

Post. cubital region

Post. brachial region

Post. brachial region

Vertebral region

Intrascapular region

Post. cubital region (Elbow)

Lumbar region

Post. antebrachial region

Sacral region

Ant. antebrachial region

Gluteal region

Palm of hand

Post. femoral region

Post. region of knee

Popliteal fossa

Post. crural region

Ant. crural region

Dorsum of foot

Calcaneal region

Sole of foot

Fig. 330. Regions of the body outlined. Dorsal view.

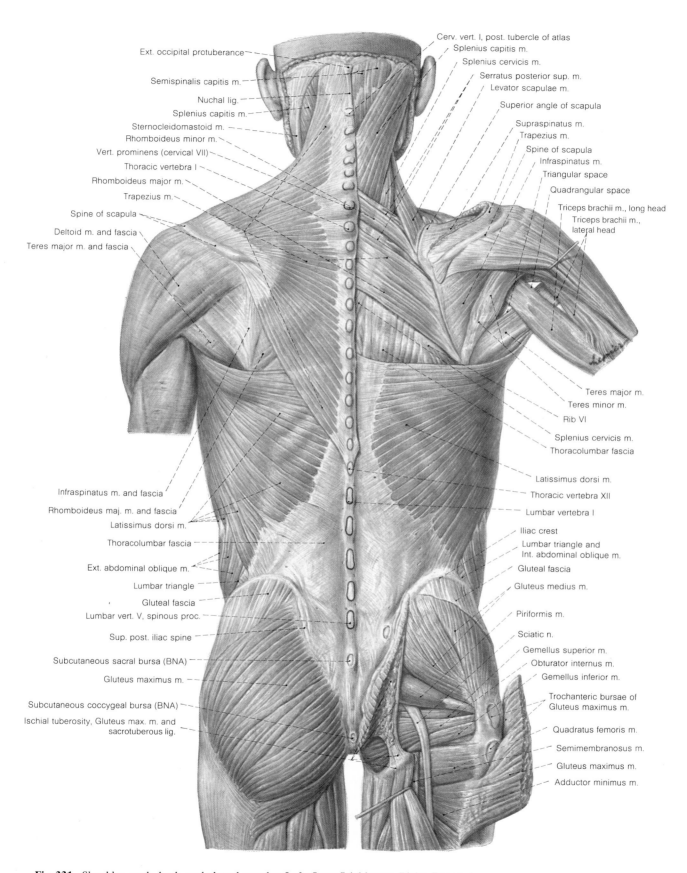

Ext. occipital protuberance

Semispinalis capitis m.

Nuchal lig.

Splenius capitis m.

Sternocleidomastoid m.

Rhomboideus minor m.

Vert. prominens (cervical VII)

Thoracic vertebra I

Rhomboideus major m.

Trapezius m.

Spine of scapula

Deltoid m. and fascia

Teres major m. and fascia

Infraspinatus m. and fascia

Rhomboideus maj. m. and fascia

Latissimus dorsi m.

Thoracolumbar fascia

Ext. abdominal oblique m.

Lumbar triangle

Gluteal fascia

Lumbar vert. V, spinous proc.

Sup. post. iliac spine

Subcutaneous sacral bursa (BNA)

Gluteus maximus m.

Subcutaneous coccygeal bursa (BNA)

Ischial tuberosity, Gluteus max. m. and sacrotuberous lig.

Cerv. vert. I, post. tubercle of atlas

Splenius capitis m.

Splenius cervicis m.

Serratus posterior sup. m.

Levator scapulae m.

Superior angle of scapula

Supraspinatus m.

Trapezius m.

Spine of scapula

Infraspinatus m.

Triangular space

Quadrangular space

Triceps brachii m., long head

Triceps brachii m., lateral head

Teres major m.

Teres minor m.

Rib VI

Splenius cervicis m.

Thoracolumbar fascia

Latissimus dorsi m.

Thoracic vertebra XII

Lumbar vertebra I

Iliac crest

Lumbar triangle and Int. abdominal oblique m.

Gluteal fascia

Gluteus medius m.

Piriformis m.

Sciatic n.

Gemellus superior m.

Obturator internus m.

Gemellus inferior m.

Trochanteric bursae of Gluteus maximus m.

Quadratus femoris m.

Semimembranosus m.

Gluteus maximus m.

Adductor minimus m.

Fig. 331. Shoulder, neck, back, and gluteal muscles. Left: Superficial layers. Right: Deeper layers.

Muscles of the Back (Figs. 331, 332, 338)

Name	Origin	Insertion
1. Trapezius muscle A flat triangular muscle (see also Fig. 7); tendinous tissue in region where the cervical and the thoracic spinous processes meet	Medial third of superior nuchal line; external occipital protuberance; cervical spinous processes via the nuchal ligament; spines of thoracic vertebrae and their supraspinous ligaments	Lateral third of clavicle acromion; spine of scapula

Nerve: Spinal accessory nerve plus C 3, 4

Function: Cranial fibers elevate the scapula, the caudal depress it; the middle fibers pull the scapula dorsally, suspend the shoulder girdle, help rotate the scapula. Normal tension helps maintain the square shoulder. When the accessory is cut the shoulder droops.

Name	Origin	Insertion
2. Latissimus dorsi muscle A large triangular muscle	By way of the thoracolumbar fascia (aponeurosis), from the 6 caudal thoraci, all lumbar spines, sacrum, and external lip of iliac crest. Muscular slips from 3 or 4 caudal ribs and inferior angle of scapula	By a flat tendon to floor of intertubercular sulcus of humerus, ventral to Teres major insertion; Latissimus dorsi bursa between tendons

Nerve: Thoracodorsal nerve of the brachial plexus (C 6, 7, 8)

Function: Extends and adducts the humerus and rotates it medially. Draws the arm and shoulder downward and backward

Name	Origin	Insertion
3. Rhomboideus major muscle	Spines of the 2nd to 5th thoracic vertebrae	Medial border of scapula, caudal to the spine of the scapula
4. Rhomboideus minor muscle	Spines of 7th cervical and 1st thoracic vertebra; the nuchal ligament	Medial border of scapula, cranial to the spine of the scapula

Nerve: For both: Dorsal scapular nerve from the brachial plexus (C 4, 5)

Function: Draws the scapula upward and medially. Holds scapula to trunk along with the Serratus anterior muscle

Name	Origin	Insertion
5. Levator scapulae muscle Borders the Scalenus posterior muscle ventrally	The posterior tubercles of the transverse processes of the upper 4 cervical vertebrae	Superior angle of the scapula (and the immediate adjacent region) to the base of the spine of the scapula

Nerve: Cervical plexus and the dorsal scapular nerve (C 3, 4)

Function: Pulls the scapula upward and medially (along with the Trapezius muscle). If the scapula is fixed, it pulls the neck laterally

Name	Origin	Insertion
6. Serratus posterior superior muscle A thin, quadrilateral muscle	Nuchal ligament, spinous processes of 7th cervical and the first 2 or 3 thoracic vertebrae	Ribs 2–5, lateral to their angles
7. Serratus posterior inferior muscle (more broad than above)	By way of thoracolumbar fascia from last 2 thoracic and upper 2 lumbar spinous processes	Inferior borders of last 4 ribs, lateral to their angels

Nerve: For both: Intercostal nerves (superior T 1–4; inferior T 9–12)

Function: Serratus posterior superior muscle elevates first 4 ribs, assists in inspiration.
Serratus posterior inferior muscle pulls last 4 ribs caudally, helps in expiration

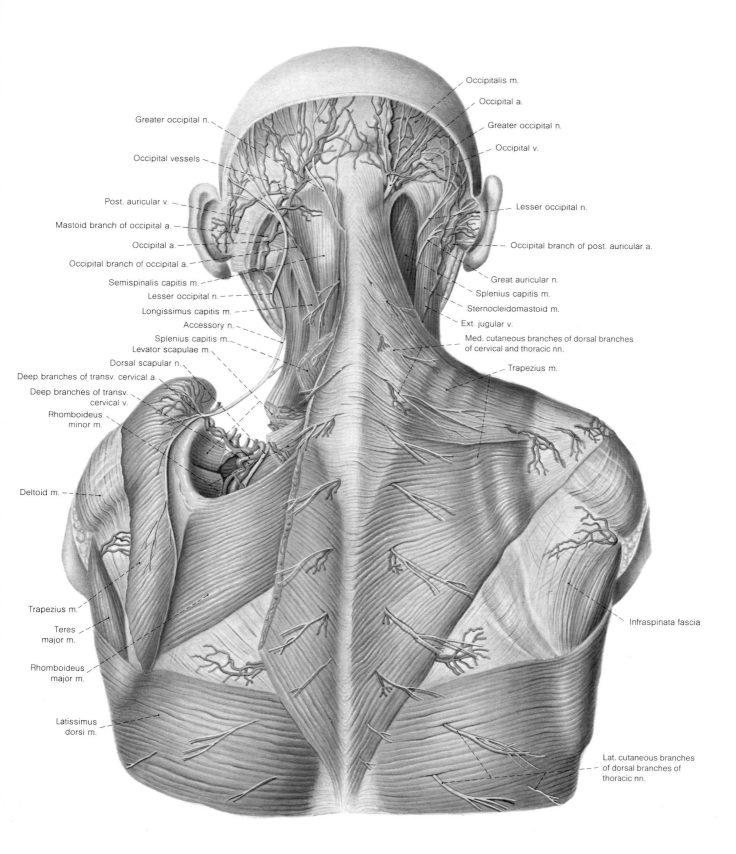

Occipitalis m.

Occipital a.

Greater occipital n.

Occipital v.

Greater occipital n.

Occipital vessels

Lesser occipital n.

Post. auricular v.

Mastoid branch of occipital a.

Occipital branch of post. auricular a.

Occipital a.

Occipital branch of occipital a.

Great auricular n.

Semispinalis capitis m.

Splenius capitis m.

Lesser occipital n.

Sternocleidomastoid m.

Longissimus capitis m.

Ext. jugular v.

Accessory n.

Med. cutaneous branches of dorsal branches of cervical and thoracic nn.

Splenius capitis m.

Levator scapulae m.

Trapezius m.

Dorsal scapular n.

Deep branches of transv. cervical a.

Deep branches of transv. cervical v.

Rhomboideus minor m.

Deltoid m.

Trapezius m.

Teres major m.

Rhomboideus major m.

Infraspinata fascia

Latissimus dorsi m.

Lat. cutaneous branches of dorsal branches of thoracic nn.

Fig. 332. Superficial and middle layer of nerves and vessels of the upper back and neck. On the left side, the trapezius, sternocleidomastoid, splenius capitis and levator scapulae muscles were divided.

227

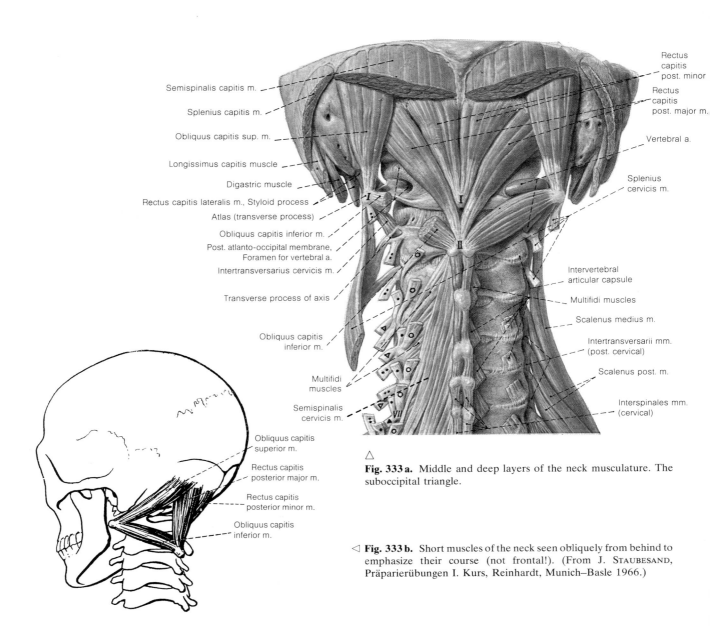

Semispinalis capitis m.

Splenius capitis m.

Obliquus capitis sup. m.

Longissimus capitis muscle

Digastric muscle

Rectus capitis lateralis m., Styloid process

Atlas (transverse process)

Obliquus capitis inferior m.

Post. atlanto-occipital membrane, Foramen for vertebral a.

Intertransversarius cervicis m.

Transverse process of axis

Obliquus capitis inferior m.

Multifidi muscles

Semispinalis cervicis m.

Rectus capitis post. minor

Rectus capitis post. major m.

Vertebral a.

Splenius cervicis m.

Intervertebral articular capsule

Multifidi muscles

Scalenus medius m.

Intertransversarii mm. (post. cervical)

Scalenus post. m.

Interspinales mm. (cervical)

Fig. 333 a. Middle and deep layers of the neck musculature. The suboccipital triangle.

Obliquus capitis superior m.

Rectus capitis posterior major m.

Rectus capitis posterior minor m.

Obliquus capitis inferior m.

◁ **Fig. 333 b.** Short muscles of the neck seen obliquely from behind to emphasize their course (not frontal!). (From J. Staubesand, Präparierübungen I. Kurs, Reinhardt, Munich–Basle 1966.)

Short Suboccipital Muscles

Name	Origin	Insertion
1. Rectus capitis posterior major muscle	Spinous process of the axis (II)	Inferior nuchal line (of occipital bone)
2. Rectus capitis posterior minor muscle	Posterior tubercle of atlas (I)	Medial part of the inferior nuchal line of the occipital bone
3. Rectus capitis lateralis muscle	Transverse process of the atlas	Jugular process of the occipital bone
4. Obliquus capitis superior muscle	Transverse process of the atlas	Occipital bone, above the inferior nuchal line
5. Obliquus capitis inferior muscle	Spinous process of the axis (II)	Transverse process of the atlas

Nerve: Suboccipital nerve (dorsal branch of the first cervical nerve)

Function: Extend and rotate head. The Rectus capitis posterior major and Obliquus capitis inferior muscles turn the head to the same side; the Rectus capitis lateralis bends the head laterally (unilateral innervation)

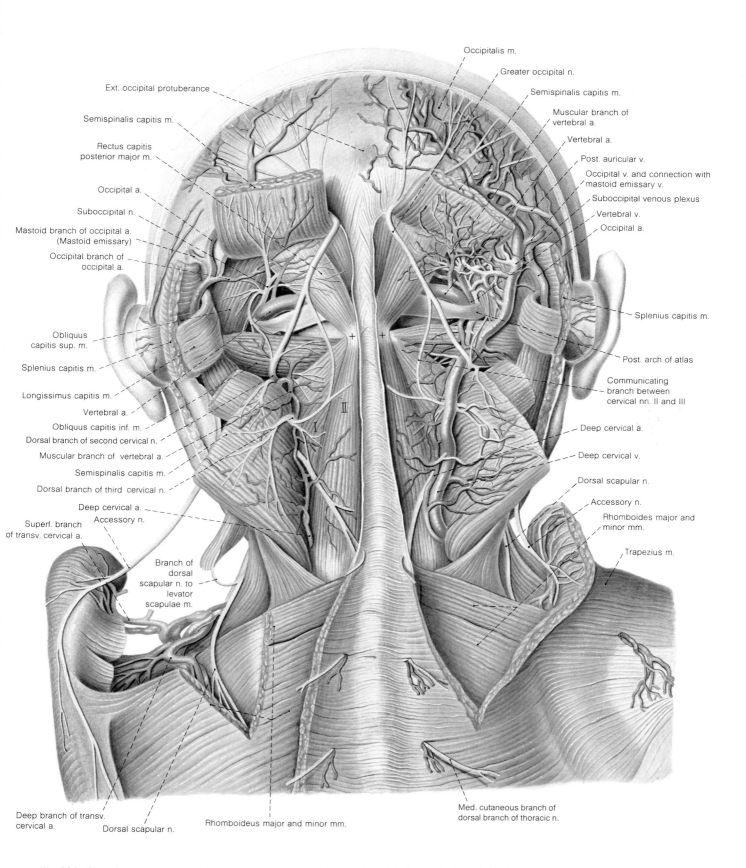

Occipitalis m.

Greater occipital n.

Semispinalis capitis m.

Muscular branch of vertebral a.

Vertebral a.

Post. auricular v.

Occipital v. and connection with mastoid emissary v.

Suboccipital venous plexus

Vertebral v.

Occipital a.

Splenius capitis m.

Post. arch of atlas

Communicating branch between cervical nn. II and III

Deep cervical a.

Deep cervical v.

Dorsal scapular n.

Accessory n.

Rhomboides major and minor mm.

Trapezius m.

Ext. occipital protuberance

Semispinalis capitis m.

Rectus capitis posterior major m.

Occipital a.

Suboccipital n.

Mastoid branch of occipital a. (Mastoid emissary)

Occipital branch of occipital a.

Obliquus capitis sup. m.

Splenius capitis m.

Longissimus capitis m.

Vertebral a.

Obliquus capitis inf. m.

Dorsal branch of second cervical n.

Muscular branch of vertebral a.

Semispinalis capitis m.

Dorsal branch of third cervical n.

Deep cervical a.

Accessory n.

Superf. branch of transv. cervical a.

Branch of dorsal scapular n. to levator scapulae m.

Deep branch of transv. cervical a.

Dorsal scapular n.

Rhomboideus major and minor mm.

Med. cutaneous branch of dorsal branch of thoracic n.

Fig. 334. Deep layer of nerves and vessels of upper back, neck and suboccipital triangle. I = Multifidus m.; II = Semispinalis cervicis m. + + = Spinous process of axis.

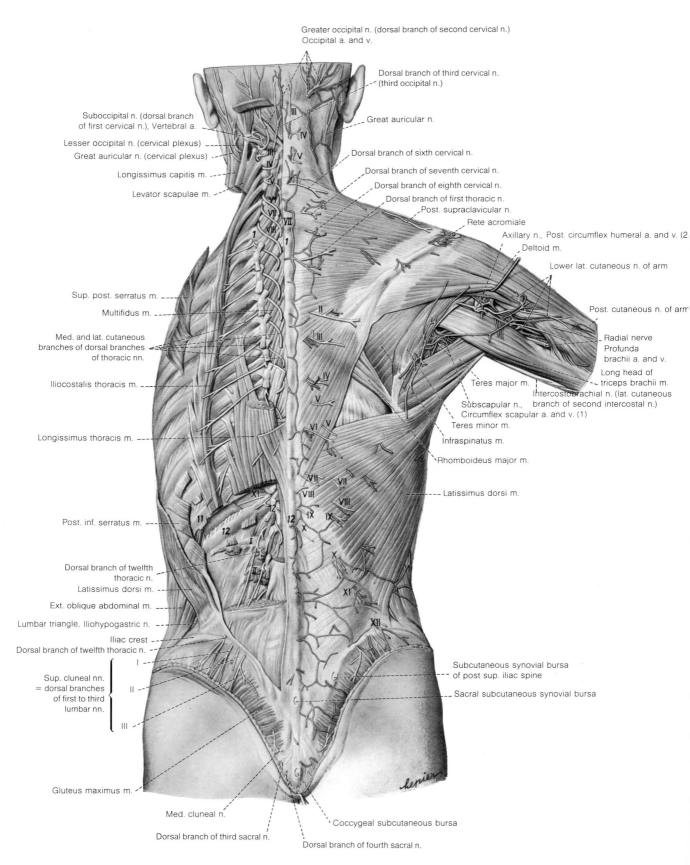

Greater occipital n. (dorsal branch of second cervical n.)
Occipital a. and v.

Dorsal branch of third cervical n.
(third occipital n.)

Suboccipital n. (dorsal branch
of first cervical n.), Vertebral a.

Great auricular n.

Lesser occipital n. (cervical plexus)

Great auricular n. (cervical plexus)

Dorsal branch of sixth cervical n.

Longissimus capitis m.

Dorsal branch of seventh cervical n.

Levator scapulae m.

Dorsal branch of eighth cervical n.

Dorsal branch of first thoracic n.

Post. supraclavicular n.

Rete acromiale

Axillary n., Post. circumflex humeral a. and v. (2

Deltoid m.

Lower lat. cutaneous n. of arm

Sup. post. serratus m.

Post. cutaneous n. of arm

Multifidus m.

Radial nerve
Profunda
brachii a. and v.

Med. and lat. cutaneous
branches of dorsal branches
of thoracic nn.

Long head of
triceps brachii m.

Intercostobrachial n. (lat. cutaneous
branch of second intercostal n.)

Iliocostalis thoracis m.

Teres major m.

Subscapular n.,
Circumflex scapular a. and v. (1)

Teres minor m.

Longissimus thoracis m.

Infraspinatus m.

Rhomboideus major m.

Latissimus dorsi m.

Post. inf. serratus m.

Dorsal branch of twelfth
thoracic n.

Latissimus dorsi m.

Ext. oblique abdominal m.

Subcutaneous synovial bursa
of post sup. iliac spine

Lumbar triangle, Iliohypogastric n.

Sacral subcutaneous synovial bursa

Iliac crest

Dorsal branch of twelfth thoracic n.

Sup. cluneal nn.
= dorsal branches
of first to third
lumbar nn.

Gluteus maximus m.

Med. cluneal n.

Coccygeal subcutaneous bursa

Dorsal branch of third sacral n.

Dorsal branch of fourth sacral n.

Fig. 335. Nerves and vessels of nucha and back. Superficial layer on the right side, deep layer on the left. Nerves and vessels of the triangular (1) and quadrangular (2) spaces of the axilla.

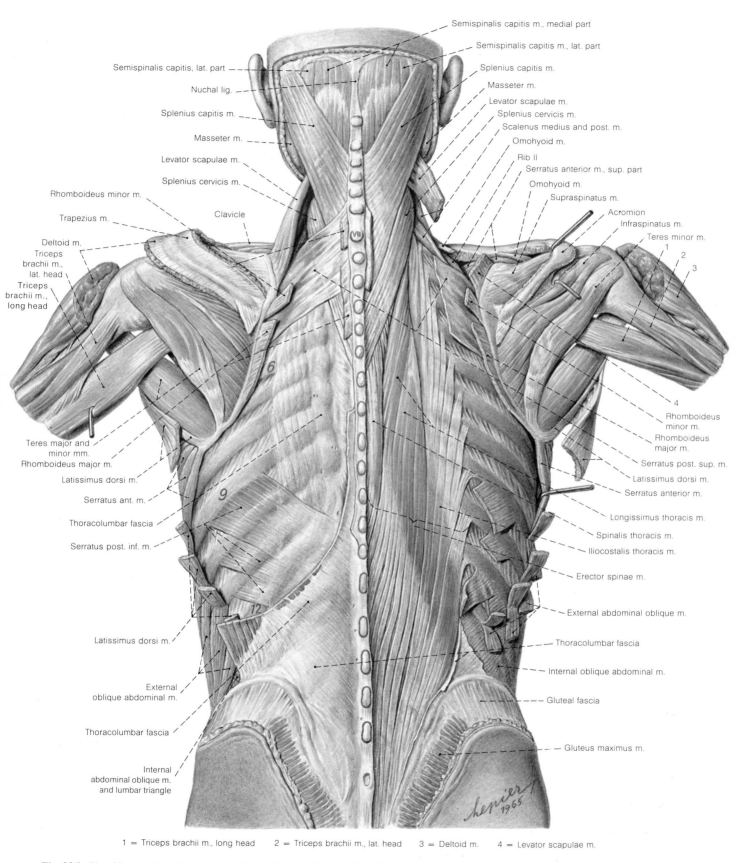

Semispinalis capitis m., medial part
Semispinalis capitis m., lat. part
Splenius capitis m.
Masseter m.
Levator scapulae m.
Splenius cervicis m.
Scalenus medius and post. m.
Omohyoid m.
Rib II
Serratus anterior m., sup. part
Omohyoid m.
Supraspinatus m.
Acromion
Infraspinatus m.
Teres minor m.
Rhomboideus minor m.
Rhomboideus major m.
Serratus post. sup. m.
Latissimus dorsi m.
Serratus anterior m.
Longissimus thoracis m.
Spinalis thoracis m.
Iliocostalis thoracis m.
Erector spinae m.
External abdominal oblique m.
Thoracolumbar fascia
Internal oblique abdominal m.
Gluteal fascia
Gluteus maximus m.

Semispinalis capitis, lat. part
Nuchal lig.
Splenius capitis m.
Masseter m.
Levator scapulae m.
Splenius cervicis m.
Rhomboideus minor m.
Trapezius m.
Clavicle
Deltoid m.
Triceps brachii m., lat. head
Triceps brachii m., long head
Teres major and minor mm.
Rhomboideus major m.
Latissimus dorsi m.
Serratus ant. m.
Thoracolumbar fascia
Serratus post. inf. m.
Latissimus dorsi m.
External oblique abdominal m.
Thoracolumbar fascia
Internal abdominal oblique m. and lumbar triangle

1 = Triceps brachii m., long head 2 = Triceps brachii m., lat. head 3 = Deltoid m. 4 = Levator scapulae m.

Fig. 336. Shoulder, neck, and back musculature. Deeper layers of long back muscles.

The Erector Spinae Muscles (Sacrospinalis) (Figs. 336, 337)

Name	Origin	Insertion

1. Iliocostalis muscle (lateral column): Ileum to ribs to ribs (red lines)

		Origin	Insertion
a–c continuous without sharp delineations	a) *Lumbar section:* Iliocostalis lumborum muscle	As the Erector spinae muscle joins with the Longissimus muscle from the external lip of the iliac crest	The angles of ribs 5 to 12 Cranial: tendinous Caudal: fleshy
	b) *Dorsal section:* Iliocostalis thoracic muscle	Individual slips from the 12th to the 7th ribs	By thin tendons on angles of the upper 6 ribs and to the transverse process of the 7 th cervical vertebrae
	c) *Cervical section:* Iliocostalis cervicis muscle	Cranial and middle ribs (2nd to 6th)	Transverse processes of the 4th to the 7th cervical vertebrae

2. Longissimus muscle (intermediate column, the longest). Sacrum to transverse process to transverse process (black lines)

		Origin	Insertion
	a) *Longissimus thoracis muscle* blends with Longissimus cervicis and then with the Spinalis muscle	As the Erector spinae muscle joins with the Iliocostalis muscle from the sacrum and transverse processes of lumbar vertebrae (tendinous) with some slips from transverse processes of thoracic vertebrae	*Cranial:* rounded tendon *Caudal:* fleshy *Medial:* Accessory processes of upper lumbar vertebrae; transverse processes of thoracic vertebrae *Lateral:* Slips to costal processes of lumbar vertebrae and all ribs between the angles and tubercles
	b) *Longissimus cervicis muscle*	Transverse processes of upper 4 or 5 thoracic vertebrae	Transverse processes of 2nd to 6th cervical vertebrae (tendinous)
	c) *Longissimus capitis muscle*	Transverse processes of the upper thoracic vertebrae and the transverse and articular processes of middle and lower cervical vertebrae	Dorsal margin of the mastoid process of the temporal bone

Nerve: Dorsal branches of cervical, thoracic and lumbar nerves

3. Spinalis muscles (medial column); Spinous process to spinous process (blue lines)

Name	Origin	Insertion
Spinalis thoracis muscle (continuation of Sacrospinalis muscle)	Spinous processes of the caudal thoracic vertebrae (blending with the Longissimus muscle)	Spinous process of 3rd to 9th thoracic vertebrae
Spinalis cervicis muscle (inconstant)	Lower 2 cervical and first 2 thoracic spinous processes	Spinous processes of axis and 2nd and 3rd vertebrae
Spinalis capitis muscle (Rarely a separate muscle, usually fused with the Semispinalis capitis muscle)	Spinous processes of the lower cervical and upper thoracic vertebrae	With Semispinalis capitis muscle between the superior and inferior nuchal line on the occipital bone

Nerve: Dorsal branches of all spinal nerves (cervical, thoracic, and lumbar)

Function: Muscles of both sides, acting together, extend the vertebral column and assist in maintaining erect posture. Muscles of one side, acting alone, bend vertebral column to the side

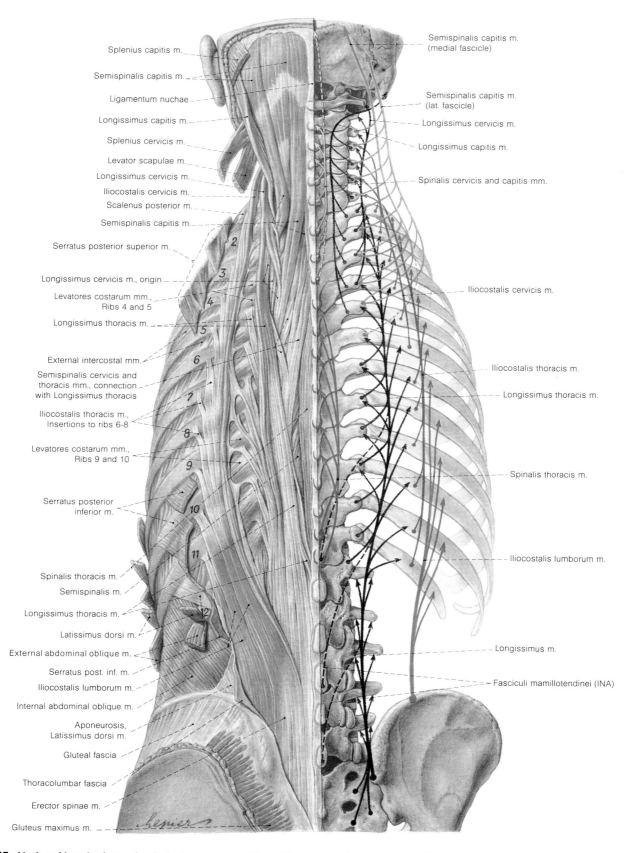

Fig. 337. Neck and long back muscles. Left: Deeper layers. Right: Diagram of origins, course, and insertion of the back muscles. Outline of spinous processus of: lumbar vertebrae, bright blue; the thoracic vertebrae, red; the cervical vertebrae, green. The longissimus muscle column, black.

Deep Layer of Back Muscles, Transversospinal Muscles (Fig. 338)

Name	Origin	Insertion
1. Semispinalis thoracis muscle **Semispinalis cervicis muscle** (without separate boundaries)	Pass obliquely upward and medially from the transverse process to the spinous processes, hence the name transversospinal. Absent in the lumbar vertebrae	
	Transverse processes of all thoracic vertebrae	Spinous processes 4 to 6 segments higher than their origin, including the spine of the axis
Semispinalis capitis muscle (transversoccipital, largest muscle in back of neck with 1 or 2 conspicuous tendinous intersections)	Transverse processes of 3 cervical and 5 or 6 thoracic vertebrae	Between the superior and inferior nuchal line

Nerve: Dorsal branches of the cervical and thoracic nerves

Function: Extend vertebral column (especially the cervical vertebrae) and head, bending the head backwards. Unilateral innervation draws the muscle of the head toward the opposing side. Together, with the Sternocleidomastoid muscle, supports the head

Name	Origin	Insertion
2. Multifidi muscles (spans 2 or 3 vertebrae)	Dorsal surface of the sacrum; transverse processes of lumbar, thoracic, and lower cervical vertebrae	Spinous process of lumbar, thoracic, and cervical vertebrae up to the axis
3. Rotatores cervicis muscles The short rotator muscles link adjacent vertebrae; the long ones skip one vertebra **Rotatores thoracis muscles** **Rotatores lumborum muscles**	Transverse process of the cervical vertebrae Transverse process of thoracic vertebrae Transverse process of the lumbar vertebrae	Roots of the spinous processes of the adjacent or the second vertebra above

Nerve: Dorsal branches of the spinal nerves: cervical, thoracic and lumbar nerves

Function: Also of the transversospinal group. When acting bilaterally, they all extend the vertebral column. When acting individually and unilaterally they bend the vertebral column to the side and rotate the vertebrae

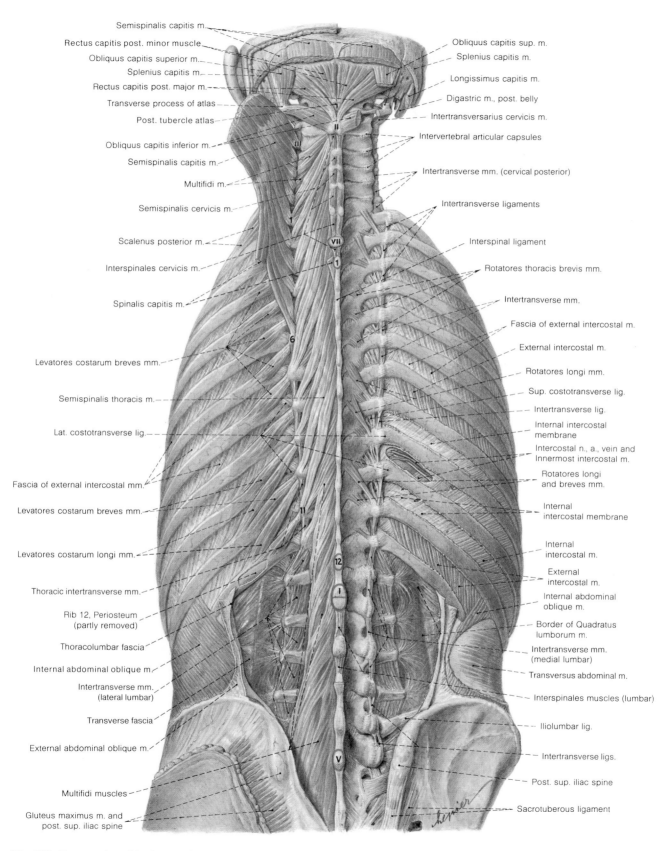

Semispinalis capitis m.
Rectus capitis post. minor muscle
Obliquus capitis superior m.
Splenius capitis m.
Rectus capitis post. major m.
Transverse process of atlas
Post. tubercle atlas
Obliquus capitis inferior m.
Semispinalis capitis m.
Multifidi m.
Semispinalis cervicis m.
Scalenus posterior m.
Interspinales cervicis m.
Spinalis capitis m.
Levatores costarum breves mm.
Semispinalis thoracis m.
Lat. costotransverse lig.
Fascia of external intercostal mm.
Levatores costarum breves mm.
Levatores costarum longi mm.
Thoracic intertransverse mm.
Rib 12, Periosteum
(partly removed)
Thoracolumbar fascia
Internal abdominal oblique m.
Intertransverse mm.
(lateral lumbar)
Transverse fascia
External abdominal oblique m.
Multifidi muscles
Gluteus maximus m. and
post. sup. iliac spine

Obliquus capitis sup. m.
Splenius capitis m.
Longissimus capitis m.
Digastric m., post. belly
Intertransversarius cervicis m.
Intervertebral articular capsules
Intertransverse mm. (cervical posterior)
Intertransverse ligaments
Interspinal ligament
Rotatores thoracis brevis mm.
Intertransverse mm.
Fascia of external intercostal m.
External intercostal m.
Rotatores longi mm.
Sup. costotransverse lig.
Intertransverse lig.
Internal intercostal
membrane
Intercostal n., a., vein and
Innermost intercostal m.
Rotatores longi
and breves mm.
Internal
intercostal membrane
Internal
intercostal m.
External
intercostal m.
Internal abdominal
oblique m.
Border of Quadratus
lumborum m.
Intertransverse mm.
(medial lumbar)
Transversus abdominal m.
Interspinales muscles (lumbar)
Iliolumbar lig.
Intertransverse ligs.
Post. sup. iliac spine
Sacrotuberous ligament

Fig. 338. Deep neck and back musculature. Transversospinal group.

235

Intertransversarii Muscles (Figs. 338, 339)

Name	Origin	Insertion
Lateral lumbar intertransversarii muscles	Costal processes of lumbar vertebrae	Costal processes of lumbar vertebrae
Medial lumbar intertransversarii muscles	Mammillary processes of lumbar vertebrae	Accessory and mammillary processes of lumbar vertebrae
Intertransversarii thoracis muscles	Transverse processes of thoracic vertebrae	Transverse process of thoracic vertebrae
Posterior cervical intertransversarii muscles	Posterior tubercles of cervical vertebrae	Posterior tubercles of cervical vertebrae
Anterior cervical intertransversarii muscles	Anterior tubercles of cervical vertebrae	Anterior tubercles of cervical vertebrae

Innervation: Dorsal and ventral branches of spinal nerves

Function: if contracting on one side: lateral bending;
                  if contracting on both sides: erection of vertebral column

Levatores Costarum Muscles (Figs. 338, 339)

Name	Origin	Insertion
Levatores costarum brevis muscles	Transverse processes of 7th to 11th thoracic vertebrae	Next lower rib
Levatores costarum longi muscles (absent in middle thoracic region)	Transverse processes of upper and lower thoracic vertebrae	Second lower rib

Innervation: Dorsal branch of cervical nerve VIII and dorsal branches of thoracic nerves

Function: In contrast to their names they act less upon the ribs, but they assist in erection, lateral bending and rotation of the vertebral column

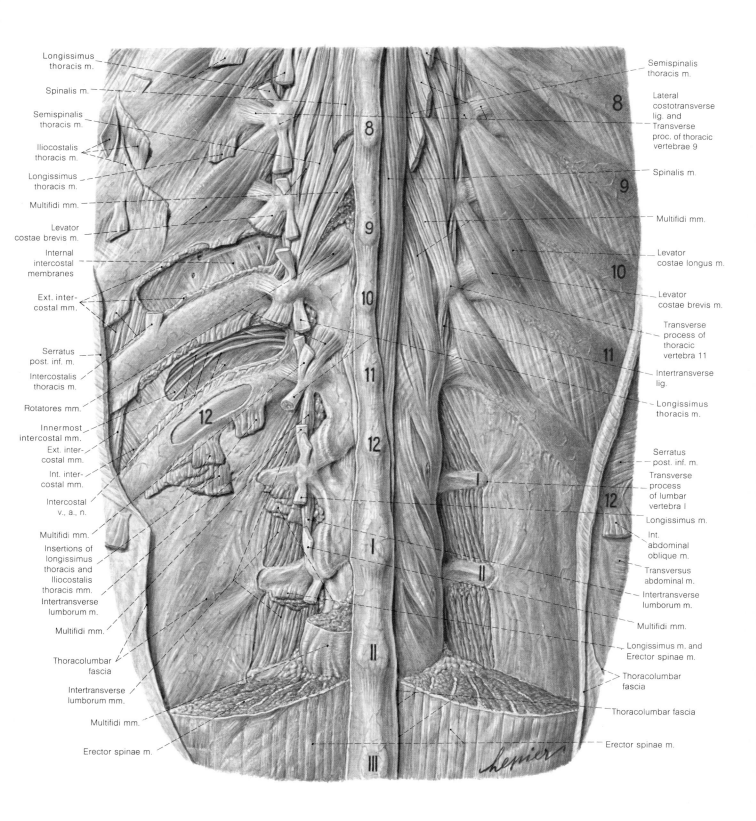

Longissimus thoracis m.

Spinalis m.

Semispinalis thoracis m.

Iliocostalis thoracis m.

Longissimus thoracis m.

Multifidi mm.

Levator costae brevis m.

Internal intercostal membranes

Ext. intercostal mm.

Serratus post. inf. m.

Intercostalis thoracis m.

Rotatores mm.

Innermost intercostal mm.

Ext. intercostal mm.

Int. intercostal mm.

Intercostal v., a., n.

Multifidi mm.

Insertions of longissimus thoracis and Iliocostalis thoracis mm.

Intertransverse lumborum m.

Multifidi mm.

Thoracolumbar fascia

Intertransverse lumborum mm.

Multifidi mm.

Erector spinae m.

Semispinalis thoracis m.

Lateral costotransverse lig. and Transverse proc. of thoracic vertebrae 9

Spinalis m.

Multifidi mm.

Levator costae longus m.

Levator costae brevis m.

Transverse process of thoracic vertebra 11

Intertransverse lig.

Longissimus thoracis m.

Serratus post. inf. m.

Transverse process of lumbar vertebra I

Longissimus m.

Int. abdominal oblique m.

Transversus abdominal m.

Intertransverse lumborum m.

Multifidi mm.

Longissimus m. and Erector spinae m.

Thoracolumbar fascia

Thoracolumbar fascia

Erector spinae m.

Fig. 339. Deep back muscles: Rotatores, Multifidi, and Levator costae. The spinous processes of the vertebral column were designated in the thoracic region with Arabic numerals 8–12; in the lumbar region with Roman numerals I–III. The first two transverse processes of the lumbar vertebrae are also labeled I and II. The ribs 8–12 on the right are shown with Arabic numerals.

237

Summary Table of the Structural Characteristics of "Typical" Vertebrae

	7 cervical vertebrae*	12 thoracic vertebrae	5 lumbar vertebrae	Sacrum (5 vertebrae)
End surfaces of vertebral bodies	rectangular, small	triangular	bean-shaped, large	fused
Vertebral foramen	large, triangular	round	small, triangular	sacral canal
Joint surfaces (joint processes)	oblique toward dorsal, like shingles	frontally positioned	sagitally positioned	crista sacralis intermedia
Transverse processes	transverse process	club-shaped with transverse costal facets	mammillary and accessory process	crista sacralis lateralis
Spinous processes	horizontal, short, bifurcated	steeply caudalward directed	horizontal, laterally flattened, massive	crista sacralis mediana
Rudiments of ribs	ventral part of transverse process and dorsal tubercle	small, because of developed ribs	costal processes	lateral parts
Characterizing feature	transverse foramen	superior and inferior costal facet	mammillary and accessory processes	synostosis of vertebrae

* The first two cervical vertebrae, atlas and axis (epistropheus), are not "typical" cervical vertebrae; they have peculiar structural characteristics.

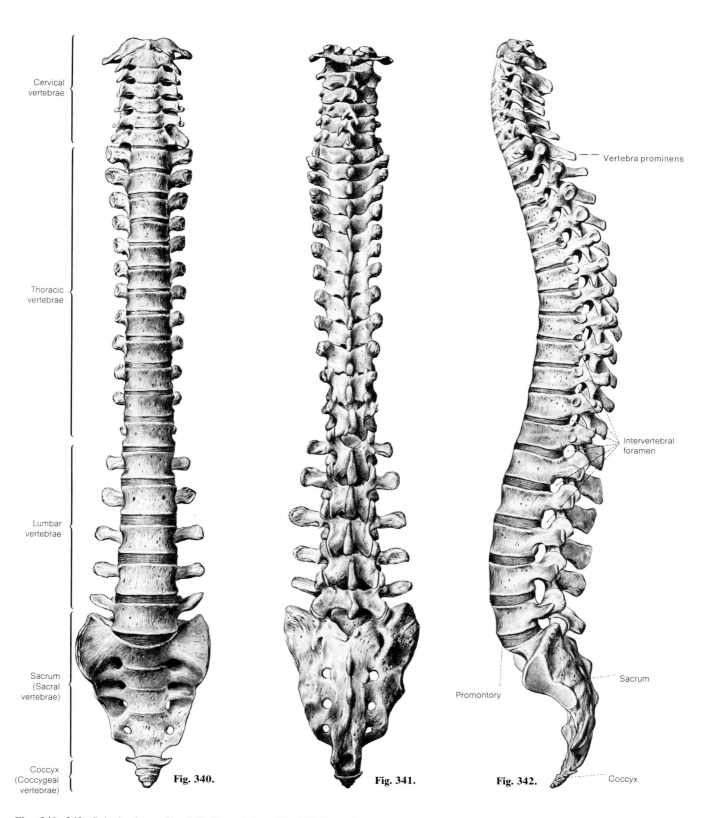

Cervical
vertebrae

Thoracic
vertebrae

Lumbar
vertebrae

Sacrum
(Sacral
vertebrae)

Coccyx
(Coccygeal
vertebrae)

Vertebra prominens

Intervertebral
foramen

Promontory

Sacrum

Coccyx

Fig. 340.

Fig. 341.

Fig. 342.

Figs. 340–342. Spinal column. Fig. 340. Ventral view. Fig. 341. Dorsal view. Fig. 342. Left lateral view. The transverse costal facet is missing on the 10th thoracic vertebra.

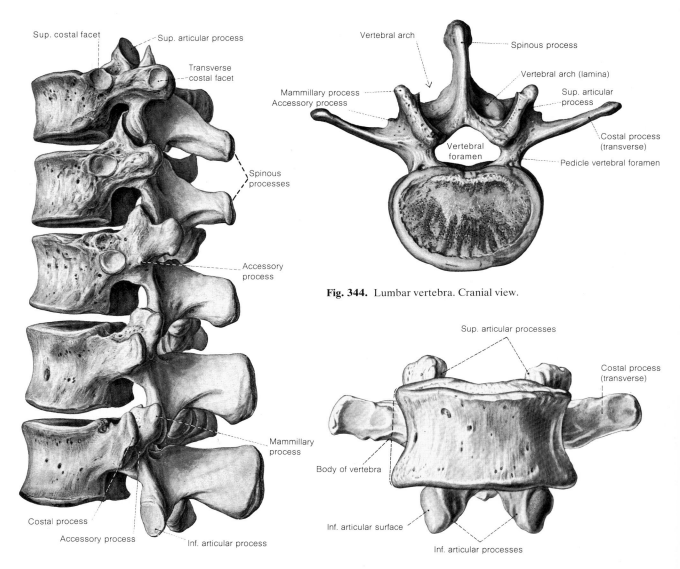

Fig. 343. The last three thoracic vertebrae, X–XII, and the first two lumbar vertebrae, I and II. Left lateral view.

Fig. 344. Lumbar vertebra. Cranial view.

Fig. 345. Lumbar vertebra. Ventral view.

NOTE: The increase in size of the body of the more caudal vertebrae. The two lower vertebrae of Fig. 343 are lumbar. They have no articular surfaces for ribs, but the rib rudiments, costal processes, are present. The transverse process is divided into an upper mammillary and a small lower process called the accessory. The articular surfaces of the articular processes are, on the thoracic vertebrae, directed ventrally and dorsally; on the lumbar vertebrae, sagittally (ante- and retroflexion are possible). The spinous processes of the lumbar vertebrae are massive and somewhat quadrilateral and extend more horizontal than those of the thoracic.

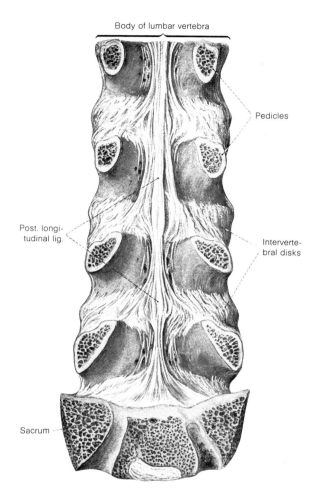

Body of lumbar vertebra

Pedicles

Post. longi-
tudinal lig.

Interverte-
bral disks

Sacrum

Fig. 346. Posterior longitudinal ligament and intervertebral disks. Vertebral canal opened by removing the vertebral arches from the dorsal side. Region of the lumbar portion of the spine and the sacrum.

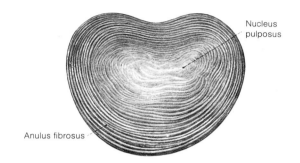

Nucleus
pulposus

Anulus fibrosus

Fig. 347. Articulating surface view of an isolated intervertebral disk. Lumbar vertebra.

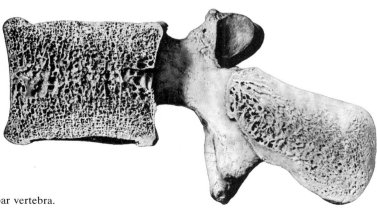

Fig. 348. Sagittal longitudinal section through a lumbar vertebra.

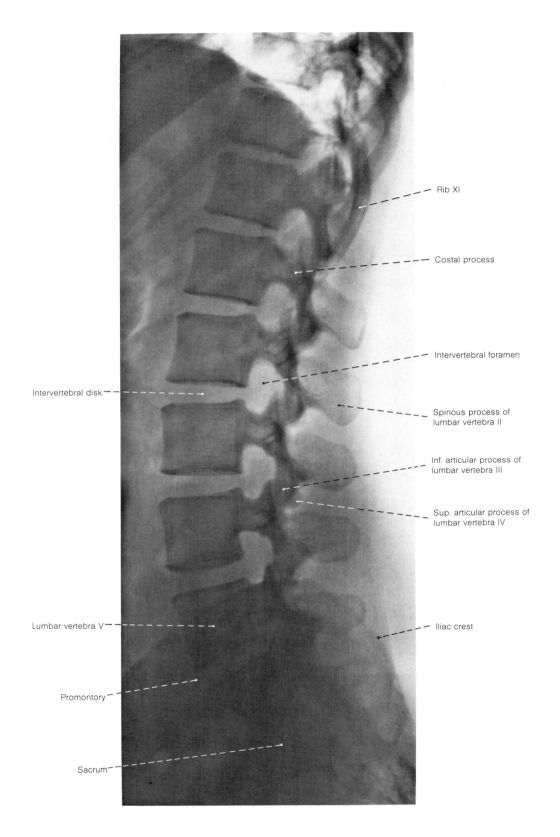

Rib XI

Costal process

Intervertebral foramen

Spinous process of
lumbar vertebra II

Inf. articular process of
lumbar vertebra III

Sup. articular process of
lumbar vertebra IV

Iliac crest

Intervertebral disk

Lumbar vertebra V

Promontory

Sacrum

Fig. 349. Left lateral X-ray film of the lumbar vertebral column. (From L. Wicke: Atlas der Röntgenanatomie, 2nd ed. Urban & Schwarzenberg, Munich–Vienna–Baltimore 1980.)

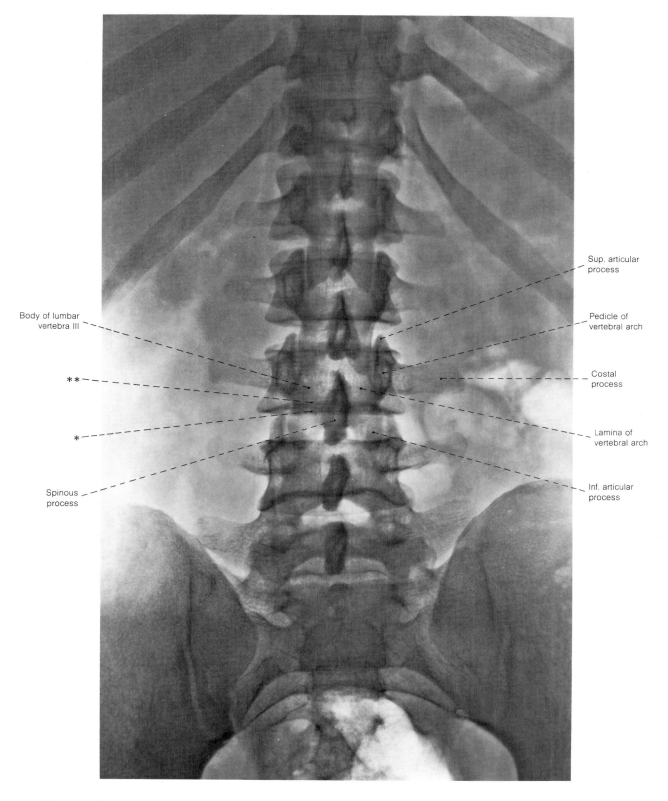

Sup. articular
process

Pedicle of
vertebral arch

Body of lumbar
vertebra III

Costal
process

**

Lamina of
vertebral arch

*

Spinous
process

Inf. articular
process

Fig. 350. X-ray film of lumbar spine (a.p. projection). (From L. Wicke: Atlas der Röntgenanatomie, 2nd ed. Urban & Schwarzenberg, Munich–Vienna–Baltimore.) * Posterior margin; ** Anterior margin.

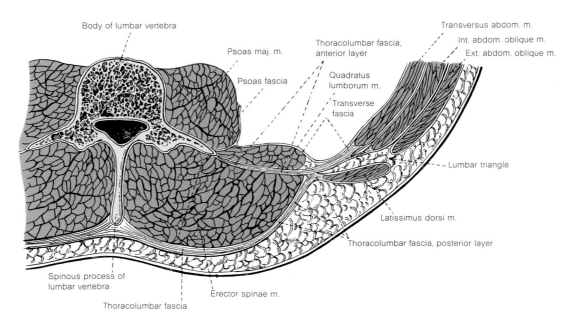

Body of lumbar vertebra

Psoas maj. m.

Thoracolumbar fascia,
anterior layer

Transversus abdom. m.

Int. abdom. oblique m.

Ext. abdom. oblique m.

Psoas fascia

Quadratus
lumborum m.

Transverse
fascia

Lumbar triangle

Latissimus dorsi m.

Thoracolumbar fascia, posterior layer

Spinous process of
lumbar vertebra

Erector spinae m.

Thoracolumbar fascia

Fig. 351. Cross section of the back and dorsal abdominal wall in the lumbar region. The thoracolumbar fascia and transversalis fascia shown diagrammatically.

NOTE:

Thoracolumbar fascia (lumbodorsal aponeurosis): A tendinous sheath from the Transversus abdominal, the Latissimus dorsi, and the Serratus posterior inferior muscles. It is fastened to the spinous processes with the posterior layer, to the transverse processes of the lumbar vertebrae with the anterior layers, and is between the 12th rib and crista iliaca (Fig. 351).

Lumbar triangle (trigonum lumbale) is a small triangular interval of the back bordered by the External oblique abdominal muscle and by the Latissimus dorsi m. and the iliac crest. Occasionally it is the site of a hernia (Fig. 331).

Transversalis fascia: The inner surface of the peritoneal musculature is separated from the peritoneum by the transverse fascia. Among other things, it strengthens the dorsal wall of the inguinal canal. The principal outpouching of the transverse fascia is the internal spermatic fascia (tunica vaginalis communis) which invests the inner part of the spermatic cord and testis.

Intercostal vessels, intercostal nerve (ventral branch): In the middle part of Fig. 338 the intercostal artery, vein, and nerve are displayed through a window in the intercostal muscles. They run lateral to the costal sulcus: the posterior intercostal vein is above; the posterior intercostal artery, in the middle; and the intercostal nerve, below.

Lower Extremity

Joints of the Lower Extremity

Joint	Type of Joint	Possibility of Movement
Hip joint	Ball and socket joint	Flexion, Extension Adduction, Abduction Inward rotation, outward rotation
Knee joint	Pivot-hinge joint	Flexion, extension, inward and outward rotation only possible in flexed position
Ankle joint talocrural articulation	Hinge joint	Plantar flexion Dorsiflexion
Subtalar joint	Gliding joint	Supination Pronation
Metatarsophalangeal joints	Candyloid joints	Sliding movements of toes against metatarsals
Toe joints interphalangeal joints	Hinge joints	Flexion, Extension

Pelvis and Hip Joint

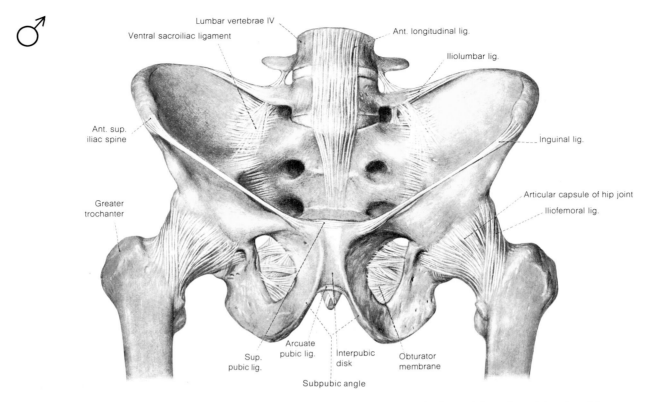

Fig. 352. Male pelvis with ligaments. Ventral view. Note also here the differences in the form of the male and female pelvis.

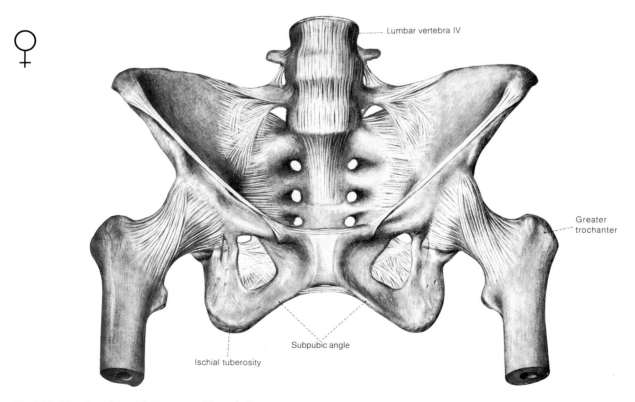

Fig. 353. Female pelvis with ligaments. Ventral view.

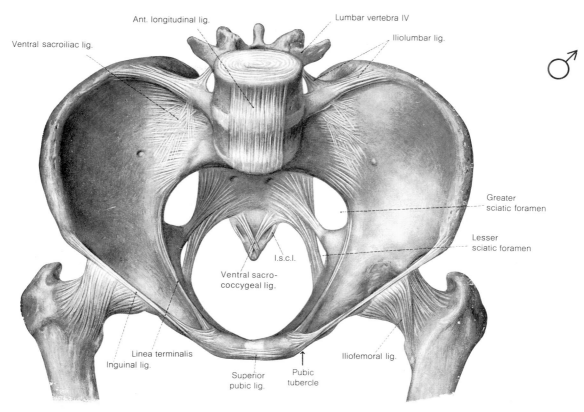

Fig. 354. Male pelvis with ligaments. The inclination of the pelvis corresponds to upright posture. Ventral superior view. Anterior superior iliac spine and upper border of the symphysis pubis are located in an approximate frontal plane. The aperture of the lesser pelvis is heart-shaped. l.s.c.l. = lateral sacrococcygeal ligament.

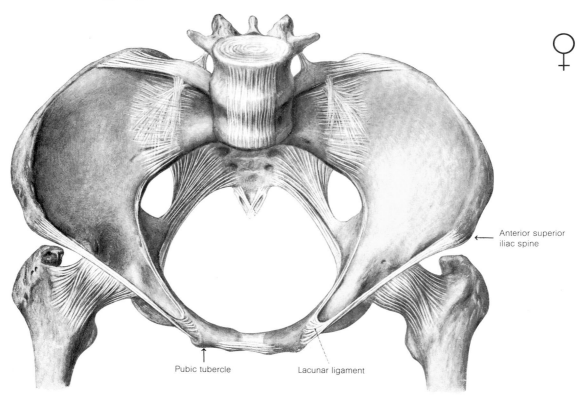

Fig. 355. Female pelvis with ligaments. Ventral superior view. The iliac alae are broader than in the male pelvis. Aperture of the lesser pelvis is transverseoval. Transverse diameter of aperture is longer than sagittal diameter.

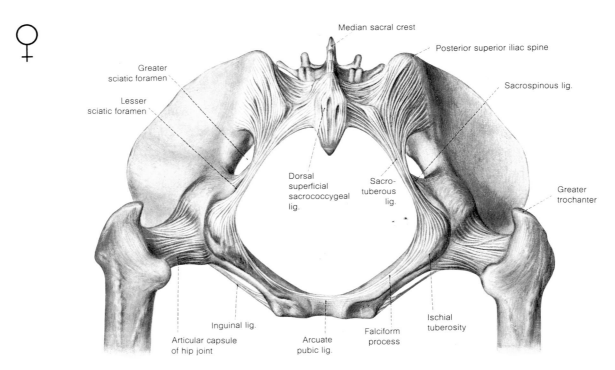

Fig. 356. Female pelvis with ligaments. Caudal view.

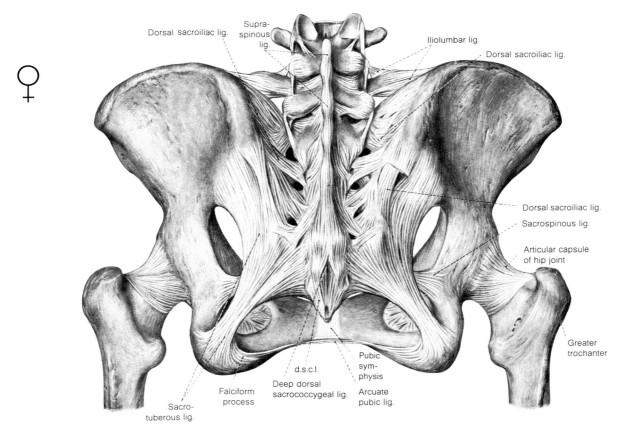

Fig. 357. Female pelvis with ligaments. Dorsal view. On the right, a portion of the superficial layer of the dorsal sacroiliac ligament has been removed. d.s.c.l. = dorsal superficial sacrococcygeal ligament.

248

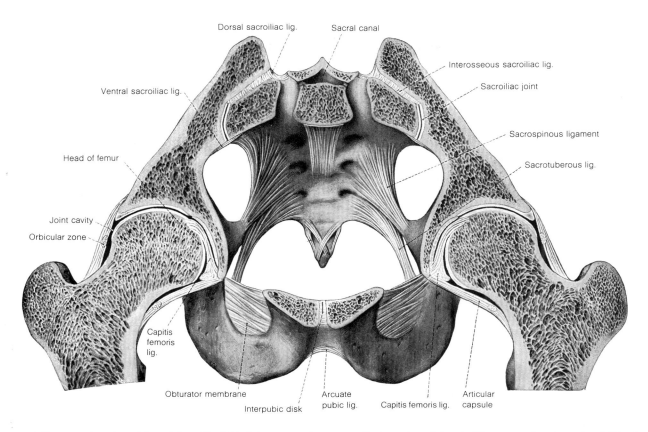

Dorsal sacroiliac lig.

Sacral canal

Interosseous sacroiliac lig.

Sacroiliac joint

Ventral sacroiliac lig.

Sacrospinous ligament

Sacrotuberous lig.

Head of femur

Joint cavity

Orbicular zone

Capitis femoris lig.

Obturator membrane

Interpubic disk

Arcuate pubic lig.

Capitis femoris lig.

Articular capsule

Fig. 358. Frontal section of the pelvis and both hip joints, somewhat perpendicular to the pelvic axis. The preparation shows, in addition to the hip joints, the symphysis pubis with its articular space, the sacroiliac articulations, the pelvic view of the sacrospinous and sacrotuberous ligaments.

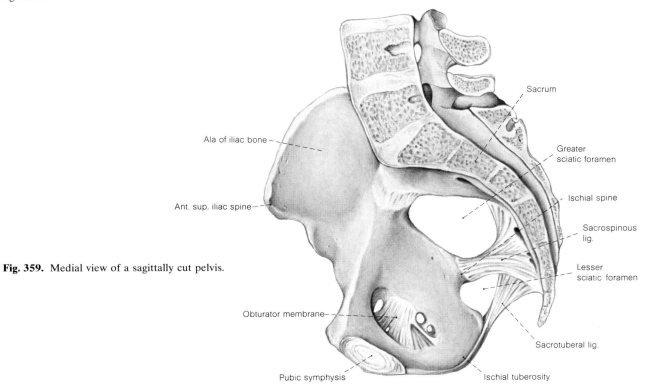

Sacrum

Ala of iliac bone

Greater sciatic foramen

Ischial spine

Ant. sup. iliac spine

Sacrospinous lig.

Lesser sciatic foramen

Fig. 359. Medial view of a sagittally cut pelvis.

Obturator membrane

Sacrotuberal lig.

Pubic symphysis

Ischial tuberosity

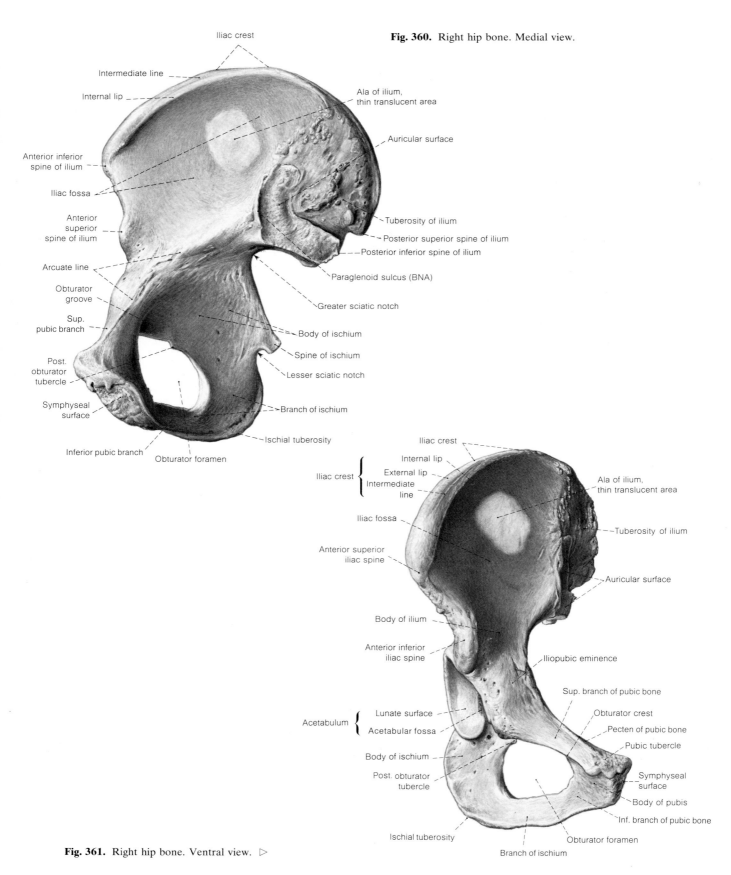

Iliac crest

Intermediate line

Internal lip

Fig. 360. Right hip bone. Medial view.

Ala of ilium,
thin translucent area

Auricular surface

Anterior inferior
spine of ilium

Iliac fossa

Anterior
superior
spine of ilium

Arcuate line

Obturator
groove

Sup.
pubic branch

Post.
obturator
tubercle

Symphyseal
surface

Inferior pubic branch   Obturator foramen

Tuberosity of ilium

Posterior superior spine of ilium

Posterior inferior spine of ilium

Paraglenoid sulcus (BNA)

Greater sciatic notch

Body of ischium

Spine of ischium

Lesser sciatic notch

Branch of ischium

Ischial tuberosity

Iliac crest

Internal lip

Iliac crest { External lip

Intermediate
line

Iliac fossa

Anterior superior
iliac spine

Body of ilium

Anterior inferior
iliac spine

Acetabulum { Lunate surface

Acetabular fossa

Body of ischium

Post. obturator
tubercle

Ischial tuberosity

Ala of ilium,
thin translucent area

Tuberosity of ilium

Auricular surface

Iliopubic eminence

Sup. branch of pubic bone

Obturator crest

Pecten of pubic bone

Pubic tubercle

Symphyseal
surface

Body of pubis

Inf. branch of pubic bone

Obturator foramen

Branch of ischium

Fig. 361. Right hip bone. Ventral view. ▷

250

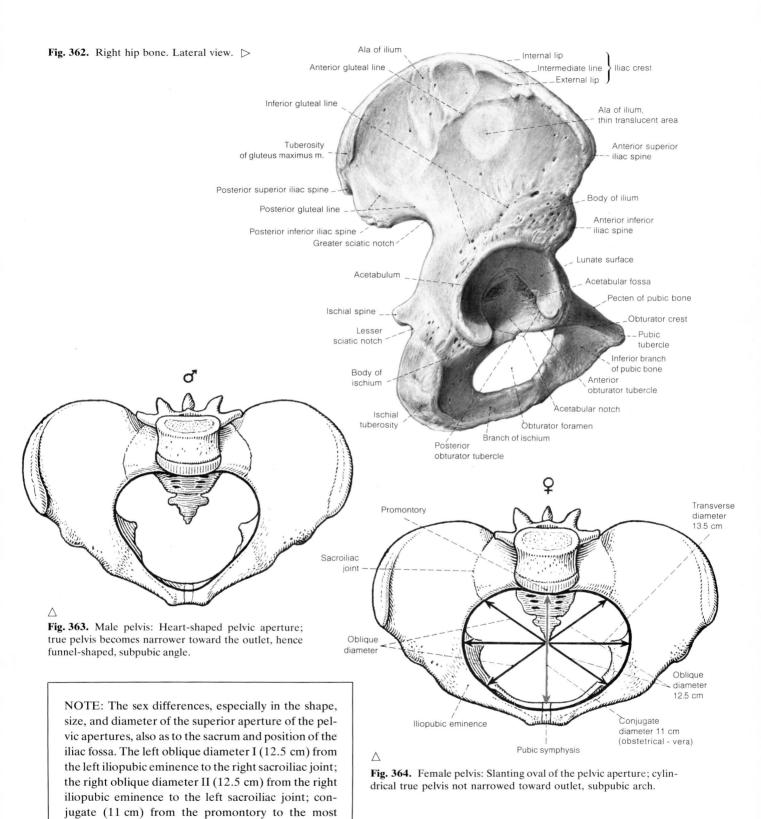

Fig. 362. Right hip bone. Lateral view. ▷

Ala of ilium

Anterior gluteal line

Inferior gluteal line

Tuberosity of gluteus maximus m.

Posterior superior iliac spine

Posterior gluteal line

Posterior inferior iliac spine

Greater sciatic notch

Acetabulum

Ischial spine

Lesser sciatic notch

Body of ischium

Ischial tuberosity

Posterior obturator tubercle

Branch of ischium

Obturator foramen

Acetabular notch

Anterior obturator tubercle

Inferior branch of pubic bone

Pubic tubercle

Obturator crest

Pecten of pubic bone

Acetabular fossa

Lunate surface

Anterior inferior iliac spine

Body of ilium

Anterior superior iliac spine

Ala of ilium, thin translucent area

Internal lip

Intermediate line

External lip

Iliac crest

♂

△ **Fig. 363.** Male pelvis: Heart-shaped pelvic aperture; true pelvis becomes narrower toward the outlet, hence funnel-shaped, subpubic angle.

NOTE: The sex differences, especially in the shape, size, and diameter of the superior aperture of the pelvic apertures, also as to the sacrum and position of the iliac fossa. The left oblique diameter I (12.5 cm) from the left iliopubic eminence to the right sacroiliac joint; the right oblique diameter II (12.5 cm) from the right iliopubic eminence to the left sacroiliac joint; conjugate (11 cm) from the promontory to the most prominent part of the posterior aspect of the symphysis of the pubic bone (red arrow).

♀

Promontory

Sacroiliac joint

Oblique diameter

Iliopubic eminence

Pubic symphysis

Transverse diameter 13.5 cm

Oblique diameter 12.5 cm

Conjugate diameter 11 cm (obstetrical - vera)

△ **Fig. 364.** Female pelvis: Slanting oval of the pelvic aperture; cylindrical true pelvis not narrowed toward outlet, subpubic arch.

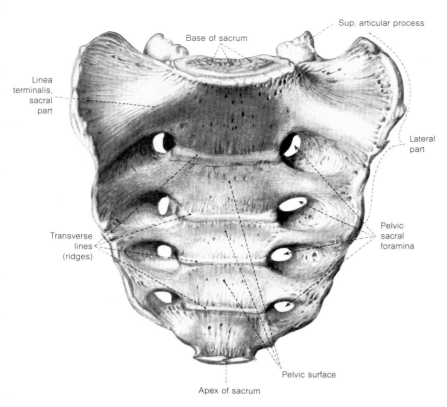

Base of sacrum

Sup. articular process

Linea terminalis, sacral part

Lateral part

Transverse lines (ridges)

Pelvic sacral foramina

Pelvic surface

Apex of sacrum

Fig. 365. The sacrum. Ventral view, pelvic surface. △

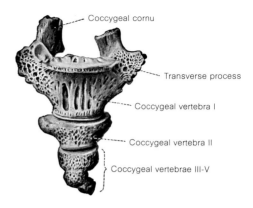

Coccygeal cornu

Transverse process

Coccygeal vertebra I

Coccygeal vertebra II

Coccygeal vertebrae III-V

Fig. 366. Coccyx. Ventral view.

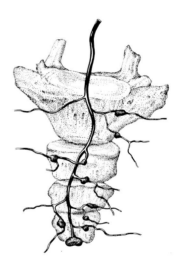

Fig. 368. Topographical relationships of the glomus coccygeum and its nodules to the medial sacral artery and its branches on the ventral side of the coccyx. (From J. Staubesand, Acta Anat. *19*, 105–131 [1953].)

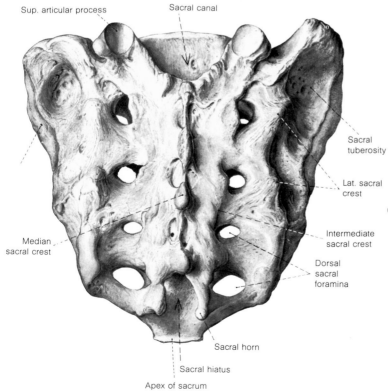

Sup. articular process

Sacral canal

Sacral tuberosity

Lat. sacral crest

Median sacral crest

Intermediate sacral crest

Dorsal sacral foramina

Sacral horn

Sacral hiatus

Apex of sacrum

Fig. 367. The sacrum. Dorsal view.

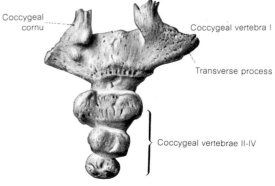

Coccygeal cornu

Coccygeal vertebra I

Transverse process

Coccygeal vertebrae II-IV

Fig. 369. Coccyx. Dorsal view.

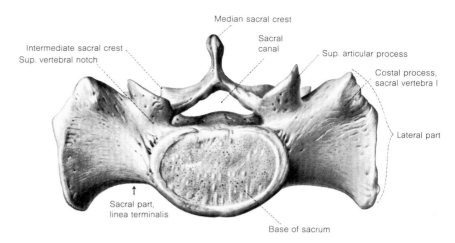

Median sacral crest

Sacral canal

Intermediate sacral crest

Sup. vertebral notch

Sup. articular process

Costal process, sacral vertebra I

Lateral part

Sacral part, linea terminalis

Base of sacrum

Fig. 370. The sacrum. Cranial view of the base.

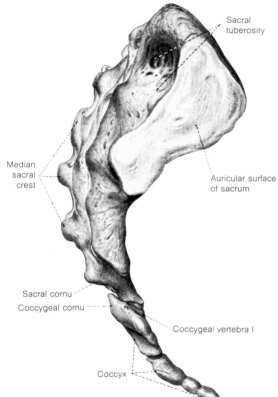

Sacral tuberosity

Auricular surface of sacrum

Median sacral crest

Sacral cornu

Coccygeal cornu

Coccygeal vertebra I

Coccyx

Fig. 371. The sacrum and coccyx. Right lateral view.

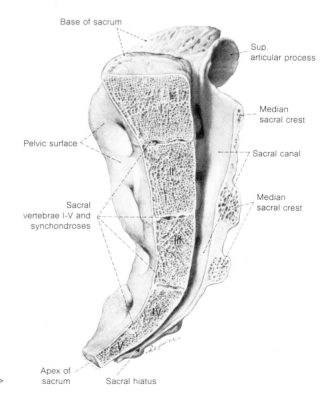

Base of sacrum

Sup. articular process

Median sacral crest

Sacral canal

Median sacral crest

Pelvic surface

Sacral vertebrae I-V and synchondroses

Apex of sacrum

Sacral hiatus

Fig. 372. The sacrum, sectioned in the median sagittal plane. ▷

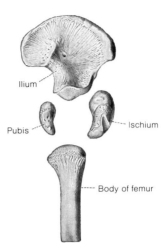

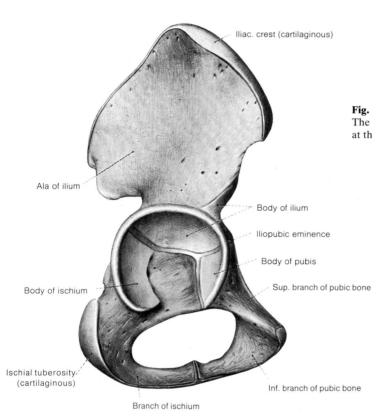

Fig. 373 b. Right hip bone and proximal part of the femur at birth. The 3 parts of the hip bone (ischium, ilium, and pubis) are not united at this stage, and the head and neck of the femur are cartilaginous.

Fig. 373 a. Hip bone of a child about 5 to 6 years old. Seen from lateral. Ilium, yellow; ischium, green; pubis, blue. The three parts first form a starlike synchondrosis. The separating cartilaginous lines are present only in the young. Later synostosis takes place when they fuse to form the hip bone in the area of the acetabulum.

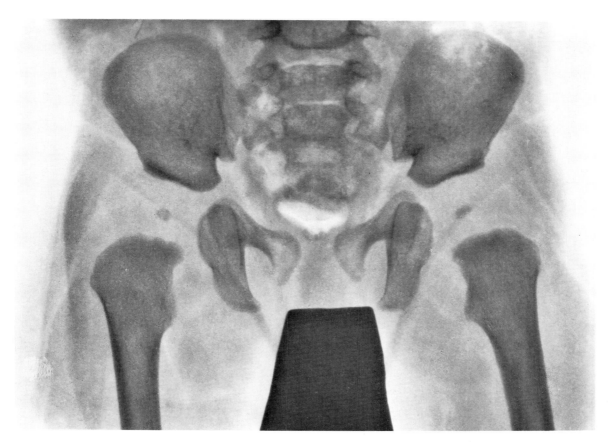

Fig.
374 a.

Figs. 374 a and b. X-ray film of an infant's pelvis with hip joints (compare with Fig. 373). From L. WICKE: Atlas der Röntgenanatomie, 2nd ed. Urban & Schwarzenberg, Munich–Vienna–Baltimore 1980.) * = Ossification centers in corresponding bones.

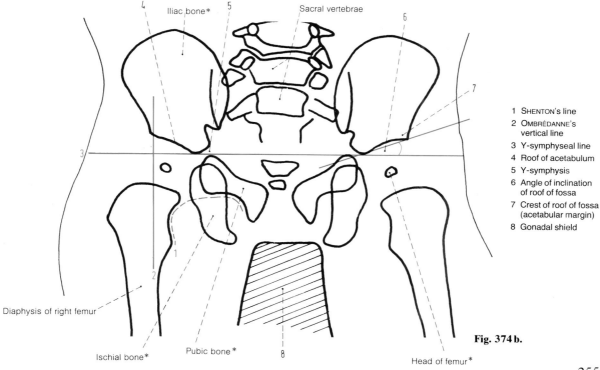

Iliac bone*

Sacral vertebrae

1 SHENTON's line
2 OMBRÉDANNE's vertical line
3 Y-symphyseal line
4 Roof of acetabulum
5 Y-symphysis
6 Angle of inclination of roof of fossa
7 Crest of roof of fossa (acetabular margin)
8 Gonadal shield

Diaphysis of right femur

Ischial bone*

Pubic bone*

Head of femur*

Fig. 374 b.

255

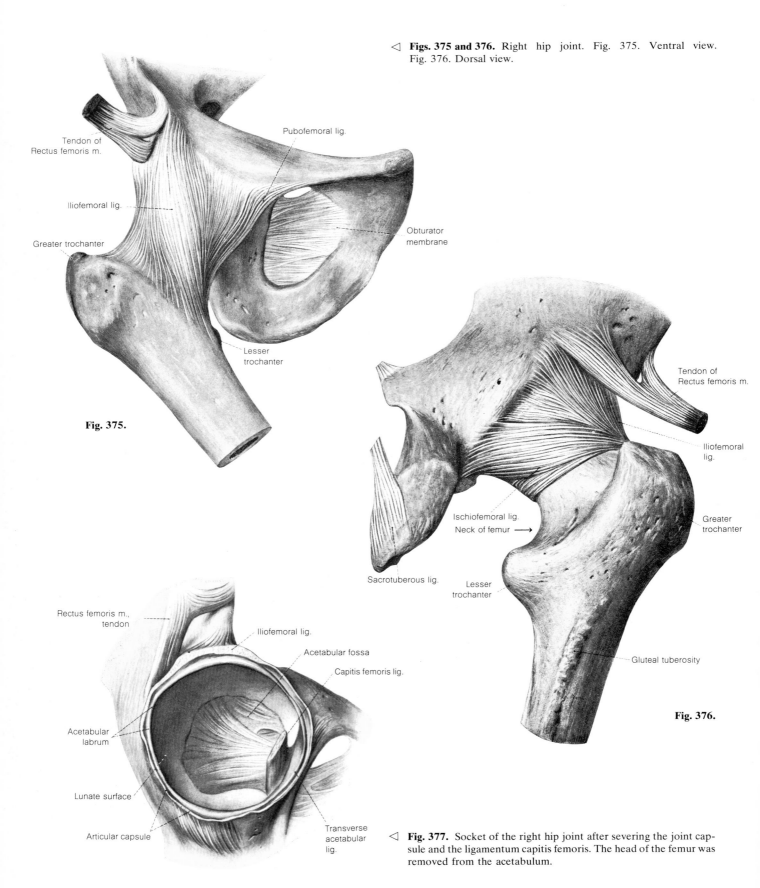

◁ **Figs. 375 and 376.** Right hip joint. Fig. 375. Ventral view. Fig. 376. Dorsal view.

Tendon of Rectus femoris m.

Pubofemoral lig.

Iliofemoral lig.

Greater trochanter

Obturator membrane

Lesser trochanter

Fig. 375.

Tendon of Rectus femoris m.

Iliofemoral lig.

Ischiofemoral lig.

Neck of femur →

Greater trochanter

Sacrotuberous lig.

Lesser trochanter

Gluteal tuberosity

Fig. 376.

Rectus femoris m., tendon

Iliofemoral lig.

Acetabular fossa

Capitis femoris lig.

Acetabular labrum

Lunate surface

Articular capsule

Transverse acetabular lig.

◁ **Fig. 377.** Socket of the right hip joint after severing the joint capsule and the ligamentum capitis femoris. The head of the femur was removed from the acetabulum.

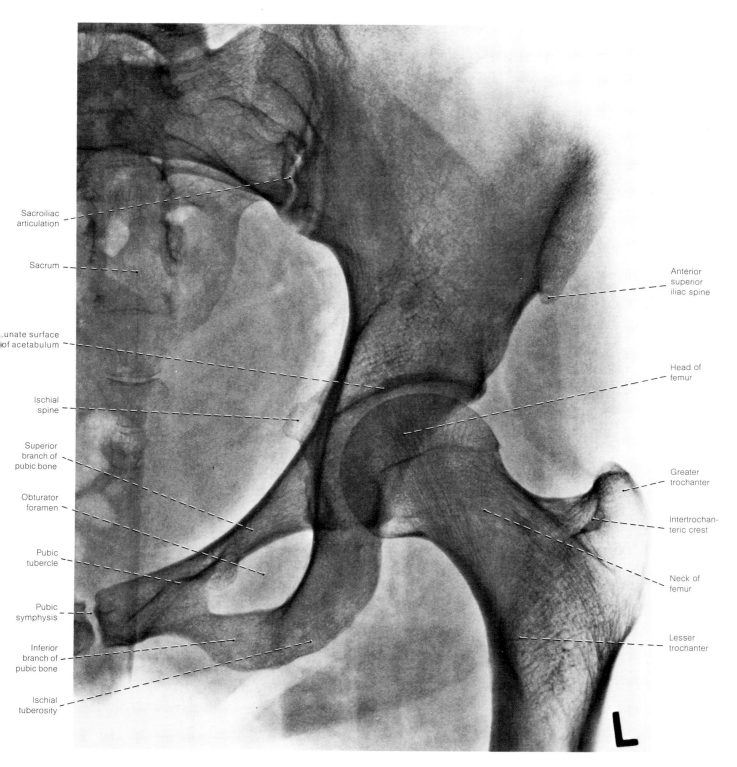

Sacroiliac
articulation

Sacrum

Lunate surface
of acetabulum

Ischial
spine

Superior
branch of
pubic bone

Obturator
foramen

Pubic
tubercle

Pubic
symphysis

Inferior
branch of
pubic bone

Ischial
tuberosity

Anterior
superior
iliac spine

Head of
femur

Greater
trochanter

Intertrochan-
teric crest

Neck of
femur

Lesser
trochanter

Fig. 378. X-ray film of the left hip joint (a.p. projection). (From L. WICKE: Atlas der Röntgenanatomie, 2nd ed. Urban & Schwarzenberg, Munich–Vienna–Baltimore 1980.)

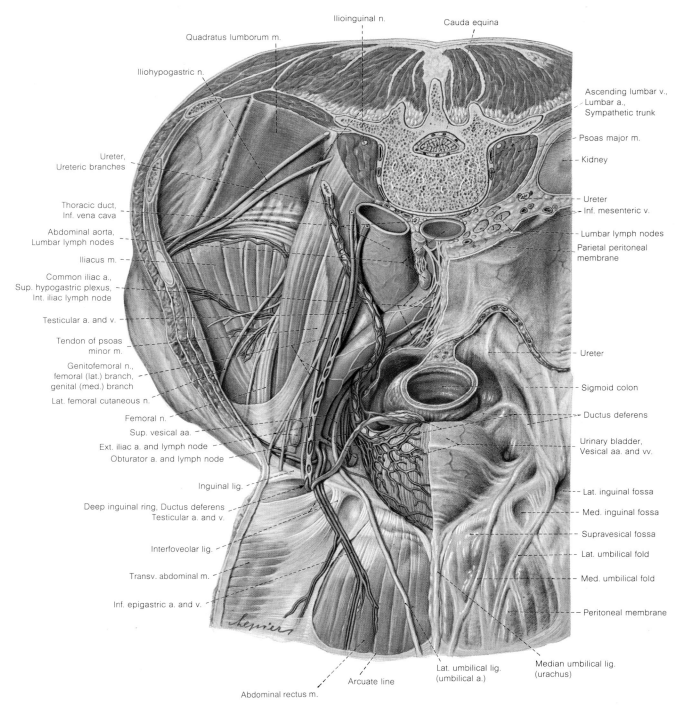

Ilioinguinal n.

Cauda equina

Quadratus lumborum m.

Iliohypogastric n.

Ascending lumbar v.,
Lumbar a.,
Sympathetic trunk

Psoas major m.

Kidney

Ureter,
Ureteric branches

Ureter
Inf. mesenteric v.

Thoracic duct,
Inf. vena cava

Lumbar lymph nodes

Abdominal aorta,
Lumbar lymph nodes

Parietal peritoneal
membrane

Iliacus m.

Common iliac a.,
Sup. hypogastric plexus,
Int. iliac lymph node

Testicular a. and v.

Ureter

Tendon of psoas
minor m.

Genitofemoral n.,
femoral (lat.) branch,
genital (med.) branch

Sigmoid colon

Lat. femoral cutaneous n.

Ductus deferens

Femoral n.

Urinary bladder,
Vesical aa. and vv.

Sup. vesical aa.

Ext. iliac a. and lymph node

Obturator a. and lymph node

Lat. inguinal fossa

Med. inguinal fossa

Inguinal lig.

Supravesical fossa

Deep inguinal ring, Ductus deferens
Testicular a. and v.

Lat. umbilical fold

Interfoveolar lig.

Med. umbilical fold

Transv. abdominal m.

Peritoneal membrane

Inf. epigastric a. and v.

Median umbilical lig.
(urachus)

Lat. umbilical lig.
(umbilical a.)

Abdominal rectus m.

Arcuate line

Fig. 379. Nerves and vessels of posterior abdominal wall, pelvis and anterior abdominal wall. The anterior abdominal wall has been deflected downward, the peritoneal membrane has been removed on the right side.

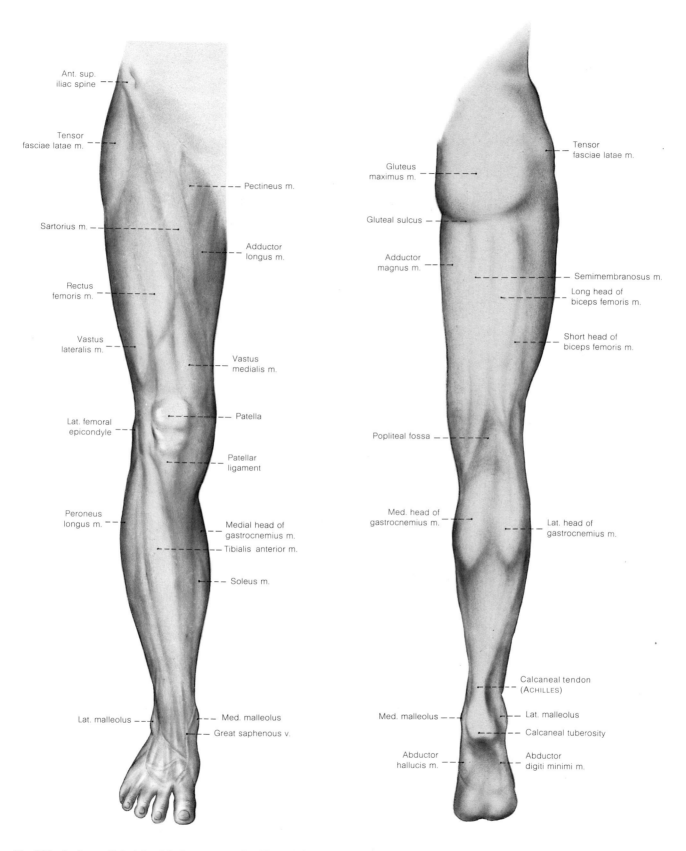

Ant. sup.
iliac spine

Tensor
fasciae latae m.

Pectineus m.

Sartorius m.

Adductor
longus m.

Rectus
femoris m.

Vastus
lateralis m.

Vastus
medialis m.

Lat. femoral
epicondyle

Patella

Patellar
ligament

Peroneus
longus m.

Medial head of
gastrocnemius m.

Tibialis anterior m.

Soleus m.

Lat. malleolus

Med. malleolus

Great saphenous v.

Gluteus
maximus m.

Tensor
fasciae latae m.

Gluteal sulcus

Adductor
magnus m.

Semimembranosus m.

Long head of
biceps femoris m.

Short head of
biceps femoris m.

Popliteal fossa

Med. head of
gastrocnemius m.

Lat. head of
gastrocnemius m.

Calcaneal tendon
(ACHILLES)

Med. malleolus

Lat. malleolus

Calcaneal tuberosity

Abductor
hallucis m.

Abductor
digiti minimi m.

Fig. 380. Surface relief of the right lower extremity. Ventral view.   **Fig. 381.** Surface relief of the right lower extremity. Dorsal view.

Nerves

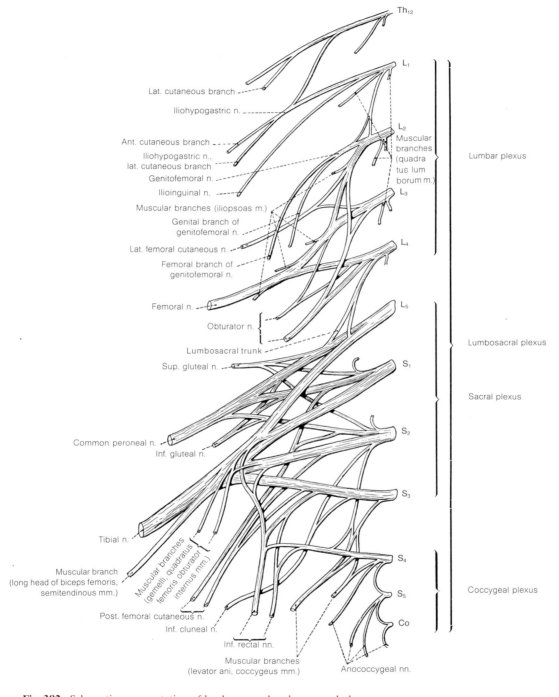

Fig. 382. Schematic representation of lumbar, sacral and coccygeal plexus.

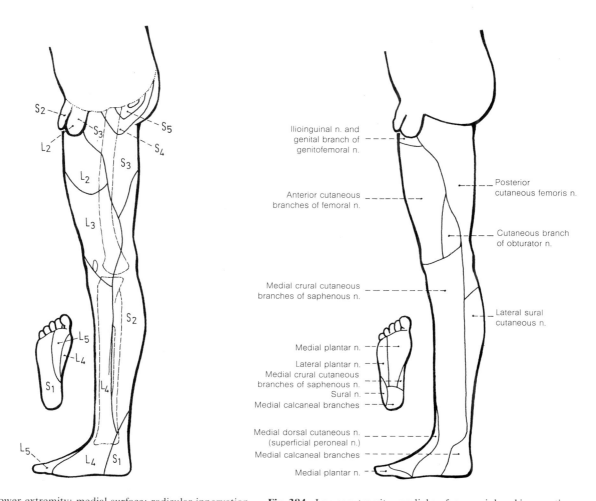

Fig. 383. Lower extremity; medial surface; radicular innervation.

Fig. 384. Lower extremity; medial surface: peripheral innervation.

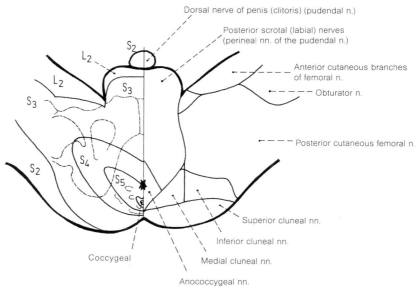

Fig. 385. Perineum. Right side of body: radicular innervation. Left side of body: peripheral innervation.

Nerve	Affected muscles	Loss of sensibility
Lumbar plexus L 1–L 4	Especially flexors of the hip joint (rotators of the hip joint), Adductors of the thigh, Extensors of the knee joint	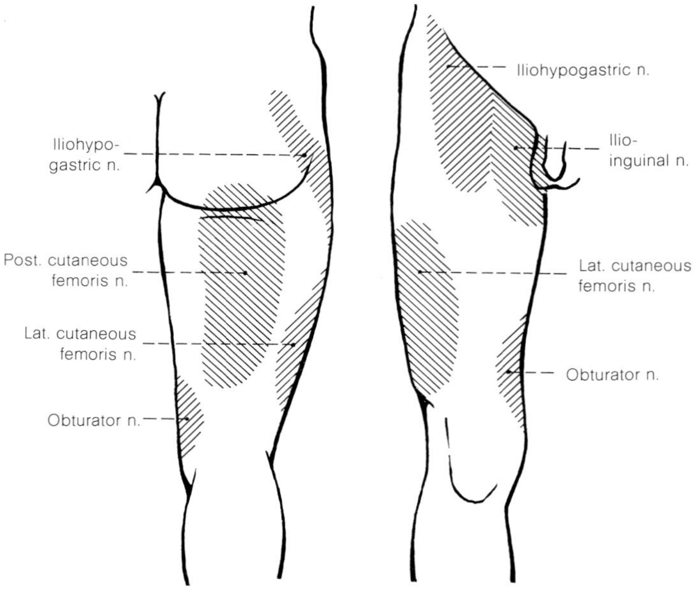
Sacral plexus L 5–S 3	Especially gluteal muscles, Ischiocrural group, Dorsal extensors and plantar flexors of foot and toes	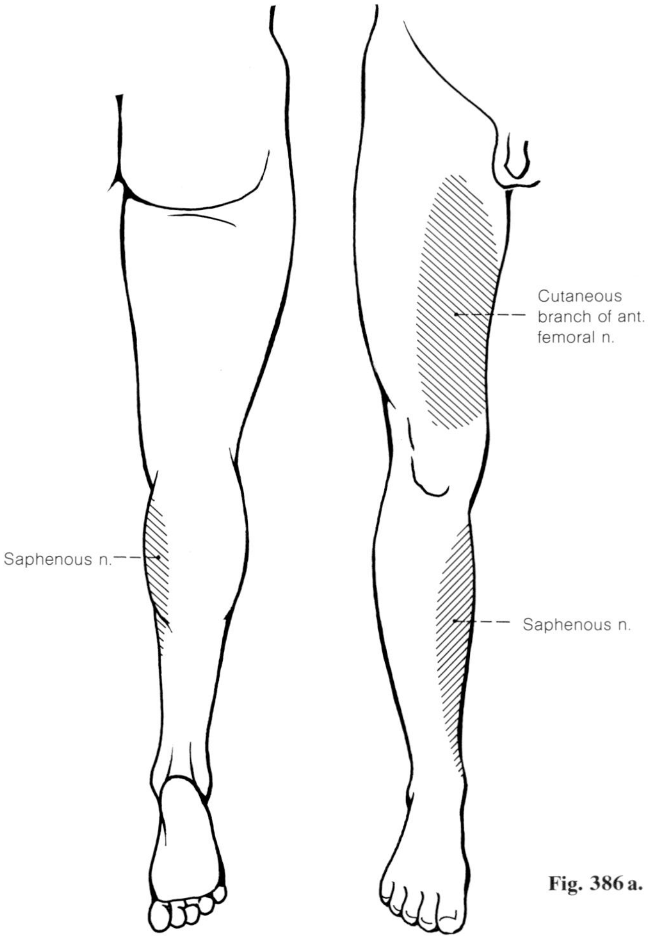
Femoral nerve L 2–L 4	Iliacus m.; pectineus m. Sartorius m; Quadriceps femoris m.	
Lateral cutaneous femoris nerve L 2–L 3	∅	
Ilioinguinal nerve L 1(–L 2)	∅	
Superior gluteal nerve L 4–S 1	Gluteus medius m. Gluteus minimus m. Tensor fasciae latae m.	

Figs. 386 a and b. Synopsis of plexus paralyses and the paralyses of single peripheral nerves in the lower extremities.

Fig. 386 a.

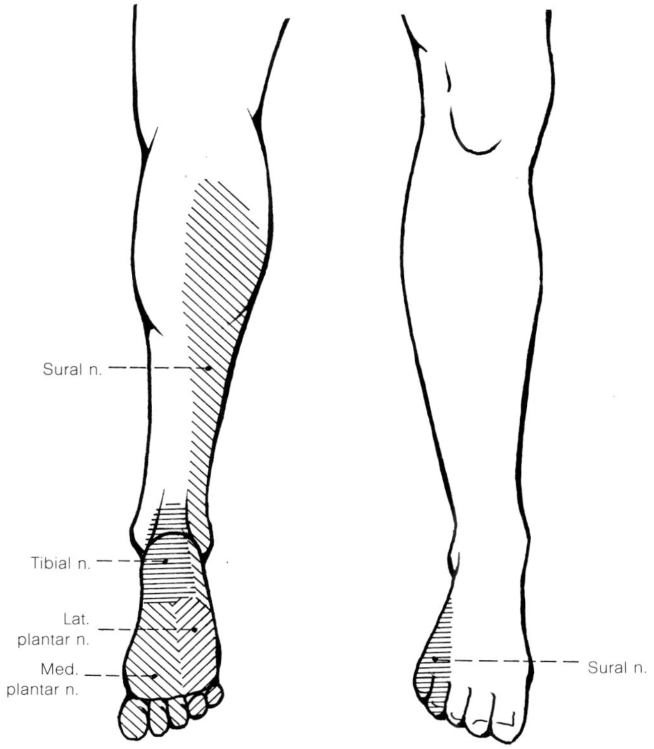

Nerve	Affected muscles	Loss of sensibility
Inf. gluteal nerve L 5–S 2	Gluteus maximus m.	
Tibial nerve L 4–S 3	Gastrocnemius m.	
	Plantaris m.	
	Soleus m.	
	Popliteus m.	
	Tibialis posterior m.	
	Flexor digitorum longus m.	
	Flexor hallucis longus m.	
	Flexor digitorum brevis m.	
	Flexor hallucis brevis m.	
	Abductor hallucis m.	
	Abductor hallucis minimi m.	
	Adductor hallucis m.	
	Quadratus plantae m.	
	Lumbricales mm.	
	Interossei mm.	
Common peroneal nerve L 4–S 2	Tibialis anterior m.	
	Extensor digitorum longus m.	
Deep peroneal nerve	Extensor hallucis longus m.	
	Peroneus tertius m.	
	Extensor digitorum brevis m.	
	Extensor hallucis brevis m.	
Superficial peroneal nerve	Peroneus longus m.	
	Peroneus brevis m.	

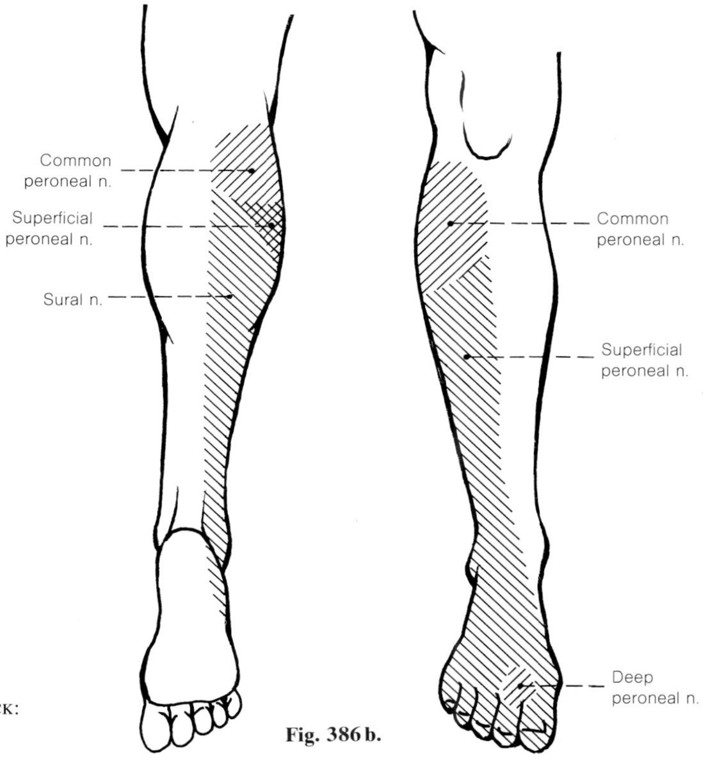

Figs. 383–386 a, b. (From M. MUMMENTHALER und H. SCHLIACK: Läsionen peripherer Nerven, 3rd ed. Thieme, Stuttgart 1977.)

Fig. 386 b.

263

Arteries

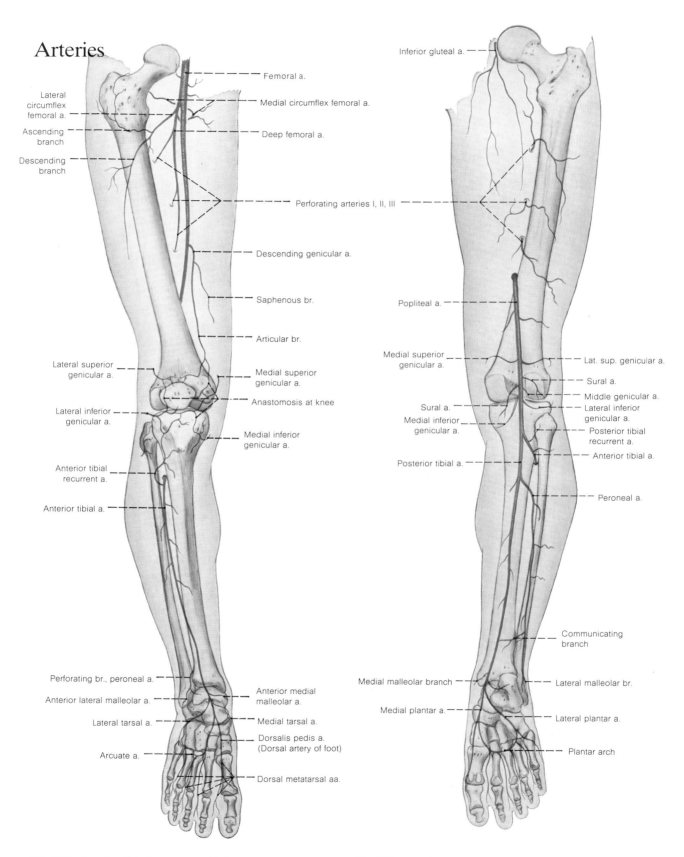

Femoral a.

Medial circumflex femoral a.

Lateral circumflex femoral a.

Deep femoral a.

Ascending branch

Descending branch

Perforating arteries I, II, III

Descending genicular a.

Saphenous br.

Articular br.

Lateral superior genicular a.

Medial superior genicular a.

Anastomosis at knee

Lateral inferior genicular a.

Medial inferior genicular a.

Anterior tibial recurrent a.

Anterior tibial a.

Perforating br., peroneal a.

Anterior lateral malleolar a.

Anterior medial malleolar a.

Lateral tarsal a.

Medial tarsal a.

Dorsalis pedis a. (Dorsal artery of foot)

Arcuate a.

Dorsal metatarsal aa.

Inferior gluteal a.

Popliteal a.

Medial superior genicular a.

Lat. sup. genicular a.

Sural a.

Middle genicular a.

Sural a.

Lateral inferior genicular a.

Medial inferior genicular a.

Posterior tibial recurrent a.

Anterior tibial a.

Posterior tibial a.

Peroneal a.

Communicating branch

Medial malleolar branch

Lateral malleolar br.

Medial plantar a.

Lateral plantar a.

Plantar arch

Fig. 387. Arteries of the lower extremity. Ventral view. (Schematic)   **Fig. 388.** Arteries of the lower extremity. Dorsal view. (Schematic)

264

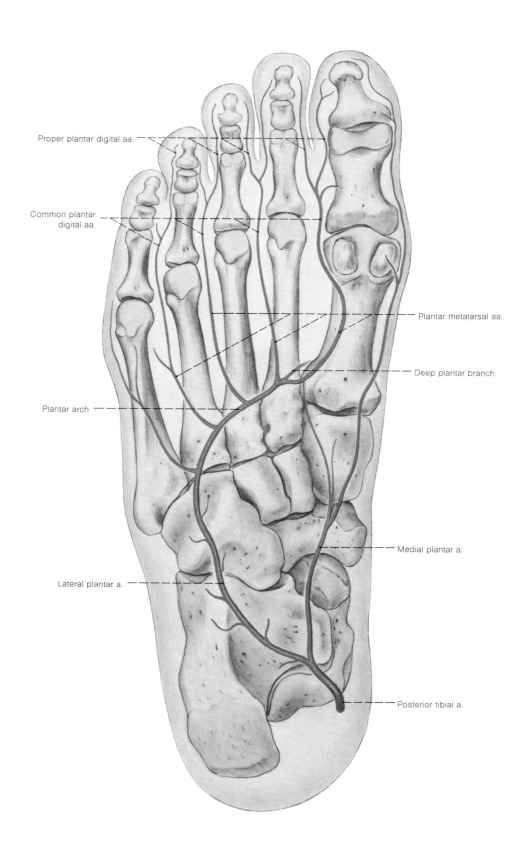

Proper plantar digital aa.

Common plantar digital aa.

Plantar metatarsal aa.

Deep plantar branch

Plantar arch

Medial plantar a.

Lateral plantar a.

Posterior tibial a.

Fig. 389. Arteries of the foot. Plantar view. (Schematic)

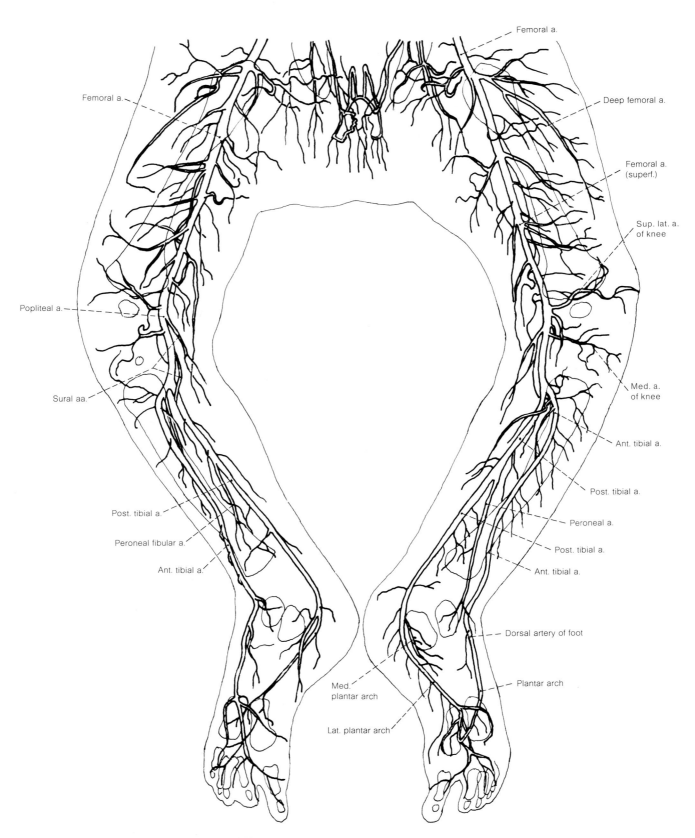

Femoral a.

Deep femoral a.

Femoral a.

Femoral a.
(superf.)

Sup. lat. a.
of knee

Popliteal a.

Med. a.
of knee

Sural aa.

Ant. tibial a.

Post. tibial a.

Peroneal a.

Post. tibial a.

Post. tibial a.

Peroneal fibular a.

Post. tibial a.

Ant. tibial a.

Ant. tibial a.

Dorsal artery of foot

Plantar arch

Med.
plantar arch

Lat. plantar arch

Fig. 390 a. Explanatory diagram for Fig. 390 b.

266

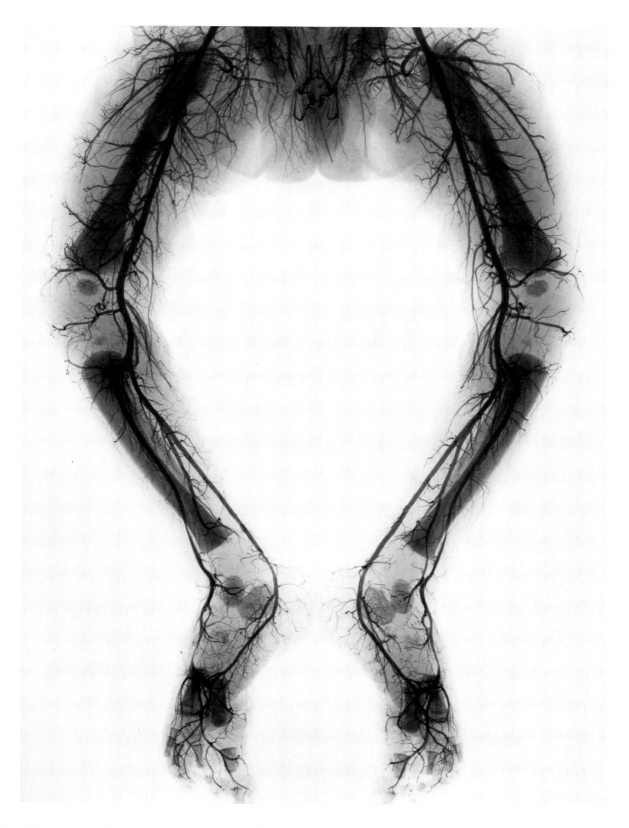

Fig. 390 b. Angiographic demonstration of the arteries of both legs (still birth). Original; Preparation injected with barium sulfate, see also Fig. 390 a. (Prof. Dr. G. W. KAUFFMANN, Zentrum Radiologie am Klinikum der Universität Freiburg i. Brsg.)

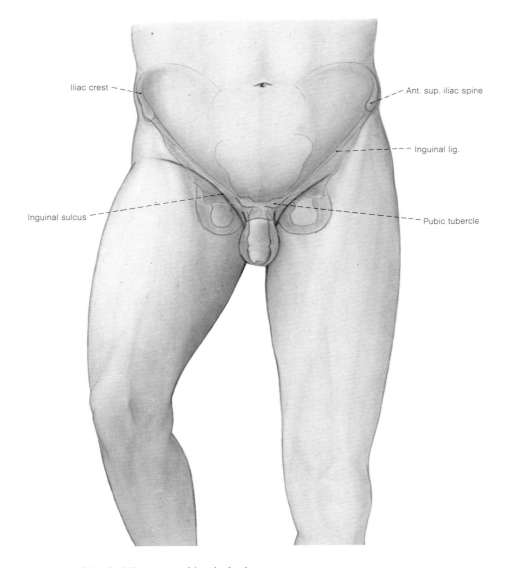

Fig. 391. Different position of inguinal ligament and inguinal sulcus.

The Lacunae of the inguinal region (compare with Fig. 392)

While the inguinal ligament extends from the superior anterior iliac spine to the pubic symphysis there are two lacunae between ligament and bone. They are separated from each other by the ileopectineal arch.

1. Lacuna musculorum, lateral, for the passage of the iliopsoas muscle and the femoral nerve to the thigh.
2. Lacuna vasorum, medial, for the passage of the femoral vessels, the femoral branch of the genitofemoral nerve, and the lymphatic vessels into the femoral trigone and from this into the pelvis.

Boundaries: above inguinal ligament, below pectineal ligament, medial lacunar ligament, lateral pectineal arch.

Topographical arrangement: medial lymphatic vessels, then the femoral vein, lateral the femoral artery.

Femoral hernia: The "internal hernial gap" is the weak site between the femoral vein and the lacunar ligament in which are located lymphatic vessels and connective tissue (femoral septum [CLOQUET]).

The "outer hernial gap" is the saphenous hiatus in the fascia lata for the entry of the great saphenous vein and the superficial lymphatic vessels. The latter cause gaps in the cribriform fascia of the hiatus.

Thigh

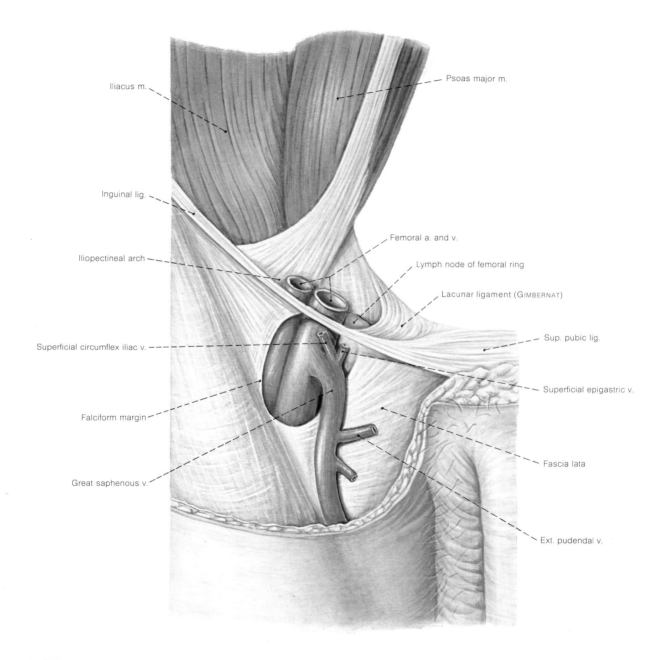

Iliacus m.

Psoas major m.

Inguinal lig.

Iliopectineal arch

Femoral a. and v.

Lymph node of femoral ring

Lacunar ligament (GIMBERNAT)

Sup. pubic lig.

Superficial circumflex iliac v.

Superficial epigastric v.

Falciform margin

Fascia lata

Great saphenous v.

Ext. pudendal v.

Fig. 392. Saphenous hiatus and femoral canal. Abdominal wall, abdominal viscera and iliac fascia have been removed to the inguinal ligament. Below the inguinal ligament, skin and lymph nodes anterior to the saphenous hiatus have been cut away.

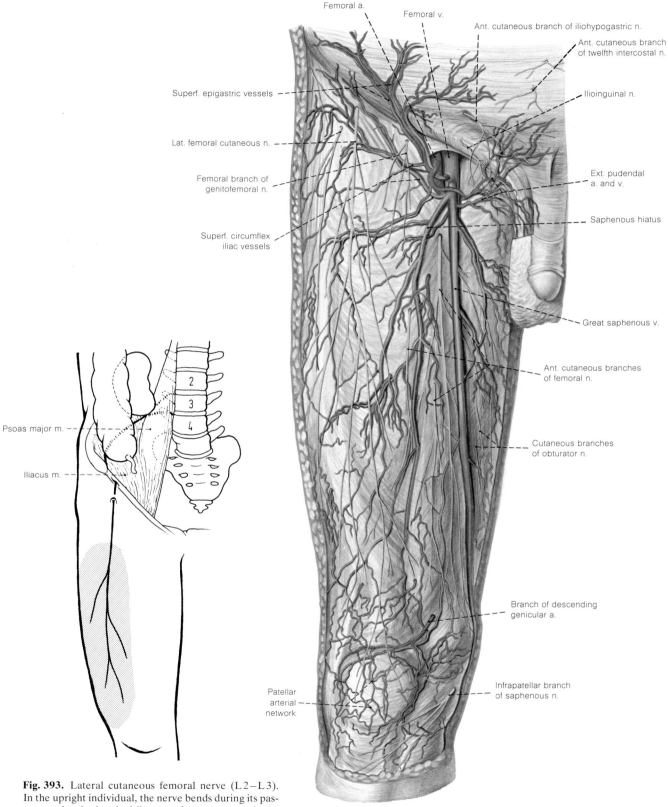

Femoral a.

Femoral v.

Ant. cutaneous branch of iliohypogastric n.

Ant. cutaneous branch of twelfth intercostal n.

Superf. epigastric vessels

Ilioinguinal n.

Lat. femoral cutaneous n.

Femoral branch of genitofemoral n.

Ext. pudendal a. and v.

Saphenous hiatus

Superf. circumflex iliac vessels

Great saphenous v.

Ant. cutaneous branches of femoral n.

Cutaneous branches of obturator n.

Psoas major m.

Iliacus m.

Branch of descending genicular a.

Patellar arterial network

Infrapatellar branch of saphenous n.

Fig. 393. Lateral cutaneous femoral nerve (L2–L3). In the upright individual, the nerve bends during its passage under the inguinal ligament from an approximate horizontal direction into an almost vertical direction. (From M. MUMMENTHALER and H. SCHLIACK: Läsionen peripherer Nerven, 3rd ed. Thieme, Stuttgart 1977.)

Fig. 394. Cutaneous nerves, superficial nerves and vessels of ventral aspect of right thigh.

270

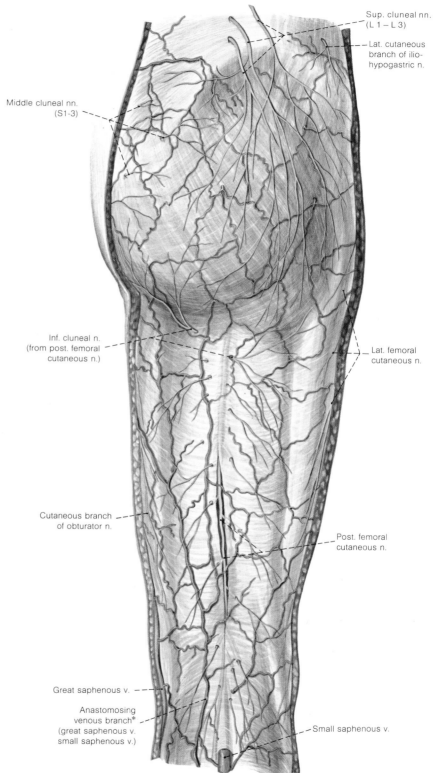

Sup. cluneal nn.
(L 1 – L 3)

Lat. cutaneous
branch of ilio-
hypogastric n.

Middle cluneal nn.
(S1-3)

Inf. cluneal n.
(from post. femoral
cutaneous n.)

Lat. femoral
cutaneous n.

Cutaneous branch
of obturator n.

Post. femoral
cutaneous n.

Great saphenous v.

Anastomosing
venous branch*
(great saphenous v.
small saphenous v.)

Small saphenous v.

Dorsal nerve
of penis

3 = lat. branch of iliohypgastric n.
4 = ant. branch of iliohypogastric n.
    and ilioinguinal n.
5 = femoral branch of genitofemoral n.
6 = genital branch of genitofemoral n.

Fig. 395. Genitofemoral nerve and sensory zones in the inguinal region. (From M. MUMMENTHALER and H. SCHLIACK: Läsionen peripherer Nerven, 3rd ed. Thieme, Stuttgart 1977.)

Fig. 396. Cutaneous nerves and veins of right gluteal region and dorsal aspect of thigh. The fascia lata has been split along the posterior femoral cutaneous nerve. * = so-called femoropopliteal vein.

271

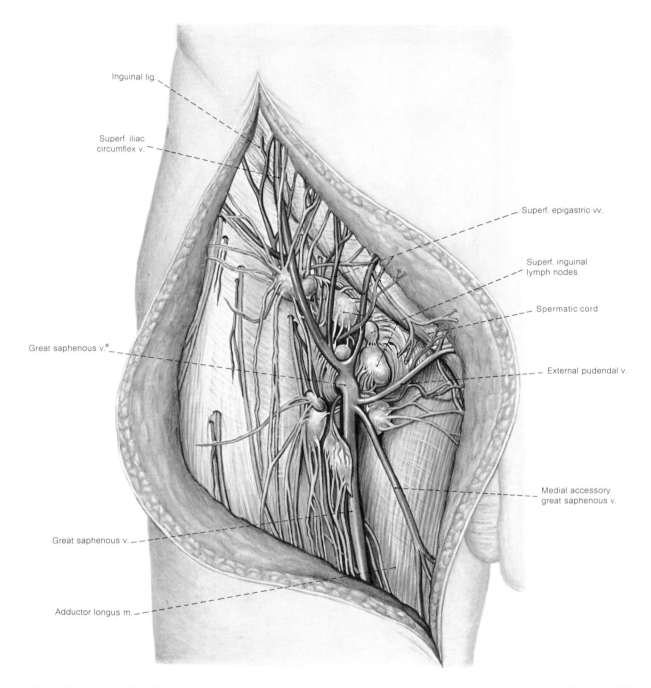

Inguinal lig.

Superf. iliac circumflex v.

Superf. epigastric vv.

Superf. inguinal lymph nodes

Spermatic cord

Great saphenous v.*

External pudendal v.

Medial accessory great saphenous v.

Great saphenous v.

Adductor longus m.

Fig. 397. Epifascial veins, lymph vessels, cutaneous nerves, and lymph nodes of the (sub.) inguinal region. After J. LANG and W. WACHSMUTH (1972) from their own preparations. * Bend before entry into femoral vein.

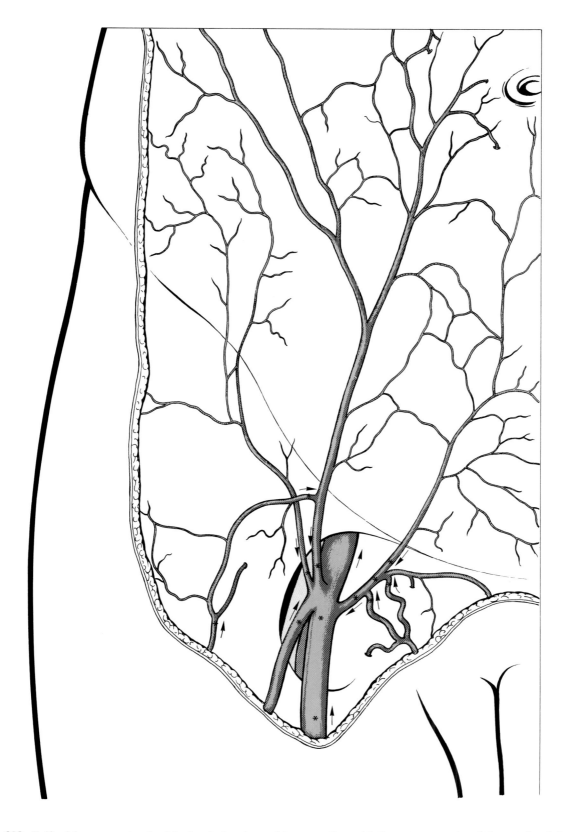

Fig. 398. Epifascial venous network of the inguinal region and its connections with the cutaneous veins of the anterior abdominal wall. Modified after an illustration from BRAUNE (1871). * Valves, →→ Direction of flow.

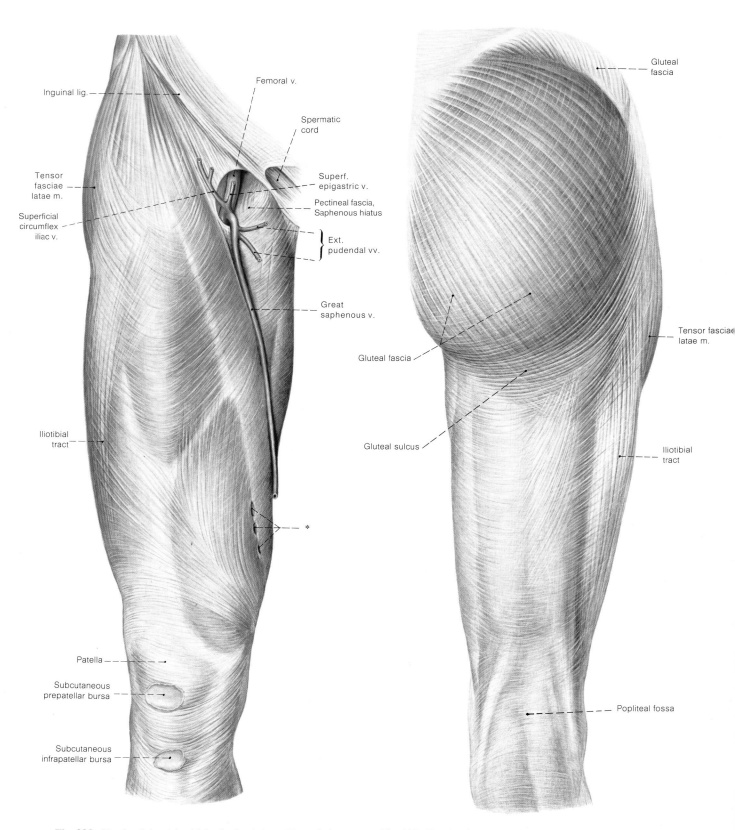

Inguinal lig.

Femoral v.

Spermatic cord

Tensor fasciae latae m.

Superf. epigastric v.

Superficial circumflex iliac v.

Pectineal fascia, Saphenous hiatus

Ext. pudendal vv.

Great saphenous v.

Iliotibial tract

*

Patella

Subcutaneous prepatellar bursa

Subcutaneous infrapatellar bursa

Gluteal fascia

Gluteal fascia

Tensor fasciae latae m.

Gluteal sulcus

Iliotibial tract

Popliteal fossa

Fig. 399. Fascia of the right thigh, the fascia lata. Ventral view.
* Gaps of the fascia for the perforating veins (DODD).

Fig. 400. Fascia of the right thigh and gluteal region. Dorsal view.

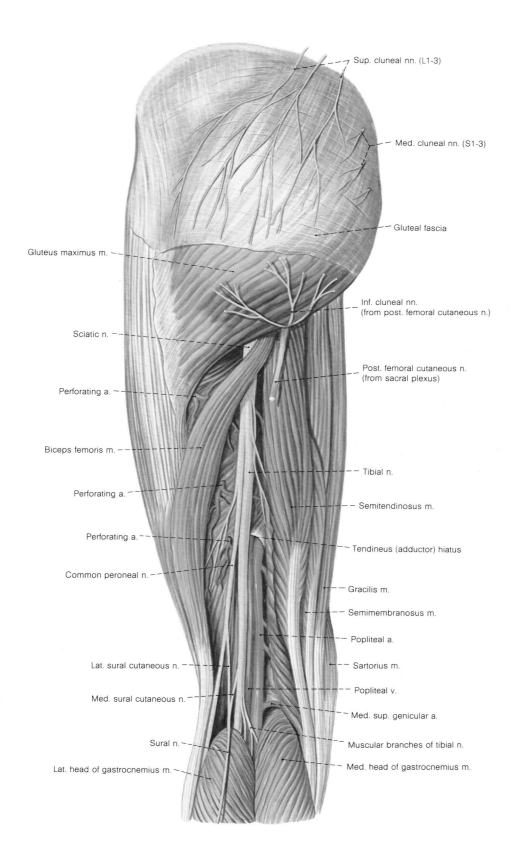

Sup. cluneal nn. (L1-3)

Med. cluneal nn. (S1-3)

Gluteal fascia

Gluteus maximus m.

Inf. cluneal nn. (from post. femoral cutaneous n.)

Sciatic n.

Post. femoral cutaneous n. (from sacral plexus)

Perforating a.

Biceps femoris m.

Tibial n.

Perforating a.

Semitendinosus m.

Perforating a.

Tendineus (adductor) hiatus

Common peroneal n.

Gracilis m.

Semimembranosus m.

Popliteal a.

Lat. sural cutaneous n.

Sartorius m.

Med. sural cutaneous n.

Popliteal v.

Med. sup. genicular a.

Sural n.

Muscular branches of tibial n.

Lat. head of gastrocnemius m.

Med. head of gastrocnemius m.

Fig. 401. Superficial nerves and vessels of the left gluteal region and dorsal aspect of thigh. Fascia lata is retained only in gluteal area; biceps femoris muscle has been pulled laterally in order to expose the sciatic nerve.

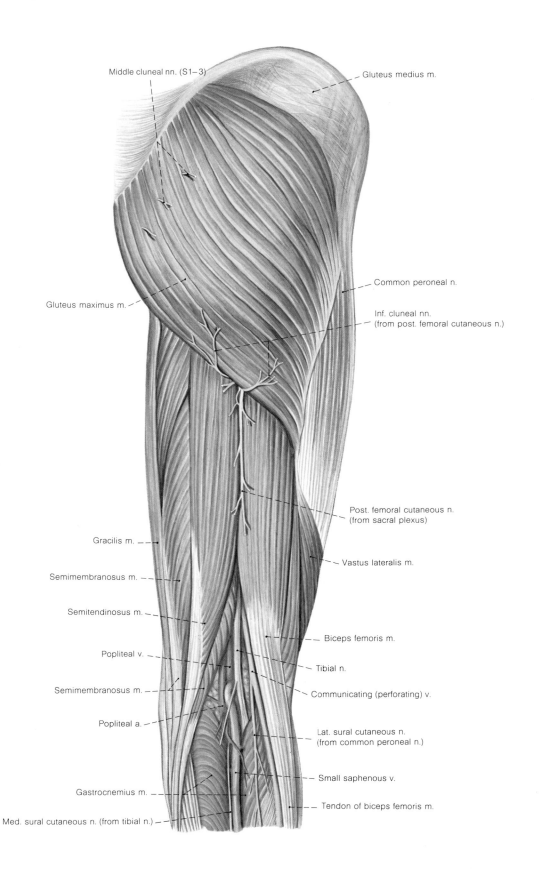

Middle cluneal nn. (S1–3)

Gluteus medius m.

Common peroneal n.

Gluteus maximus m.

Inf. cluneal nn.
(from post. femoral cutaneous n.)

Post. femoral cutaneous n.
(from sacral plexus)

Gracilis m.

Vastus lateralis m.

Semimembranosus m.

Semitendinosus m.

Biceps femoris m.

Popliteal v.

Tibial n.

Communicating (perforating) v.

Semimembranosus m.

Popliteal a.

Lat. sural cutaneous n.
(from common peroneal n.)

Small saphenous v.

Gastrocnemius m.

Tendon of biceps femoris m.

Med. sural cutaneous n. (from tibial n.)

Fig. 402. Superficial nerves and vessels of right gluteal region and dorsal aspect of thigh. Fascia lata and superior cluneal nerves have been removed.

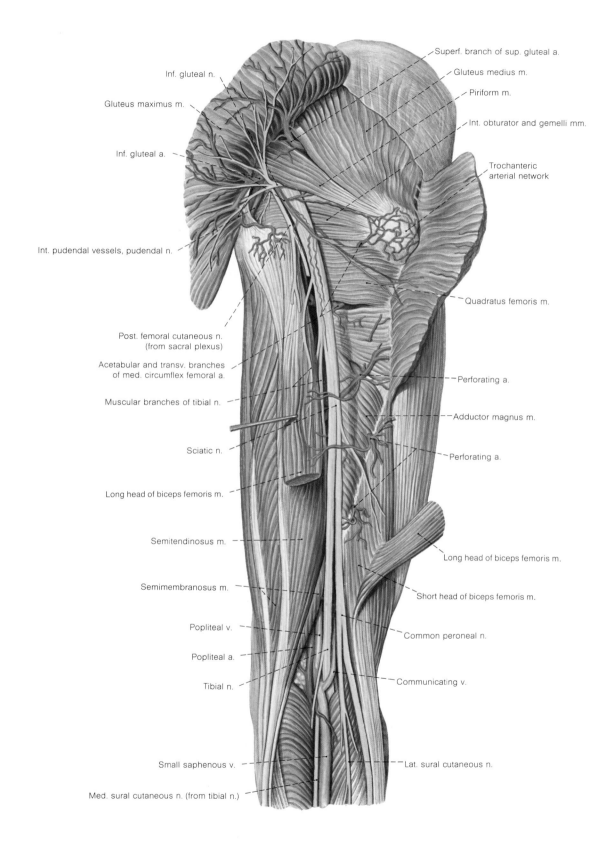

Inf. gluteal n.

Gluteus maximus m.

Inf. gluteal a.

Int. pudendal vessels, pudendal n.

Post. femoral cutaneous n. (from sacral plexus)

Acetabular and transv. branches of med. circumflex femoral a.

Muscular branches of tibial n.

Sciatic n.

Long head of biceps femoris m.

Semitendinosus m.

Semimembranosus m.

Popliteal v.

Popliteal a.

Tibial n.

Small saphenous v.

Med. sural cutaneous n. (from tibial n.)

Superf. branch of sup. gluteal a.

Gluteus medius m.

Piriform m.

Int. obturator and gemelli mm.

Trochanteric arterial network

Quadratus femoris m.

Perforating a.

Adductor magnus m.

Perforating a.

Long head of biceps femoris m.

Short head of biceps femoris m.

Common peroneal n.

Communicating v.

Lat. sural cutaneous n.

Fig. 403. Nerves and vessels of the right gluteal region and dorsal aspect of thigh, middle layer. Gluteus maximus muscle and long head of biceps muscle have been sectioned and reflected.

277

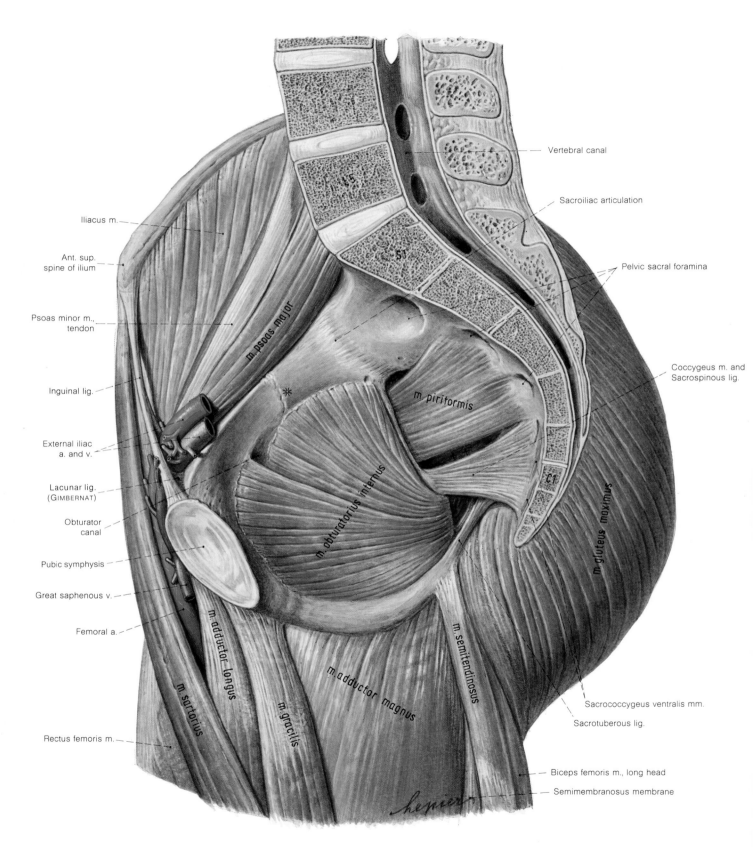

Vertebral canal

Sacroiliac articulation

Pelvic sacral foramina

Coccygeus m. and
Sacrospinous lig.

Iliacus m.

Ant. sup.
spine of ilium

Psoas minor m.,
tendon

Inguinal lig.

External iliac
a. and v.

Lacunar lig.
(GIMBERNAT)

Obturator
canal

Pubic symphysis

Great saphenous v.

Femoral a.

Rectus femoris m.

m. psoas major

m. piriformis

m. obturatorius internus

m. gluteus maximus

m. adductor longus

m. sartorius

m. gracilis

m. adductor magnus

m. semitendinosus

Sacrococcygeus ventralis mm.

Sacrotuberous lig.

Biceps femoris m., long head

Semimembranosus membrane

Fig. 404. Musculature of the true pelvis and the medial side of the thigh. The pelvis and vertebral column are cut in the midline: The viscera, fascia, and peritoneum have been removed. * Fracture of the superior branch of pubic bone.

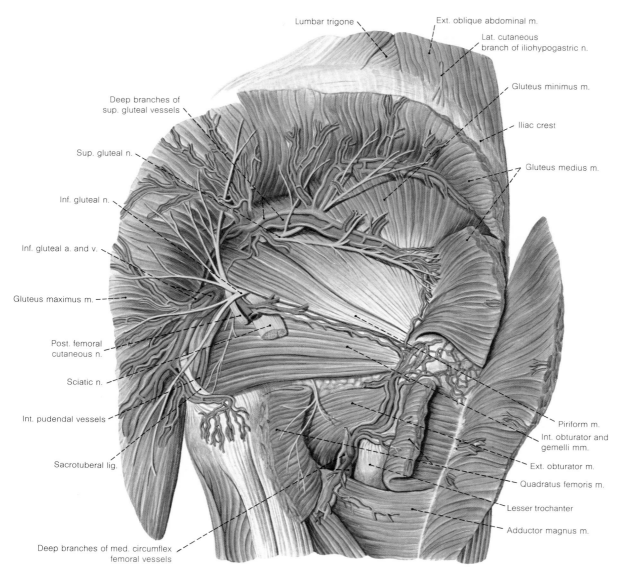

Lumbar trigone

Ext. oblique abdominal m.

Lat. cutaneous branch of iliohypogastric n.

Deep branches of sup. gluteal vessels

Gluteus minimus m.

Iliac crest

Sup. gluteal n.

Gluteus medius m.

Inf. gluteal n.

Inf. gluteal a. and v.

Gluteus maximus m.

Post. femoral cutaneous n.

Sciatic n.

Int. pudendal vessels

Piriform m.

Int. obturator and gemelli mm.

Sacrotuberal lig.

Ext. obturator m.

Quadratus femoris m.

Lesser trochanter

Adductor magnus m.

Deep branches of med. circumflex femoral vessels

Fig. 405. Deep nerves and vessels of the gluteal region. Gluteus maximus, gluteus medius, quadratus femoris muscles and sciatic nerve have been sectioned and partly removed.

M. iliopsoas (Figs. 404, 410)

Name	*Origin*	*Insertion*
Iliacus muscle	Iliac fossa, anterior inferior iliac spine, anterior capsule of hip joint	Lesser trochanter and adjacent region of the medial lip of the linea aspera
Psoas major muscle	Lateral surfaces of the 12th thoracic and 1st–4th lumbar vertebrae, costal processes of the 1st–5th (4th) lumbar vertebrae	Lesser trochanter
Psoas minor muscle	Lateral surfaces of the 12th thoracic and 1st lumbar vertebrae	Lesser trochanter, insertion often with a long tendon

Innervation: Branches of the lumbar plexus

Function: Flexion and outward rotation of hip joint, lateral binding of lumbar spine

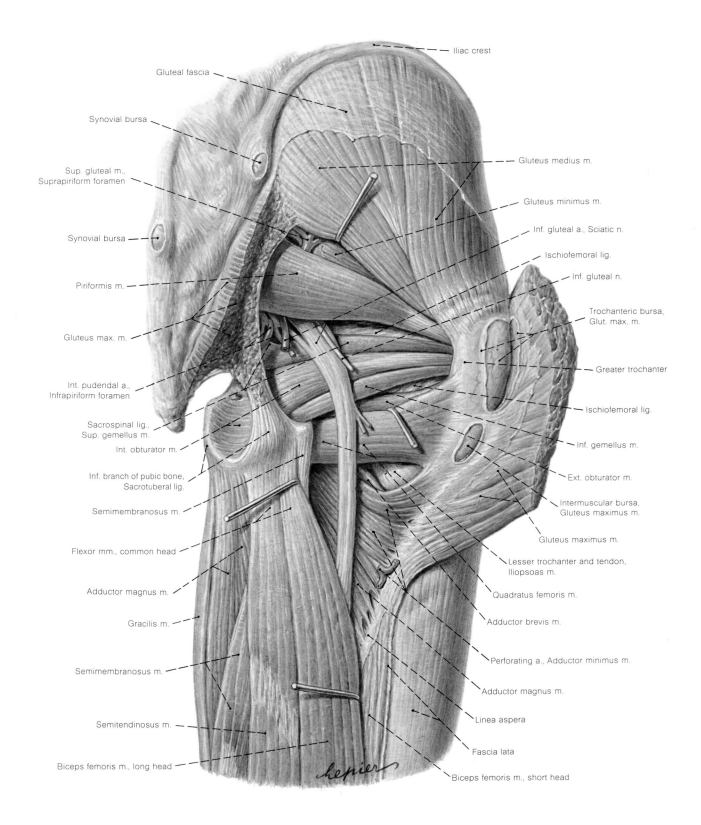

Iliac crest

Gluteal fascia

Synovial bursa

Gluteus medius m.

Sup. gluteal m.,
Suprapiriform foramen

Gluteus minimus m.

Inf. gluteal a., Sciatic n.

Synovial bursa

Ischiofemoral lig.

Inf. gluteal n.

Piriformis m.

Trochanteric bursa,
Glut. max. m.

Gluteus max. m.

Greater trochanter

Int. pudendal a.,
Infrapiriform foramen

Ischiofemoral lig.

Sacrospinal lig.,
Sup. gemellus m.

Inf. gemellus m.

Int. obturator m.

Ext. obturator m.

Inf. branch of pubic bone,
Sacrotuberal lig.

Intermuscular bursa,
Gluteus maximus m.

Semimembranosus m.

Gluteus maximus m.

Flexor mm., common head

Lesser trochanter and tendon,
Iliopsoas m.

Adductor magnus m.

Quadratus femoris m.

Gracilis m.

Adductor brevis m.

Perforating a., Adductor minimus m.

Semimembranosus m.

Adductor magnus m.

Linea aspera

Semitendinosus m.

Fascia lata

Biceps femoris m., long head

Biceps femoris m., short head

Fig. 406. Middle and deep layers of the gluteal region and a superficial layer of the flexors on the thigh. The Gluteus maximus muscle is severed and reflected.

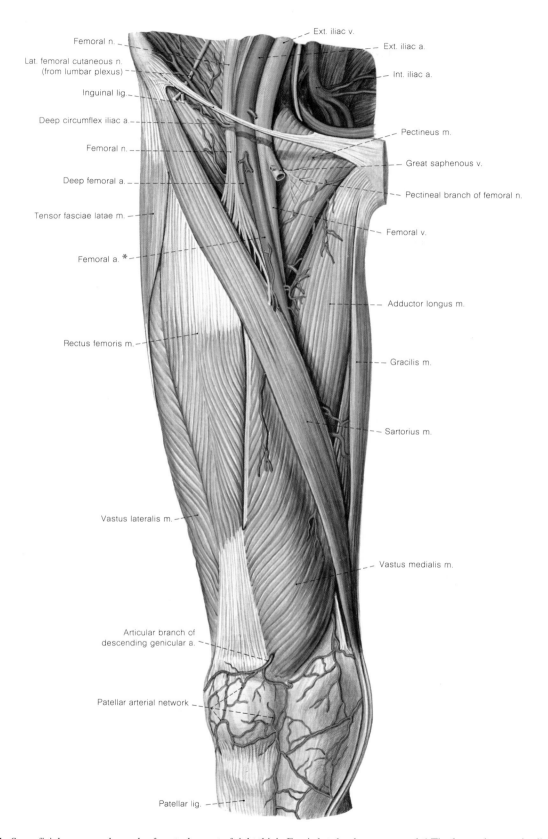

Fig. 407. Superficial nerves and vessels of ventral aspect of right thigh. Fascia lata has been removed. * The femoral artery, in clinical usage, sometimes is called superficial femoral artery.

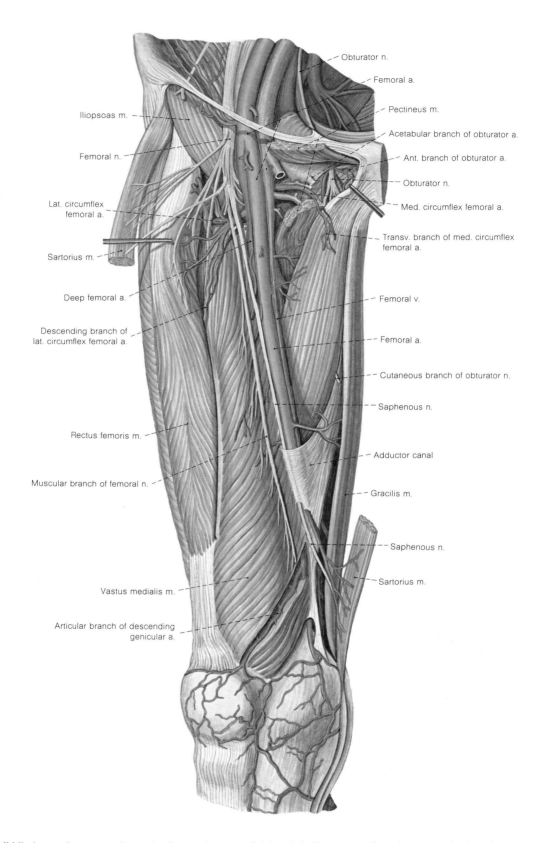

Obturator n.

Femoral a.

Pectineus m.

Acetabular branch of obturator a.

Ant. branch of obturator a.

Obturator n.

Med. circumflex femoral a.

Transv. branch of med. circumflex femoral a.

Femoral v.

Femoral a.

Cutaneous branch of obturator n.

Saphenous n.

Adductor canal

Gracilis m.

Saphenous n.

Sartorius m.

Iliopsoas m.

Femoral n.

Lat. circumflex femoral a.

Sartorius m.

Deep femoral a.

Descending branch of lat. circumflex femoral a.

Rectus femoris m.

Muscular branch of femoral n.

Vastus medialis m.

Articular branch of descending genicular a.

Fig. 408. Middle layer of nerves and vessels of ventral aspect of right thigh. Sartorius and pectineus muscles have been sectioned and partially removed.

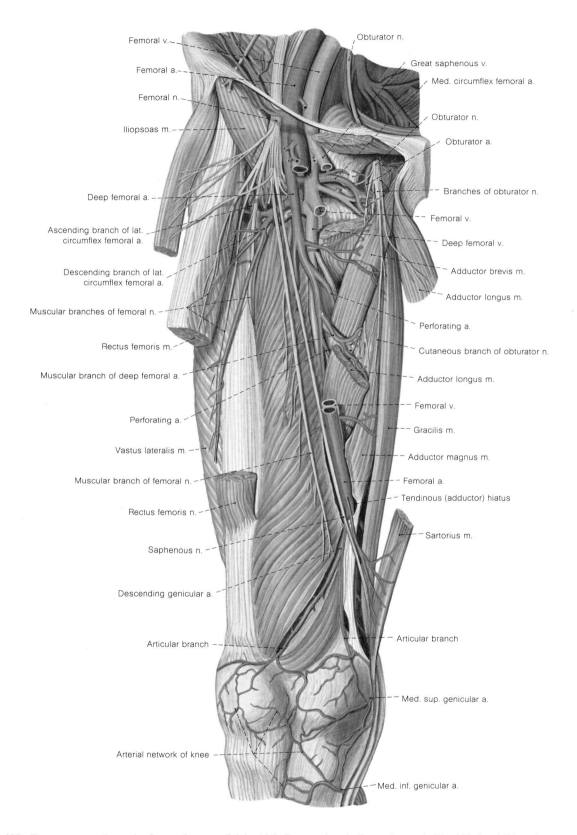

Femoral v.

Femoral a.

Femoral n.

Iliopsoas m.

Deep femoral a.

Ascending branch of lat. circumflex femoral a.

Descending branch of lat. circumflex femoral a.

Muscular branches of femoral n.

Rectus femoris m.

Muscular branch of deep femoral a.

Perforating a.

Vastus lateralis m.

Muscular branch of femoral n.

Rectus femoris n.

Saphenous n.

Descending genicular a.

Articular branch

Arterial network of knee

Obturator n.

Great saphenous v.

Med. circumflex femoral a.

Obturator n.

Obturator a.

Branches of obturator n.

Femoral v.

Deep femoral v.

Adductor brevis m.

Adductor longus m.

Perforating a.

Cutaneous branch of obturator n.

Adductor longus m.

Femoral v.

Gracilis m.

Adductor magnus m.

Femoral a.

Tendinous (adductor) hiatus

Sartorius m.

Articular branch

Med. sup. genicular a.

Med. inf. genicular a.

Fig. 409. Deep nerves and vessels of ventral aspect of right thigh. Preparation similar to the one in Fig. 408. In addition, the rectus femoris and adductor longus muscles have been sectioned and partially removed; the vastus medialis muscle has been split in order to expose the descending genicular artery.

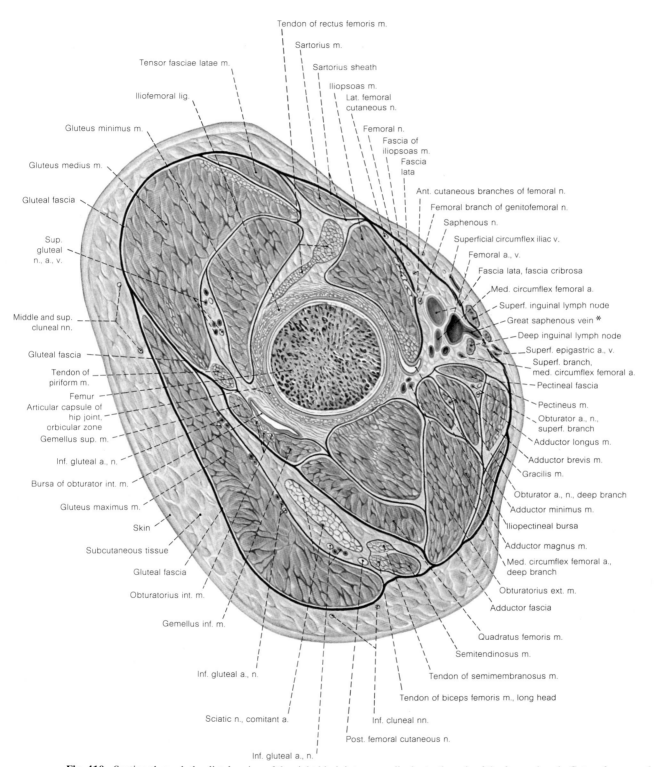

Tendon of rectus femoris m.
Sartorius m.
Tensor fasciae latae m.
Sartorius sheath
Iliopsoas m.
Iliofemoral lig.
Lat. femoral cutaneous n.
Gluteus minimus m.
Femoral n.
Fascia of iliopsoas m.
Gluteus medius m.
Fascia lata
Gluteal fascia
Ant. cutaneous branches of femoral n.
Femoral branch of genitofemoral n.
Saphenous n.
Sup. gluteal n., a., v.
Superficial circumflex iliac v.
Femoral a., v.
Fascia lata, fascia cribrosa
Med. circumflex femoral a.
Superf. inguinal lymph node
Great saphenous vein *
Middle and sup. cluneal nn.
Deep inguinal lymph node
Superf. epigastric a., v.
Gluteal fascia
Superf. branch, med. circumflex femoral a.
Tendon of piriform m.
Pectineal fascia
Femur
Pectineus m.
Articular capsule of hip joint, orbicular zone
Obturator a., n., superf. branch
Gemellus sup. m.
Adductor longus m.
Inf. gluteal a., n.
Adductor brevis m.
Gracilis m.
Bursa of obturator int. m.
Obturator a., n., deep branch
Gluteus maximus m.
Adductor minimus m.
Iliopectineal bursa
Skin
Subcutaneous tissue
Adductor magnus m.
Gluteal fascia
Med. circumflex femoral a., deep branch
Obturatorius int. m.
Obturatorius ext. m.
Adductor fascia
Gemellus inf. m.
Quadratus femoris m.
Semitendinosus m.
Inf. gluteal a., n.
Tendon of semimembranosus m.
Sciatic n., comitant a.
Tendon of biceps femoris m., long head
Inf. cluneal nn.
Post. femoral cutaneous n.
Inf. gluteal a., n.

Fig. 410. Section through the distal region of the right hip joint perpendicular to the axis of the femoral neck. Cut surface seen from distal. In Figs. 410 and 411 the fasciae are shown in black, tendons and ligaments in violet. (Figs. 410 and 411 from PERNKOPF: Atlas der topographischen und angewandten Anatomie des Menschen, Vol. 2, 2nd ed. [Ed. H. FERNER]. Urban & Schwarzenberg, Munich–Vienna–Baltimore 1980.)

284

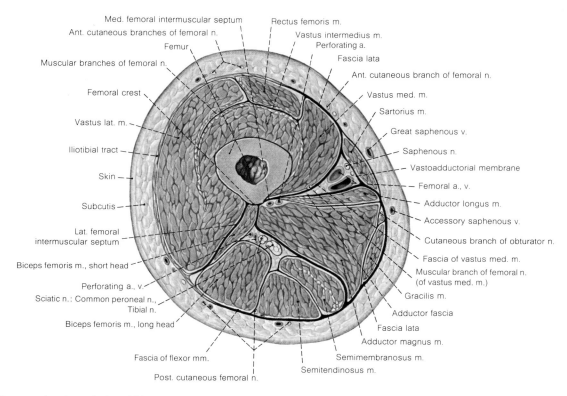

Fig. 411 a. Cross section through the middle third of the right thigh. Sectioned surface seen from distal.

Med. femoral intermuscular septum
Ant. cutaneous branches of femoral n.
Femur
Muscular branches of femoral n.
Femoral crest
Vastus lat. m.
Iliotibial tract
Skin
Subcutis
Lat. femoral intermuscular septum
Biceps femoris m., short head
Perforating a., v.
Sciatic n.: Common peroneal n.,
Tibial n.
Biceps femoris m., long head
Fascia of flexor mm.
Post. cutaneous femoral n.

Rectus femoris m.
Vastus intermedius m.
Perforating a.
Fascia lata
Ant. cutaneous branch of femoral n.
Vastus med. m.
Sartorius m.
Great saphenous v.
Saphenous n.
Vastoadductorial membrane
Femoral a., v.
Adductor longus m.
Accessory saphenous v.
Cutaneous branch of obturator n.
Fascia of vastus med. m.
Muscular branch of femoral n. (of vastus med. m.)
Gracilis m.
Adductor fascia
Fascia lata
Adductor magnus m.
Semimembranosus m.
Semitendinosus m.

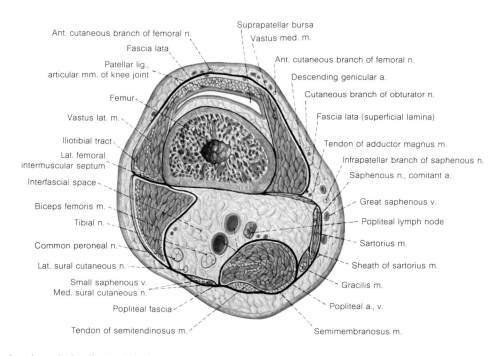

Fig. 411 b. Cross section through the distal third of the right thigh. Sectioned surface seen from distal.

Ant. cutaneous branch of femoral n.
Fascia lata
Patellar lig., articular mm. of knee joint
Femur
Vastus lat. m.
Iliotibial tract
Lat. femoral intermuscular septum
Interfascial space
Biceps femoris m.
Tibial n.
Common peroneal n.
Lat. sural cutaneous n.
Small saphenous v.
Med. sural cutaneous n.
Popliteal fascia
Tendon of semitendinosus m.

Suprapatellar bursa
Vastus med. m.
Ant. cutaneous branch of femoral n.
Descending genicular a.
Cutaneous branch of obturator n.
Fascia lata (superficial lamina)
Tendon of adductor magnus m.
Infrapatellar branch of saphenous n.
Saphenous n., comitant a.
Great saphenous v.
Popliteal lymph node
Sartorius m.
Sheath of sartorius m.
Gracilis m.
Popliteal a., v.
Semimembranosus m.

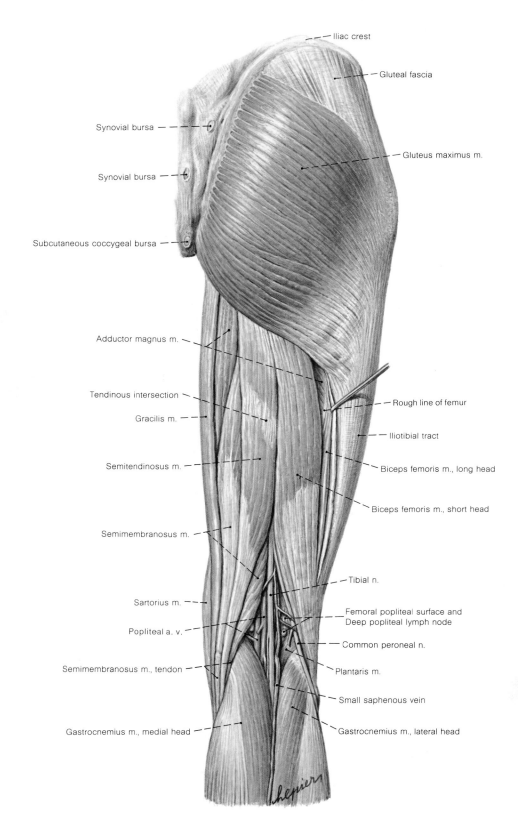

Iliac crest

Gluteal fascia

Synovial bursa

Gluteus maximus m.

Synovial bursa

Subcutaneous coccygeal bursa

Adductor magnus m.

Rough line of femur

Tendinous intersection

Gracilis m.

Iliotibial tract

Biceps femoris m., long head

Semitendinosus m.

Biceps femoris m., short head

Semimembranosus m.

Tibial n.

Sartorius m.

Femoral popliteal surface and
Deep popliteal lymph node

Popliteal a. v.

Common peroneal n.

Semimembranosus m., tendon

Plantaris m.

Small saphenous vein

Gastrocnemius m., medial head

Gastrocnemius m., lateral head

Fig. 412. Superficial layer of dorsal hip and thigh muscles, including the popliteal fossa.

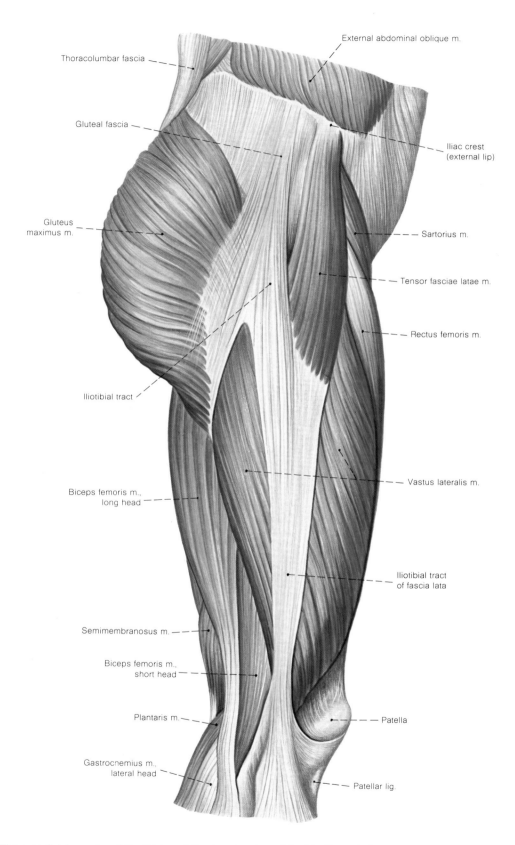

Thoracolumbar fascia

External abdominal oblique m.

Gluteal fascia

Iliac crest
(external lip)

Gluteus
maximus m.

Sartorius m.

Tensor fasciae latae m.

Rectus femoris m.

Iliotibial tract

Biceps femoris m.,
long head

Vastus lateralis m.

Iliotibial tract
of fascia lata

Semimembranosus m.

Biceps femoris m.,
short head

Plantaris m.

Patella

Gastrocnemius m.,
lateral head

Patellar lig.

Fig. 413. The superficial muscles of the thigh and the dorsal region of the hip. Lateral view.

Dorsal Hip Muscles (Figs. 399–406, 412, 413, 418, 419)

Name	Origin	Insertion
1. Gluteus maximus muscle (powerful, with coarse fasciculi)	Posterior gluteal line of the ileum; posterior aspect of sacrum, side of coccyx, sacro-tuberous ligament	Gluteal tuberosity of femur and iliotibial tract of fascia lata

Nerve: Inferior gluteal nerve (L 5; S 1, 2)

Function: Extensor and powerful lateral rotator of thigh; inferior fibers assist in adduction of thigh; balances trunk on femur; fibers to iliotibial tract braces knee joint

2. Gluteus medius muscle	External aspect of ilium; between anterior and posterior gluteal lines; gluteal apo-neurosis	Oblique ridge on lateral surface of greater trochanter of femur

Nerve: Superior gluteal nerve (L 4, 5; S 1)

Function: Abducts femur, posterior fibers extend and rotate laterally, anterior fibers flex and rotate medially

3. Gluteus minimus muscle	Outer aspect of ilium between anterior and inferior gluteal lines	Tip (tendinous) of greater trochanter of femur and capsule of hip joint

Nerve: Superior gluteal nerve (L 4, 5; S 1)

Function: Rotates thigh medially, abducts femur and, to some extent, flexes it

4. Piriformis muscle	Pelvic surface of sacrum, lateral to sacral foramina 2, 3, and 4	A long tendon to upper border of greater trochanter of the femur

Nerve: Sciatic nerve or direct branches from the sacral plexus (S 1, 2)

Function: Rotates femur laterally; assists in abduction

5. Internal obturator muscle	Margin of obturator foramen; obturator membrane	Medial surface of greater trochanter of femur, proximal to trochanteric fossa
6. Superior gemellus muscle	Ischial spine	With tendon of Internal obturator muscle to greater trochanter
7. Inferior gemellus muscle	Ischial tuberosity	

Nerve: Direct branches from the sacral plexus

Function: Rotates femur laterally, Internal obturator muscle extends and abducts when femur is flexed

8. Quadratus femoris muscle	Lateral border of ischial tuberosity	Quadrate line of femur extending down to intertrochanteric crest

Nerve: Sciatic nerve, branch from sacral plexus (L 4, 5; S 1)

Function: Rotates femur laterally and helps in adduction

9. Tensor fasciae latae muscle	Iliac crest; anterior superior iliac spine	Iliotibial tract of fascia lata

Nerve: Superior gluteal nerve (L 4, 5; S 1)

Function: Tenses fascia lata; assists in flexion, abduction, and medial rotation of femur

Anterior Muscles of the Thigh (Figs. 407–409, 414–417)

Name	Origin	Insertion
Sartorius muscle	Anterior superior iliac spine	Medial margin of tibial tuberosity

Nerve: Femoral nerve (L 2, 3)

Function: Flexes, laterally rotates, abducts thigh; flexes leg; rotates leg medially in knee joint when leg is flexed

Quadriceps femoris muscle (Extensor muscles)

Name	Origin	Insertion
Rectus femoris muscle (operates 2 joints) Straight (anterior) head	Tendon from anterior inferior spine of ileum	The common tendon of the Quadriceps femoris muscle (which is the most powerful muscle in the entire human body) attaches to the cranial, medial, and lateral margins of the patella and, through intermediation of the patellar ligament, is inserted on the tibial tuberosity
Reflected (posterior head)	Cranial margin of acetabulum	
Vastus medialis muscle	Medial lip of linea aspera; intertrochanteric line (distal end thicker than proximal)	
Vastus lateralis muscle	Lateral lip of linea aspera as far proximally as greater trochanter	
Vastus intermedius muscle	Anterior and lateral surfaces of the shaft of the femur; lateral intermuscular septum	
Articularis genus muscle	From anterior surface of femur	Synovial membrane of knee joint

Nerve: Femoral nerve (L 2, 3, 4)

Function: Extends leg. Rectus femoris aids in flexion of hip joint; Articularis genus muscle draws articular capsule proximally

Medial Muscles of the Thigh (Adductors) (Figs. 407–409, 414–417)

Name	Origin	Insertion
1. Pectineus muscle	Pecten of pubic bone	Pectineal line of femur

Nerve: Femoral nerve (L 2, 3) and the accessory obturator nerve

Function: Adducts the thigh; also aids in flexion and lateral rotation in the hip joint

2. Adductor longus muscle	Tendon from the border of superior and inferior pubic branches near symphysis	Middle third of medial lip of linea aspera

Nerve: Obturator nerve

Function: Adducts, aids flexion, and rotates thigh laterally

3. Gracilis muscle (forms middle tendon of pes anserinus)	Flat tendon from inferior branch of pubis near symphysis	Long tendon on medial borders of the shaft of the tibia near the tibial tuberosity (pes anserinus)

Nerve: Obturator nerve (L 3, 4)

Function: Adducts thigh, aids in flexion of the knee; rotates the leg medially

4. Adductor brevis muscle	Inferior pubic branch	Proximal third of medial lip of linea aspera; and pectineal line

Nerve: Obturator nerve (L 3, 4)

Function: Adducts thigh, aids in flexion and in lateral rotation of the thigh

5. Adductor magnus muscle* (This and also the Adductor brevis muscle, lie in deeper layers than 1 to 3 above)	Lower part of inferior pubic branch; branch of ischium; ischial tuberosity	Fleshy: proximal $^2/_3$ of linea aspera, medial lip, gluteal tuberosity Tendinous: Medial epicondyle of femur *(hiatus tendineus)*

Nerve: Obturator (L 3, 4) nerve and sciatic (L 4, 5; S 1) nerve

Function: Powerful adductor of thigh; aids in flexion and assists in lateral rotation in hip joint. Lower portion of muscle extends the thigh and rotates it medially

6. Obturator externus muscle	Medial margin of obturator foramen; outer surface of obturator membrane	Trochanteric fossa of femur

Nerve: Obturator nerve (L 3, 4)

Function: Rotates femur laterally; also aids in flexing the hip joint

---

* The proximal, almost transverse part of the Adductor magnus muscle was formerly called (BNA) the Adductor minimus muscle. It works somewhat irregularly from the main muscle and aids in the lateral rotation of the hip joint.

The Posterior Muscles of the Thigh (Hamstring Muscles) (Flexors) (Figs. 401–403, 418, 419)

Name	Origin	Insertion
1. Biceps femoris muscle		
Long head – operates 2 joints	Ischial tuberosity (short tendon fuses with Semitendinosus muscle)	Head of fibula by strong tendon, lateral condyle of tibia (small slip)
Short head – operates 1 joint	Distal half of lateral lip of linea aspera	

Nerve: *Long head:* Tibial nerve (S 1–3). *Short head:* Common peroneal nerve (L 5; S 1, 2)

Function: Both heads flex the leg, then rotate it laterally; long head also extends the thigh

2. Semitendinosus muscle (forms the 3rd tendon of the pes anserinus) (operates 2 joints)	Short tendon from ischial tuberosity, fused with the long head of the biceps femoris muscle	Long tendon; the terminal ramification (pes anserinus) of the tendon takes place on medial margin of the tuberosity of the tibia

Nerve: Tibial nerve (L 4, 5; S 1, 2)

Function: Extends thigh; flexes the leg (medial rotation)

3. Semimembranosus muscle (operates 2 joints)	Ischial tuberosity (by broad tendon; in the inner space with No. 1 and No. 2 above and the Adductor magnus muscle)	Thick, short tendon on medial condyle of the tibia (via oblique popliteal ligament, to lateral condyle of the femur)

Nerve: Tibial nerve (L 5; S 1, 2)

Function: Flexes the leg, medial rotation of the flexed leg; extends the thigh

---

I. **Greater sciatic foramen** (foramen ischiadicum majus). Boundaries: Greater sciatic notch (incisura ischiadica major), sacrospinal and sacrotuberous ligaments. The Piriformis muscle passes through this foramen.

   1. **Caudal to the Piriformis muscle** (the infrapiriform foramen) is the passage for the sciatic nerve (n. ischiadicus), inferior gluteal vessels, the posterior femoral cutaneous nerve, the internal pudendal vessels, the pudendal nerve.

   2. **Cranial to the Piriformis muscle** (suprapiriform foramen) is the passage of superior gluteal vessels and superior gluteal nerve.

II. **Lesser sciatic foramen** (foramen ischiadicum minus). Boundaries: Lesser sciatic notch (incisura ischiadica minor), sacrospinal and sacrotuberous ligaments transmit the internal pudendal vessels and nerve and the tendon of the Obturator internus m. and its nerve in the pudendal canal (ALCOCK's). The pudendal canal lies in the deep ischiorectal fossa and is formed from the fascia of the Obturator internus muscle.

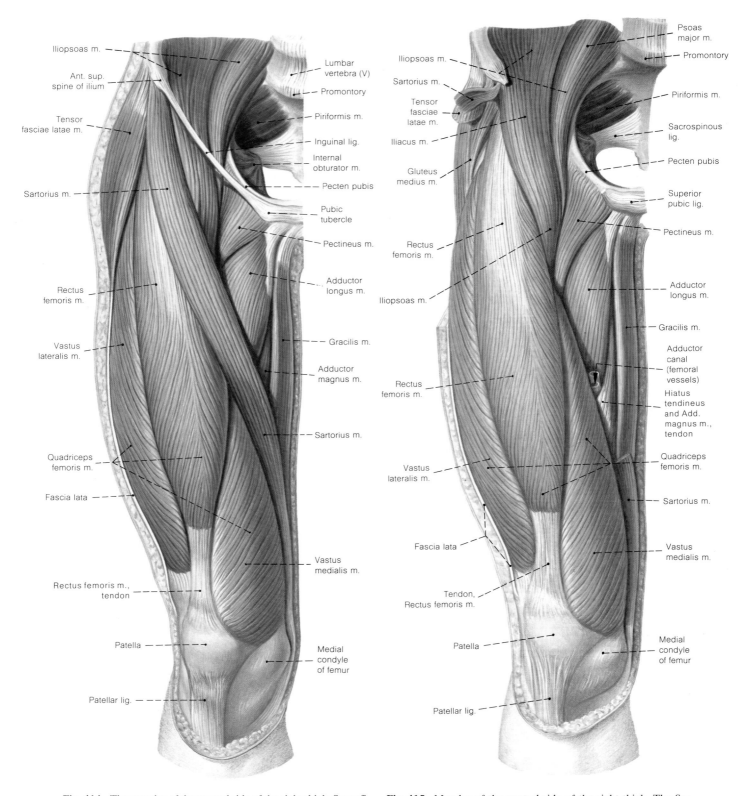

Fig. 414. The muscles of the ventral side of the right thigh. Superficial layer. The inguinal ligament is retained to show its attachments.

Fig. 415. Muscles of the ventral side of the right thigh. The Sartorius muscle and the inguinal ligament have been removed.

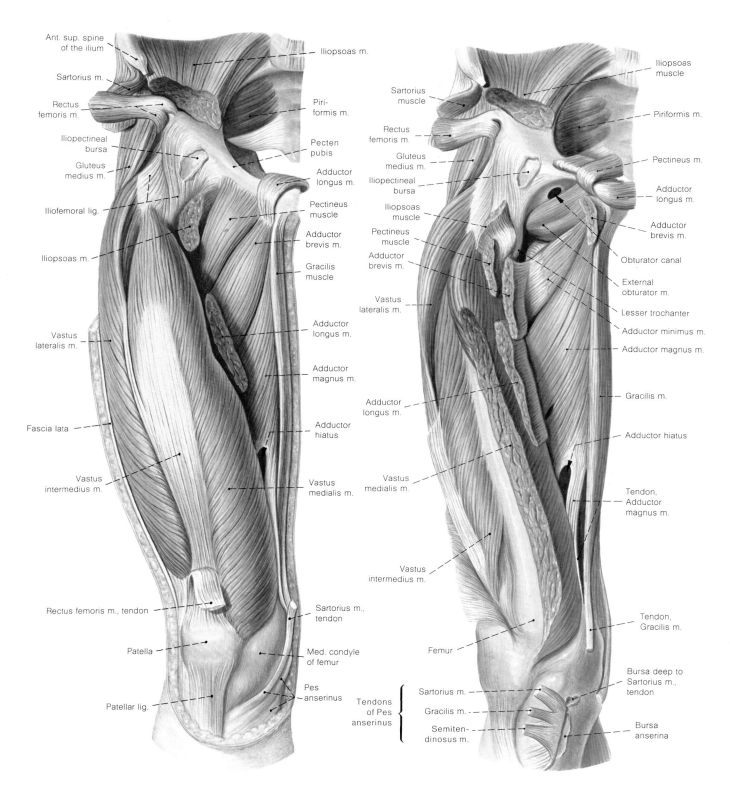

Fig. 416. Middle layer of muscles of the ventral surface of the thigh. The Sartorius, Iliopsoas, Rectus femoris, and Adductor longus muscles were partially resected.

Fig. 417. Deep layers of muscles of the ventral surface of the thigh. Preparation same as in Fig. 416; in addition, the Pectineus, Adductor brevis, Vastus medialis, and Gracilis muscles were cut.

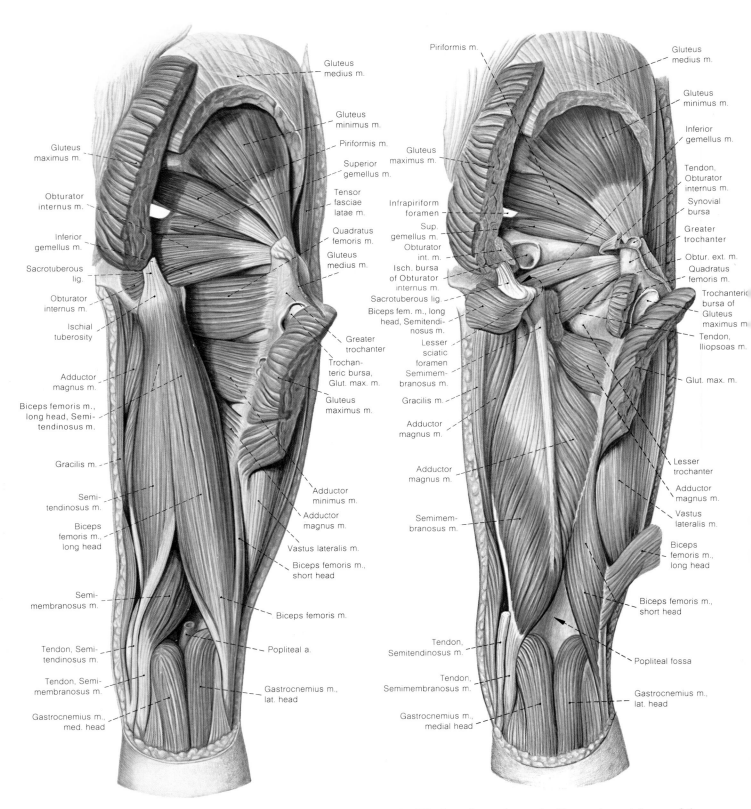

Fig. 418. Deep layer of the dorsal muscles of the hip and superficial layers of the flexors on the thigh, the muscles of the popliteal fossa. The Gluteus maximus and medius muscles were transected and reflected.

Fig. 419. Deep layer of posterior hip muscles and flexors of the thigh. Besides the Gluteus maximus and medius, the Quadratus femoris, Internal obturator, Biceps femoris (long head), and the Semitendinosus muscles were cut. (The latter was cleaned away so that only the terminal tendons remain.)

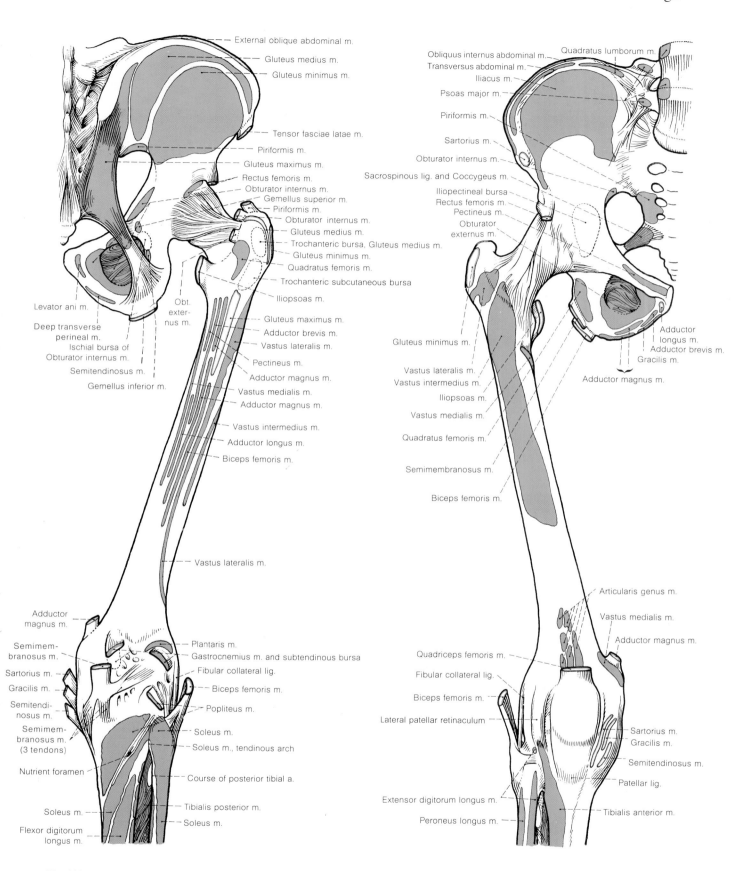

External oblique abdominal m.
Gluteus medius m.
Gluteus minimus m.

Tensor fasciae latae m.
Piriformis m.
Gluteus maximus m.
Rectus femoris m.
Obturator internus m.
Gemellus superior m.
Piriformis m.
Obturator internus m.
Gluteus medius m.
Trochanteric bursa, Gluteus medius m.
Gluteus minimus m.
Quadratus femoris m.
Trochanteric subcutaneous bursa
Iliopsoas m.
Gluteus maximus m.
Adductor brevis m.
Vastus lateralis m.
Pectineus m.
Adductor magnus m.
Vastus medialis m.
Adductor magnus m.
Vastus intermedius m.
Adductor longus m.
Biceps femoris m.

Levator ani m.
Deep transverse perineal m.
Ischial bursa of Obturator internus m.
Semitendinosus m.
Gemellus inferior m.

Obt. externus m.

Vastus lateralis m.

Adductor magnus m.
Semimembranosus m.
Sartorius m.
Gracilis m.
Semitendinosus m.
Semimembranosus m. (3 tendons)
Nutrient foramen
Soleus m.
Flexor digitorum longus m.

Plantaris m.
Gastrocnemius m. and subtendinous bursa
Fibular collateral lig.
Biceps femoris m.
Popliteus m.
Soleus m.
Soleus m., tendinous arch
Course of posterior tibial a.
Tibialis posterior m.
Soleus m.

Obliquus internus abdominal m.
Transversus abdominal m.
Iliacus m.
Psoas major m.
Piriformis m.
Sartorius m.
Obturator internus m.
Sacrospinous lig. and Coccygeus m.
Iliopectineal bursa
Rectus femoris m.
Pectineus m.
Obturator externus m.

Quadratus lumborum m.

Adductor longus m.
Adductor brevis m.
Gracilis m.
Adductor magnus m.

Gluteus minimus m.
Vastus lateralis m.
Vastus intermedius m.
Iliopsoas m.
Vastus medialis m.
Quadratus femoris m.
Semimembranosus m.
Biceps femoris m.

Articularis genus m.
Vastus medialis m.
Adductor magnus m.

Quadriceps femoris m.
Fibular collateral lig.
Biceps femoris m.
Lateral patellar retinaculum
Extensor digitorum longus m.
Peroneus longus m.

Sartorius m.
Gracilis m.
Semitendinosus m.
Patellar lig.
Tibialis anterior m.

Fig. 420. Muscle attachments mapped out on the pelvis and right lower limb, including below the knee. Dorsal view.

Fig. 421. Diagram of the muscle attachments to the pelvis and right lower limb, including below the knee. Ventral view.

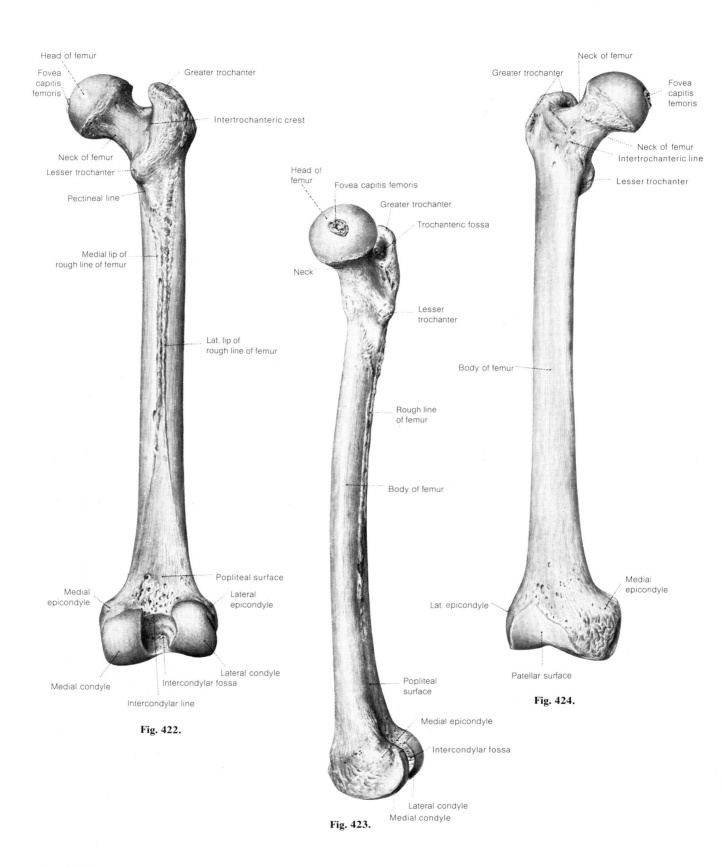

Fig. 422.

Head of femur
Fovea capitis femoris
Greater trochanter
Intertrochanteric crest
Neck of femur
Lesser trochanter
Pectineal line
Medial lip of rough line of femur
Lat. lip of rough line of femur
Popliteal surface
Medial epicondyle
Lateral epicondyle
Medial condyle
Intercondylar fossa
Lateral condyle
Intercondylar line

Fig. 423.

Head of femur
Fovea capitis femoris
Greater trochanter
Trochanteric fossa
Neck
Lesser trochanter
Rough line of femur
Body of femur
Popliteal surface
Medial epicondyle
Intercondylar fossa
Lateral condyle
Medial condyle

Fig. 424.

Neck of femur
Greater trochanter
Fovea capitis femoris
Neck of femur
Intertrochanteric line
Lesser trochanter
Body of femur
Lat. epicondyle
Medial epicondyle
Patellar surface

Figs. 422–424. Right femur. Fig. 422 Dorsal view; Fig. 423 Medial view; Fig. 424 Ventral view.

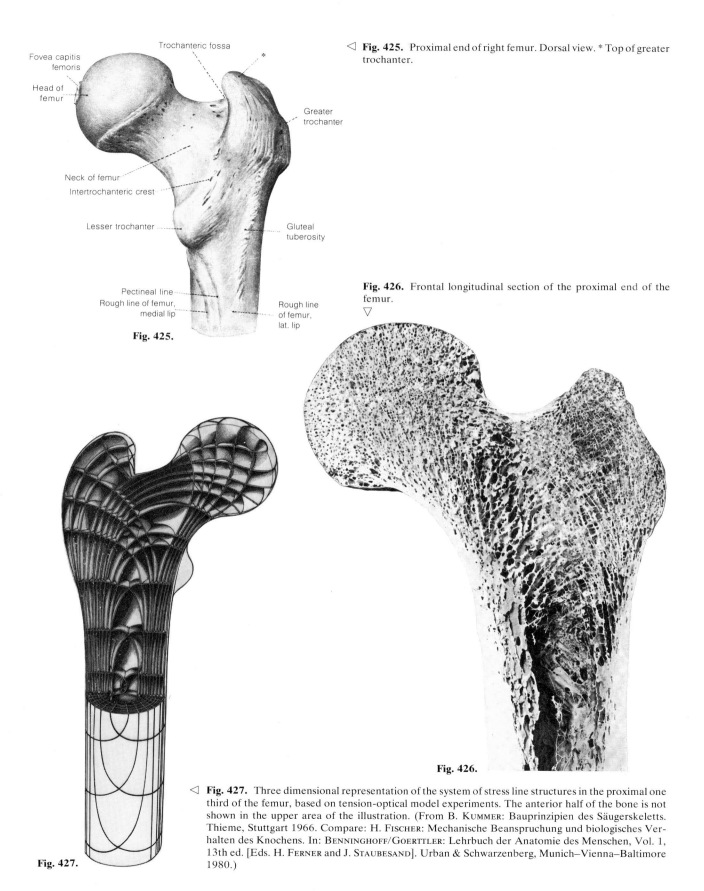

Fovea capitis femoris

Head of femur

Neck of femur

Intertrochanteric crest

Lesser trochanter

Pectineal line
Rough line of femur, medial lip

Trochanteric fossa

*

Greater trochanter

Gluteal tuberosity

Rough line of femur, lat. lip

Fig. 425.

◁ **Fig. 425.** Proximal end of right femur. Dorsal view. * Top of greater trochanter.

Fig. 426. Frontal longitudinal section of the proximal end of the femur.
▽

Fig. 426.

Fig. 427.

◁ **Fig. 427.** Three dimensional representation of the system of stress line structures in the proximal one third of the femur, based on tension-optical model experiments. The anterior half of the bone is not shown in the upper area of the illustration. (From B. KUMMER: Bauprinzipien des Säugerskeletts. Thieme, Stuttgart 1966. Compare: H. FISCHER: Mechanische Beanspruchung und biologisches Verhalten des Knochens. In: BENNINGHOFF/GOERTTLER: Lehrbuch der Anatomie des Menschen, Vol. 1, 13th ed. [Eds. H. FERNER and J. STAUBESAND]. Urban & Schwarzenberg, Munich–Vienna–Baltimore 1980.)

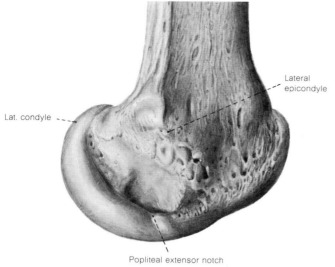

Lateral epicondyle

Lat. condyle

Popliteal extensor notch

Fig. 428. Distal end of right femur. Lateral view.

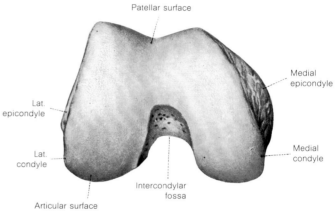

Patellar surface

Medial epicondyle

Lat. epicondyle

Medial condyle

Lat. condyle

Intercondylar fossa

Articular surface

Fig. 429. Distal end of right femur. Seen from below.

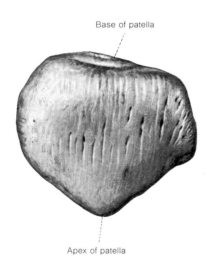

Base of patella

Apex of patella

Fig. 430. Patella. Ventral view.

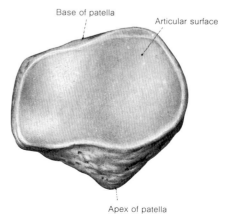

Base of patella

Articular surface

Apex of patella

Fig. 431. Patella. Dorsal view.

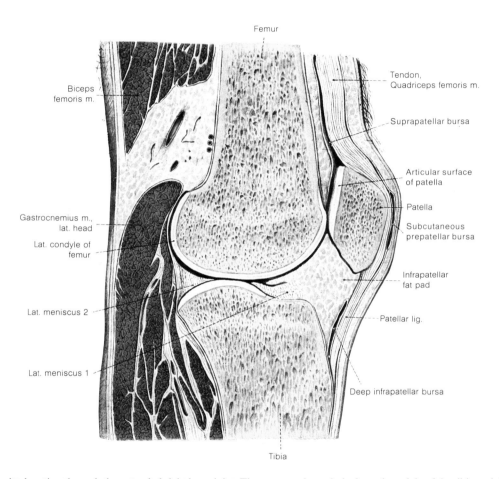

Femur

Biceps
femoris m.

Tendon,
Quadriceps femoris m.

Suprapatellar bursa

Articular surface
of patella

Patella

Gastrocnemius m.,
lat. head

Lat. condyle of
femur

Subcutaneous
prepatellar bursa

Infrapatellar
fat pad

Lat. meniscus 2

Lat. meniscus 1

Patellar lig.

Deep infrapatellar bursa

Tibia

Fig. 432. Sagittal section through the extended right knee joint. The cut goes through the lateral condyle of the tibia and the lateral meniscus. The latter was cut in two places: anterior and posterior. The congruity of the articular surfaces covered with cartilage are made possible by means of menisci, the plica alares and the fat bodies of the joint. The articular cavity is enlarged through the communication with the labyrinthine bursa.

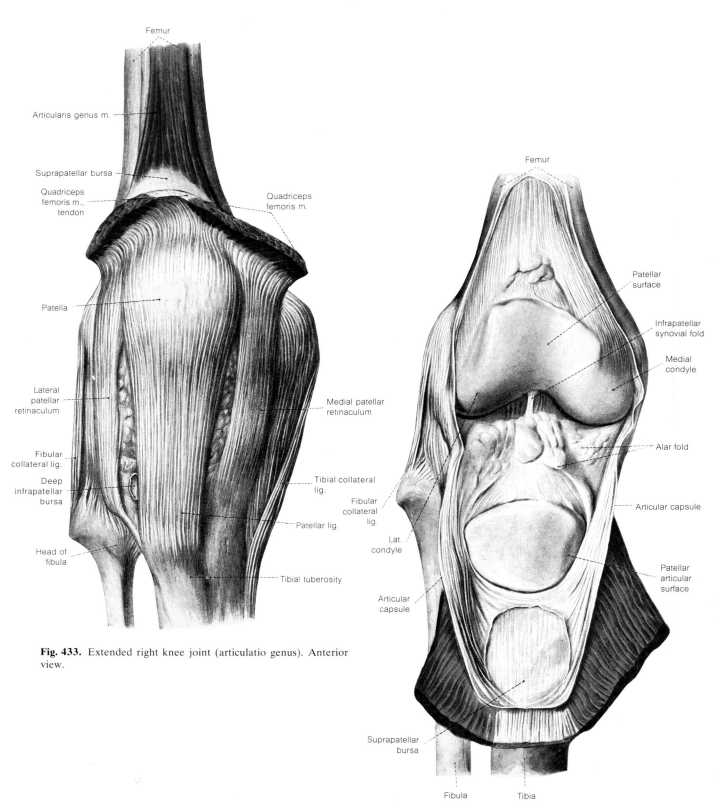

Fig. 433. Extended right knee joint (articulatio genus). Anterior view.

Fig. 434. Extended right knee joint (articulatio genus). Opened by two lateral incisions and the Quadriceps muscle with the patella pulled downward.

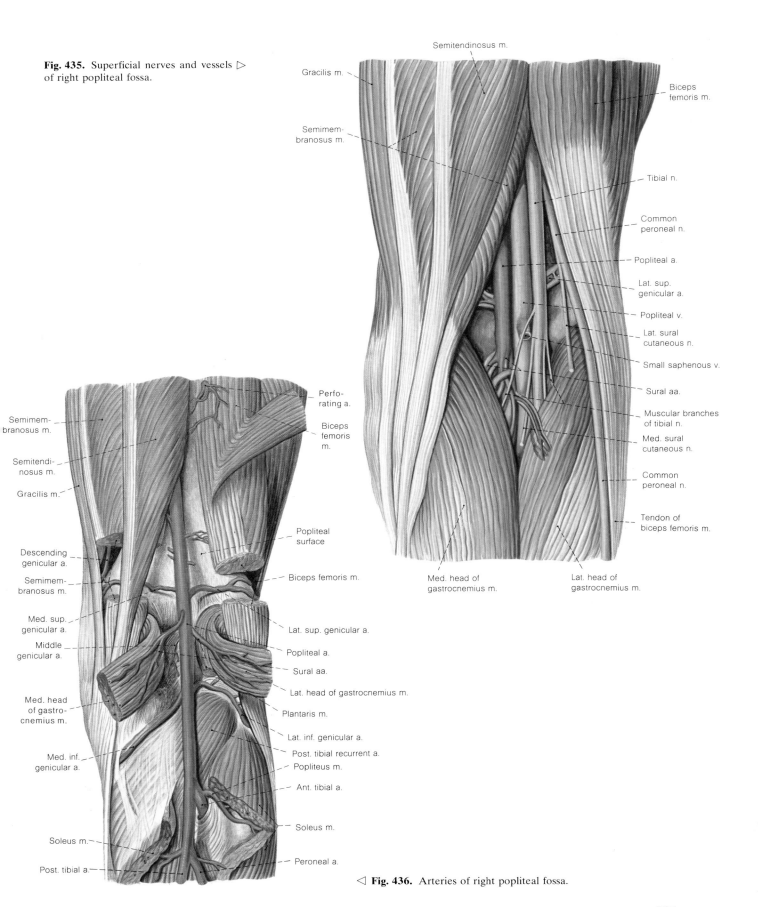

Fig. 435. Superficial nerves and vessels ▷ of right popliteal fossa.

Semitendinosus m.

Gracilis m.

Biceps femoris m.

Semimembranosus m.

Tibial n.

Common peroneal n.

Popliteal a.

Lat. sup. genicular a.

Popliteal v.

Lat. sural cutaneous n.

Small saphenous v.

Sural aa.

Muscular branches of tibial n.

Med. sural cutaneous n.

Common peroneal n.

Tendon of biceps femoris m.

Med. head of gastrocnemius m.

Lat. head of gastrocnemius m.

Semimembranosus m.

Semitendinosus m.

Gracilis m.

Perforating a.

Biceps femoris m.

Descending genicular a.

Semimembranosus m.

Med. sup. genicular a.

Middle genicular a.

Med. head of gastrocnemius m.

Med. inf. genicular a.

Popliteal surface

Biceps femoris m.

Lat. sup. genicular a.

Popliteal a.

Sural aa.

Lat. head of gastrocnemius m.

Plantaris m.

Lat. inf. genicular a.

Post. tibial recurrent a.

Popliteus m.

Ant. tibial a.

Soleus m.

Soleus m.

Post. tibial a.

Peroneal a.

◁ **Fig. 436.** Arteries of right popliteal fossa.

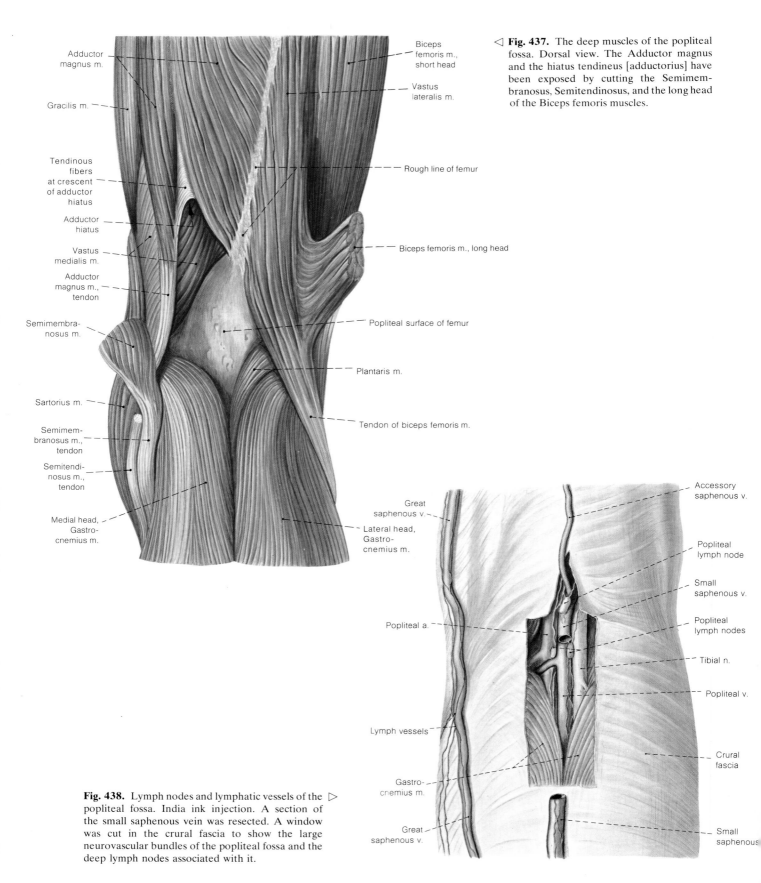

Adductor magnus m.

Gracilis m.

Tendinous fibers at crescent of adductor hiatus

Adductor hiatus

Vastus medialis m.

Adductor magnus m., tendon

Semimembranosus m.

Sartorius m.

Semimembranosus m., tendon

Semitendinosus m., tendon

Medial head, Gastrocnemius m.

Biceps femoris m., short head

Vastus lateralis m.

Rough line of femur

Biceps femoris m., long head

Popliteal surface of femur

Plantaris m.

Tendon of biceps femoris m.

Lateral head, Gastrocnemius m.

◁ **Fig. 437.** The deep muscles of the popliteal fossa. Dorsal view. The Adductor magnus and the hiatus tendineus [adductorius] have been exposed by cutting the Semimembranosus, Semitendinosus, and the long head of the Biceps femoris muscles.

Great saphenous v.

Popliteal a.

Lymph vessels

Gastrocnemius m.

Great saphenous v.

Accessory saphenous v.

Popliteal lymph node

Small saphenous v.

Popliteal lymph nodes

Tibial n.

Popliteal v.

Crural fascia

Small saphenous

Fig. 438. Lymph nodes and lymphatic vessels of the ▷ popliteal fossa. India ink injection. A section of the small saphenous vein was resected. A window was cut in the crural fascia to show the large neurovascular bundles of the popliteal fossa and the deep lymph nodes associated with it.

Muscles of the Posterior Compartment of the Leg (Figs. 437, 470, 471)

Name	Origin	Insertion
1. Gastrocnemius muscle		
Medial head	Medial condyle of femur; capsule of knee	Aponeurosis units with the tendon of the Soleus muscle to form the tendo calcaneus
Lateral head	Lateral condyle of femur; capsule of knee	
2. Soleus muscle (with Gastrocnemius, occasionally described as Triceps surae muscle)	Posterior surface of head and upper third of fibula; soleal line and middle third of medial border of tibia; tendinous arch (transverse intermuscular septum) between the tibia and fibula	
3. Plantaris muscle	Lateral condyle of femur	Posterior part of calcaneus in front or side of the calcaneal tendon (with long thin tendon)

Nerve:　　Tibial nerve

Function:　Plantar flexion of foot and tends to supinate it; Gastrocnemius muscle points the toe (with Plantaris); flexes knee; braces knee and ankle joints when standing

4. Popliteus muscle	Tendon from lateral condyle of femur; somewhat from the oblique popliteal ligament	Posterior surface of tibia, proximal to soleal line (Fig. 471)

Nerve:　　Tibial nerve

Function:　Flexes leg; rotates femur medially to help unlock dead center

---

NOTE: The oblique origin of the Soleus muscle arises through a tendinous arch of the Soleus muscle fissure, through this the popliteal vessels and tibial nerve leave the popliteal space distally and arrive in the deep region of the calf.

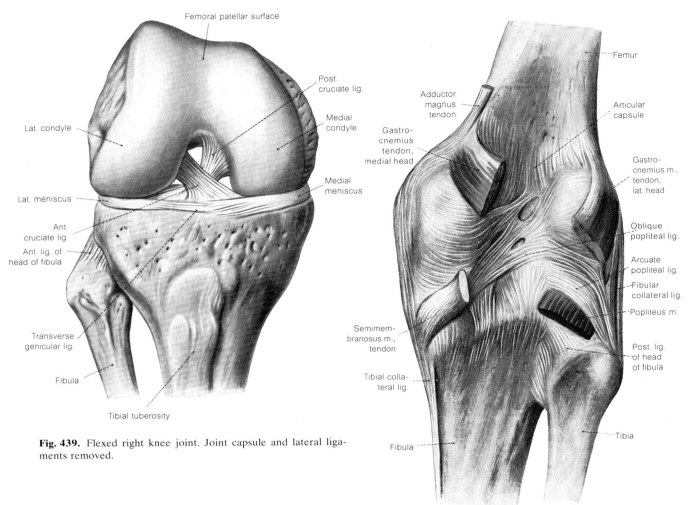

Fig. 439. Flexed right knee joint. Joint capsule and lateral ligaments removed.

Fig. 440. Extended right knee joint. Dorsal view.

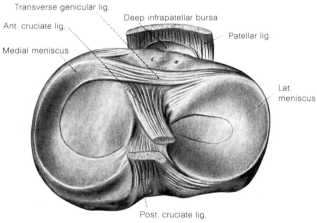

Fig. 441. Condyles of the tibia with both menisci and the origin of the cruciate ligaments (ligamenta cruciata genus) of the knee.

Fig. 442. Arterial supply of the menisci and surrounding structures. ▷ After H. Sick and J. G. Koritké: La vascularisation des ménisques de l'articulation du genou. Z. Anat. Entwickl.-Gesch. 129, 359–379 (1969).

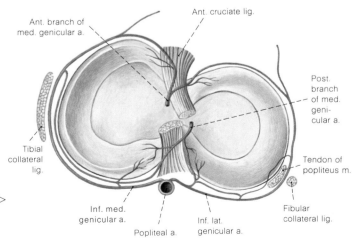

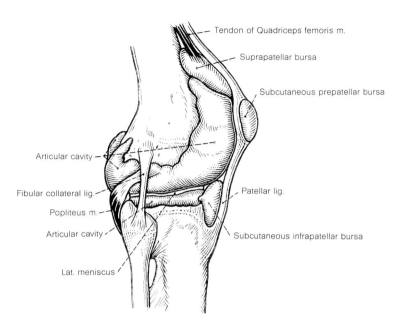

Tendon of Quadriceps femoris m.

Suprapatellar bursa

Subcutaneous prepatellar bursa

Articular cavity

Fibular collateral lig.

Popliteus m.

Articular cavity

Patellar lig.

Subcutaneous infrapatellar bursa

Lat. meniscus

Fig. 443. Joint effusion of the right knee joint. Lateral view.

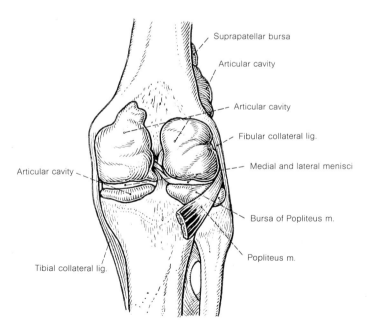

Suprapatellar bursa

Articular cavity

Articular cavity

Fibular collateral lig.

Medial and lateral menisci

Articular cavity

Bursa of Popliteus m.

Popliteus m.

Tibial collateral lig.

Fig. 444. Joint effusion of the right knee joint. Dorsal view.

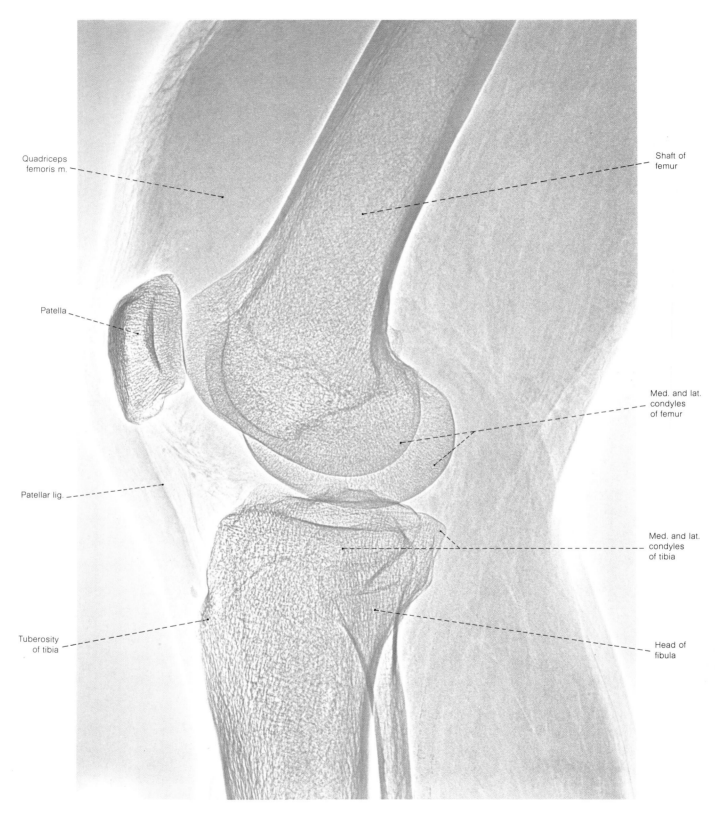

Quadriceps
femoris m.

Patella

Patellar lig.

Tuberosity
of tibia

Shaft of
femur

Med. and lat.
condyles
of femur

Med. and lat.
condyles
of tibia

Head of
fibula

Fig. 445. Xeroradiogram of the left knee joint in slight flexion (lateral view). Note the good visibility of soft tissue structures, muscles and tendons. (Photo: Prof. Dr. D. KAUFFMANN, Zentrum Radiologie am Klinikum der Universität Freiburg i. Brsg.)

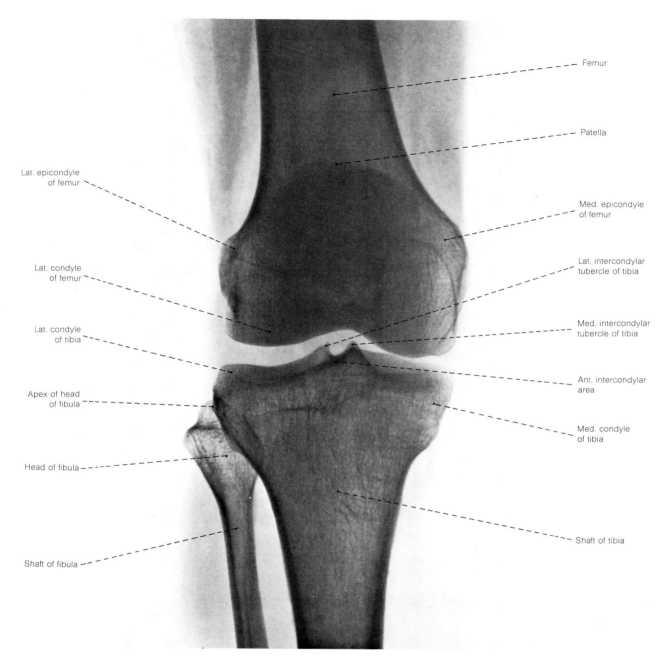

Fig. 446. X-ray film of the right knee joint (sagittal projection). (From L. WICKE: Atlas der Röntgenanatomie, 2nd ed. Urban & Schwarzenberg, Munich–Vienna–Baltimore 1980.)

◁

Xeroradiography is a roentgenologic method in which an electrostatically charged selenium surface is differentially discharged by ionizing rays. This causes an electrostatic charge image which corresponds to the image of the rays exiting from the body. By dusting with an electrically charged powder the image can be made optically visible, and can be melted by heat and thereby fixed. An important advantage of the method is that the increasingly scarce silver does not have to be used any more. Structural differences are enhanced in conventional roentgenography, in xeroradiography they are evened out, i.e., bony and soft tissue structures are easily visualized simultaneously.

307

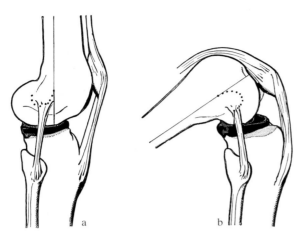

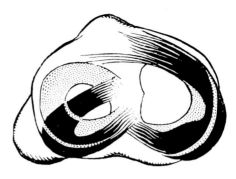

Fig. 447. Right knee joint, lateral view. a) Extended. b) Flexed. With stronger flexion, the meniscus, especially the lateral on the cartilaginous plate of the tibia (stippling) will be pushed backward.

Fig. 448. View of the left superior articular surface of the tibia. Position of meniscus in extension of knee joint, stippled; in flexion, black. Note the greater movement of the lateral meniscus. (Figs. 447 and 448 after H. VIRCHOW.) (From BENNINGHOFF/GOERTTLER: Lehrbuch der Anatomie der Menschen, Vol. 1, 13th ed. [Eds. H. FERNER and J. STAUBESAND]. Urban & Schwarzenberg, Munich–Vienna–Baltimore 1980.)

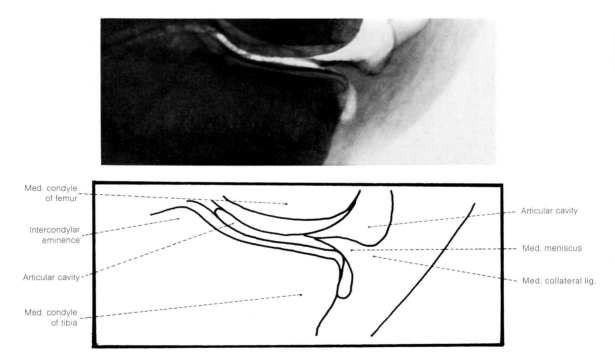

Med. condyle of femur

Intercondylar eminence

Articular cavity

Med. condyle of tibia

Articular cavity

Med. meniscus

Med. collateral lig.

Fig. 449. Arthrogram of knee joint, medial meniscus (sagittal projection). (From L. WICKE: Atlas der Röntgenanatomie, 2nd ed. Urban & Schwarzenberg, Munich–Vienna–Baltimore 1980.)

Fig. 450. Cutaneous nerves and veins of the dorsal aspect of right leg and foot. The fascia lata has been split along the small saphenous vein ▷ and the distal portion of the posterior femoral cutaneous nerve. * = clinically also called femoropopliteal vein.

Fig. 451. Cutaneous nerves and veins of the medial side of right leg and foot.

Leg

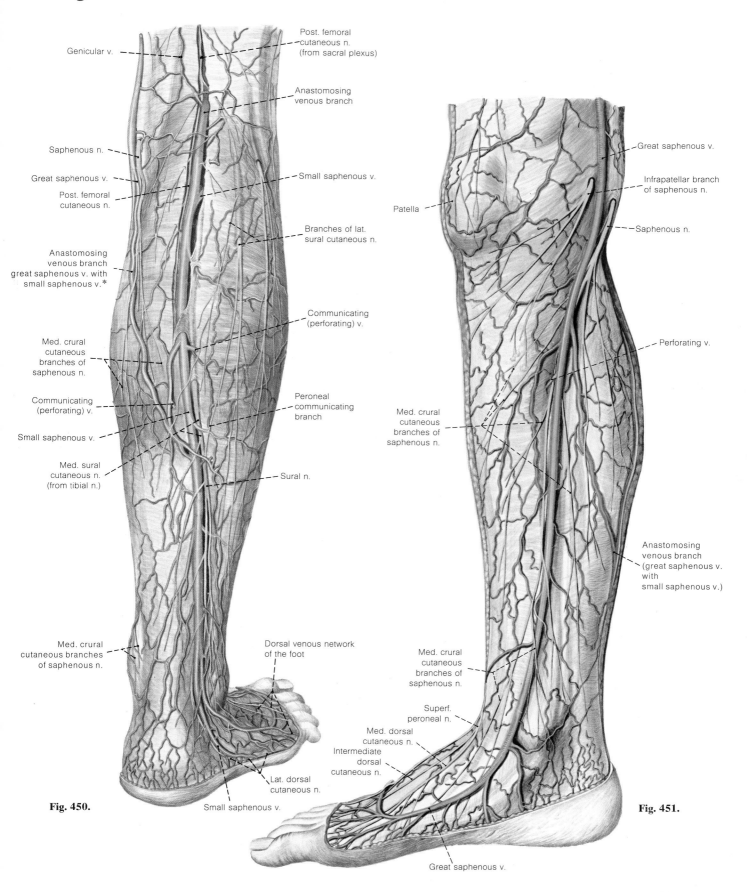

Genicular v.

Post. femoral cutaneous n. (from sacral plexus)

Anastomosing venous branch

Saphenous n.

Great saphenous v.

Post. femoral cutaneous n.

Small saphenous v.

Anastomosing venous branch great saphenous v. with small saphenous v.*

Branches of lat. sural cutaneous n.

Communicating (perforating) v.

Med. crural cutaneous branches of saphenous n.

Communicating (perforating) v.

Peroneal communicating branch

Small saphenous v.

Med. sural cutaneous n. (from tibial n.)

Sural n.

Med. crural cutaneous branches of saphenous n.

Dorsal venous network of the foot

Lat. dorsal cutaneous n.

Small saphenous v.

Fig. 450.

Great saphenous v.

Infrapatellar branch of saphenous n.

Patella

Saphenous n.

Perforating v.

Med. crural cutaneous branches of saphenous n.

Anastomosing venous branch (great saphenous v. with small saphenous v.)

Med. crural cutaneous branches of saphenous n.

Superf. peroneal n.

Med. dorsal cutaneous n.

Intermediate dorsal cutaneous n.

Great saphenous v.

Fig. 451.

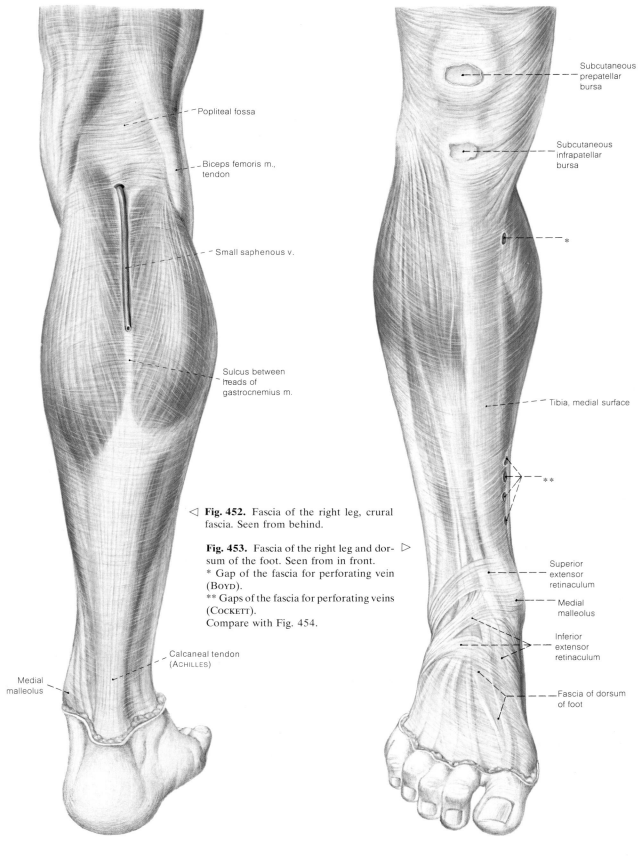

Popliteal fossa

Biceps femoris m., tendon

Small saphenous v.

Sulcus between heads of gastrocnemius m.

Medial malleolus

Calcaneal tendon (ACHILLES)

Subcutaneous prepatellar bursa

Subcutaneous infrapatellar bursa

*

Tibia, medial surface

**

Superior extensor retinaculum

Medial malleolus

Inferior extensor retinaculum

Fascia of dorsum of foot

◁ **Fig. 452.** Fascia of the right leg, crural fascia. Seen from behind.

Fig. 453. Fascia of the right leg and dorsum of the foot. Seen from in front. ▷
* Gap of the fascia for perforating vein (BOYD).
** Gaps of the fascia for perforating veins (COCKETT).
Compare with Fig. 454.

Those veins that connect superficial (= epifascial) with deep (= subfascial) ones through the fascia are called perforating veins. These anastomoses are medically important in relation to formation and treatment of varicose veins. Especially important perforating veins are named, in clinical usage, with the proper name of their first describers, e.g., DODD's perforating veins at the level of the adductor canal, BOYD's perforating vein at the level of the tuberosity of the tibia, and the three perforating veins of COCKETT at the medial side of the leg (see Fig. 454). (From R. MAY in MAY/PARTSCH/STAUBESAND [Eds.]: Venae perforantes. Urban & Schwarzenberg, Munich–Vienna–Baltimore 1981.)

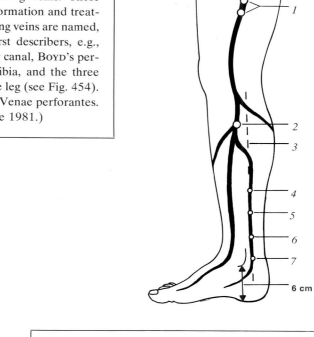

1	DODD's group	*5* COCKETT III	18.5 cm
2	BOYD's perforating v.	*6* COCKETT II	13.5 cm
3	LINTON's line	*7* COCKETT I	6–7 cm
4	24-cm-perforating v.		

△

Fig. 454. Diagram of clinically important perforating veins of the lower extremity, medial side.

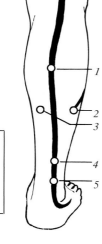

1	Gastrocnemial point
2	Lat. perforating v.
3	Soleus point
4	12-cm-perforating v.
5	BASSI's perforating v.

△

Fig. 455. Diagram of clinically important perforating veins of the dorsal side of the leg.

Fig. 456. Diagram of clinically important perforating veins in the ▷ region of the medial malleolus (= KUSTER's perforating veins). P_1 about 90° and 2.6 cm anterior to the medial malleolus, P_2 about 200° and 2.8 cm below the medial malleolus, P_3 about 180° and 3.4 cm below the medial malleolus, P_4 about 136° and 3.5 cm distal to the medial malleolus.

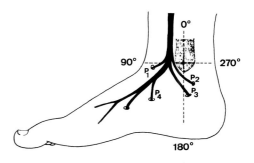

Fig. 457. Diagram of clinically important perforating veins in the ▷ region of the lateral malleolus (= KUSTER's perforating veins). P_1 about 90° and 2.6 cm in front of the lateral malleolus, P_2 about 230° and 2.8 cm below the lateral malleolus, P_3 about 180° and 3.4 cm below the lateral malleolus, P_4 about 146° and 4.4 cm distal to the lateral malleolus, P_5 about 138° at the level of the tuberosity of the metatarsal bone. (From R. MAY in MAY/PARTSCH/STAUBESAND [Eds.]: Venae perforantes. Urban & Schwarzenberg, Munich–Vienna–Baltimore 1981.)

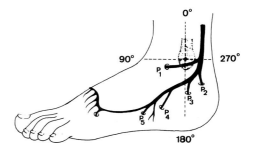

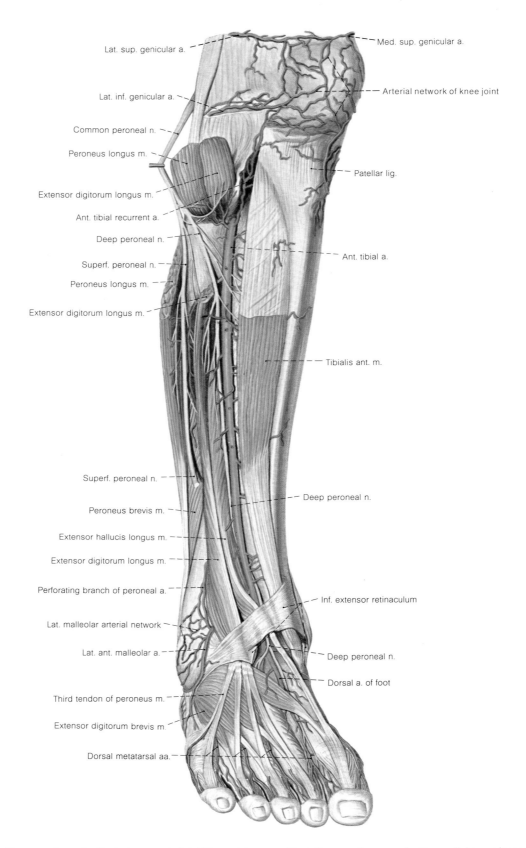

Lat. sup. genicular a.

Med. sup. genicular a.

Lat. inf. genicular a.

Arterial network of knee joint

Common peroneal n.

Peroneus longus m.

Extensor digitorum longus m.

Patellar lig.

Ant. tibial recurrent a.

Deep peroneal n.

Superf. peroneal n.

Ant. tibial a.

Peroneus longus m.

Extensor digitorum longus m.

Tibialis ant. m.

Superf. peroneal n.

Deep peroneal n.

Peroneus brevis m.

Extensor hallucis longus m.

Extensor digitorum longus m.

Perforating branch of peroneal a.

Inf. extensor retinaculum

Lat. malleolar arterial network

Lat. ant. malleolar a.

Deep peroneal n.

Dorsal a. of foot

Third tendon of peroneus m.

Extensor digitorum brevis m.

Dorsal metatarsal aa.

Fig. 458. Nerves and vessels of anterior aspect of right leg and dorsum of foot. Peroneus longus and extensor digitorum longus muscles have been sectioned in order to expose the peroneal nerve and its ramifications. The inferior extensor retinaculum has been partially removed.

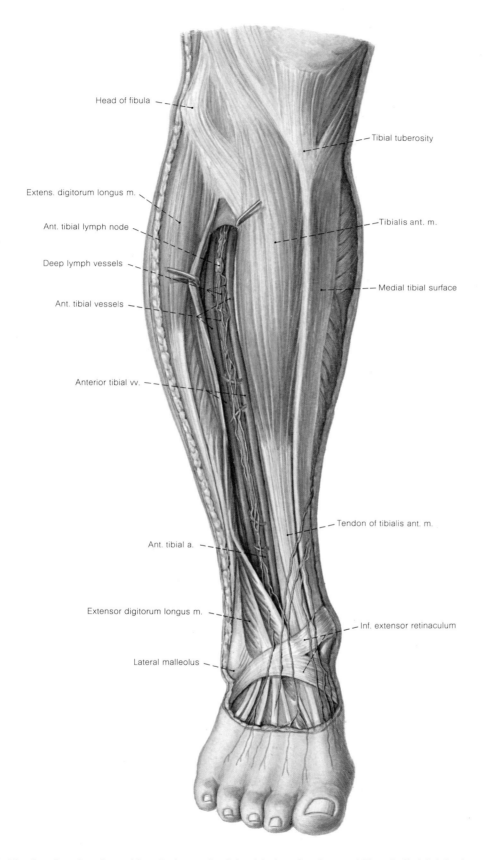

Head of fibula

Extens. digitorum longus m.

Ant. tibial lymph node

Deep lymph vessels

Ant. tibial vessels

Anterior tibial vv.

Ant. tibial a.

Extensor digitorum longus m.

Lateral malleolus

Tibial tuberosity

Tibialis ant. m.

Medial tibial surface

Tendon of tibialis ant. m.

Inf. extensor retinaculum

Fig. 459. The deep lymph nodes and lymphatic vessels of the right leg of an 8-year old boy. India ink injection. After elimination of the crural fascia and retraction of extensor muscles, the deep lymphatic vessels and a lymph node are shown where they accompany the anterior tibial vessels.

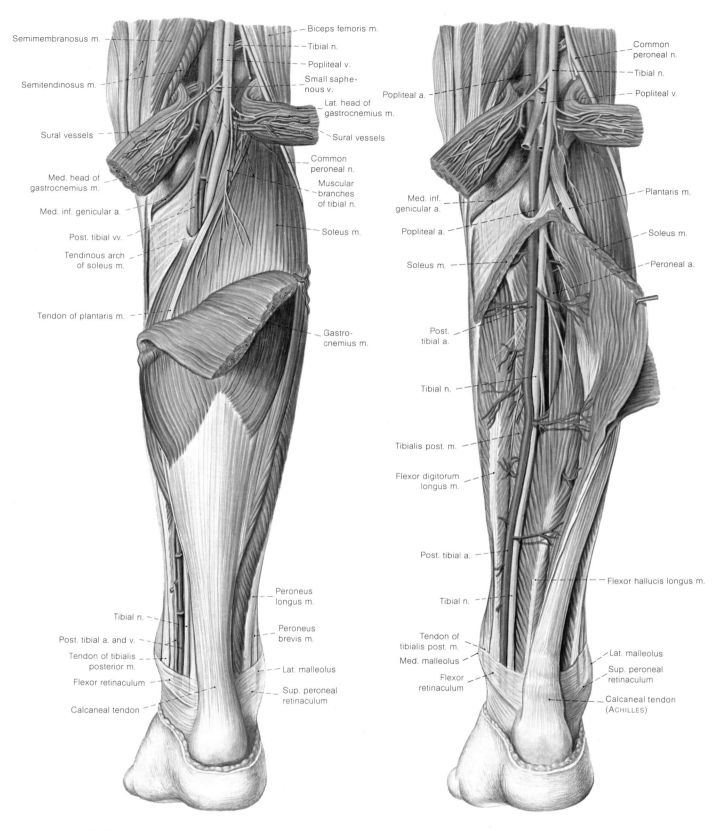

Semimembranosus m.

Semitendinosus m.

Sural vessels

Med. head of
gastrocnemius m.

Med. inf. genicular a.

Post. tibial vv.

Tendinous arch
of soleus m.

Tendon of plantaris m.

Tibial n.

Post. tibial a. and v.

Tendon of tibialis
posterior m.

Flexor retinaculum

Calcaneal tendon

Biceps femoris m.

Tibial n.

Popliteal v.

Small saphe-
nous v.

Lat. head of
gastrocnemius m.

Sural vessels

Common
peroneal n.

Muscular
branches
of tibial n.

Soleus m.

Gastro-
cnemius m.

Peroneus
longus m.

Peroneus
brevis m.

Lat. malleolus

Sup. peroneal
retinaculum

Popliteal a.

Med. inf.
genicular a.

Popliteal a.

Soleus m.

Post.
tibial a.

Tibial n.

Tibialis post. m.

Flexor digitorum
longus m.

Post. tibial a.

Tibial n.

Tendon of
tibialis post. m.

Med. malleolus

Flexor
retinaculum

Common
peroneal n.

Tibial n.

Popliteal v.

Plantaris m.

Soleus m.

Peroneal a.

Flexor hallucis longus m.

Lat. malleolus

Sup. peroneal
retinaculum

Calcaneal tendon
(ACHILLES)

Fig. 460. Superficial nerves and vessels of the dorsal aspect of the right leg.

Fig. 461. Middle layer of nerves and vessels of dorsal aspect of right leg. Preparation as in Fig. 460 but the soleus muscle has been sectioned and pulled sideward.

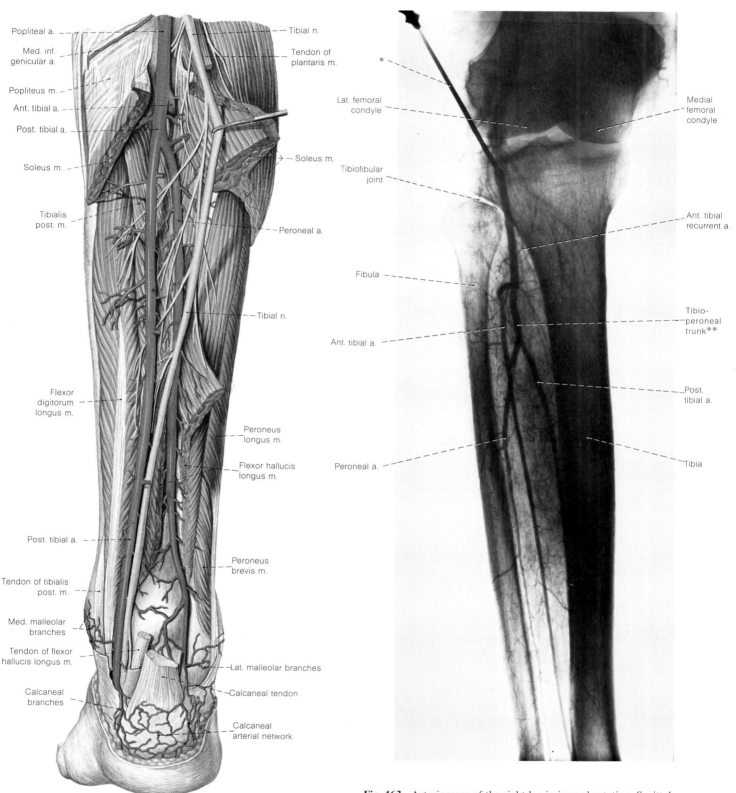

Popliteal a.

Med. inf. genicular a.

Popliteus m.

Ant. tibial a.

Post. tibial a.

Soleus m.

Tibialis post. m.

Flexor digitorum longus m.

Post. tibial a.

Tendon of tibialis post. m.

Med. malleolar branches

Tendon of flexor hallucis longus m.

Calcaneal branches

Tibial n.

Tendon of plantaris m.

Soleus m.

Peroneal a.

Tibial n.

Peroneus longus m.

Flexor hallucis longus m.

Peroneus brevis m.

Lat. malleolar branches

Calcaneal tendon

Calcaneal arterial network

Fig. 462. Deep nerves and vessels of posterior aspect of right leg.

*

Lat. femoral condyle

Tibiofibular joint

Fibula

Ant. tibial a.

Peroneal a.

Medial femoral condyle

Ant. tibial recurrent a.

Tibio-peroneal trunk**

Post. tibial a.

Tibia

Fig. 463. Arteriogram of the right leg in inward rotation. Sagittal projection. (Original: Dr. F. PLATZ, Anatomical Institute, University of Freiburg i. Brsg.) * Canula in the popliteal artery; ** clinically important.

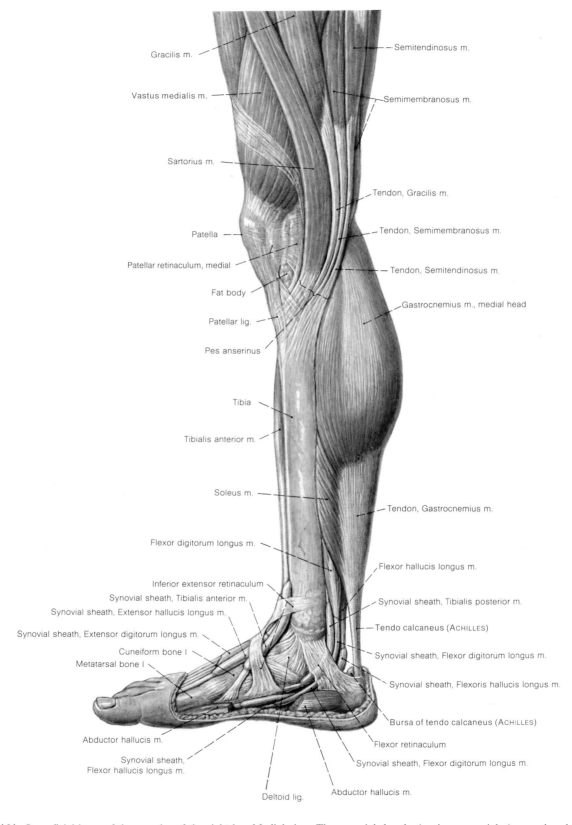

Gracilis m.

Vastus medialis m.

Sartorius m.

Patella

Patellar retinaculum, medial

Fat body

Patellar lig.

Pes anserinus

Tibia

Tibialis anterior m.

Soleus m.

Flexor digitorum longus m.

Inferior extensor retinaculum
Synovial sheath, Tibialis anterior m.
Synovial sheath, Extensor hallucis longus m.

Synovial sheath, Extensor digitorum longus m.

Cuneiform bone I
Metatarsal bone I

Abductor hallucis m.

Synovial sheath,
Flexor hallucis longus m.

Deltoid lig.

Semitendinosus m.

Semimembranosus m.

Tendon, Gracilis m.

Tendon, Semimembranosus m.

Tendon, Semitendinosus m.

Gastrocnemius m., medial head

Tendon, Gastrocnemius m.

Flexor hallucis longus m.

Synovial sheath, Tibialis posterior m.

Tendo calcaneus (ACHILLES)

Synovial sheath, Flexor digitorum longus m.

Synovial sheath, Flexoris hallucis longus m.

Bursa of tendo calcaneus (ACHILLES)

Flexor retinaculum

Synovial sheath, Flexor digitorum longus m.

Abductor hallucis m.

Fig. 464. Superficial layer of the muscles of the right leg. Medial view. The synovial sheaths (vaginae synoviales) are colored blue.

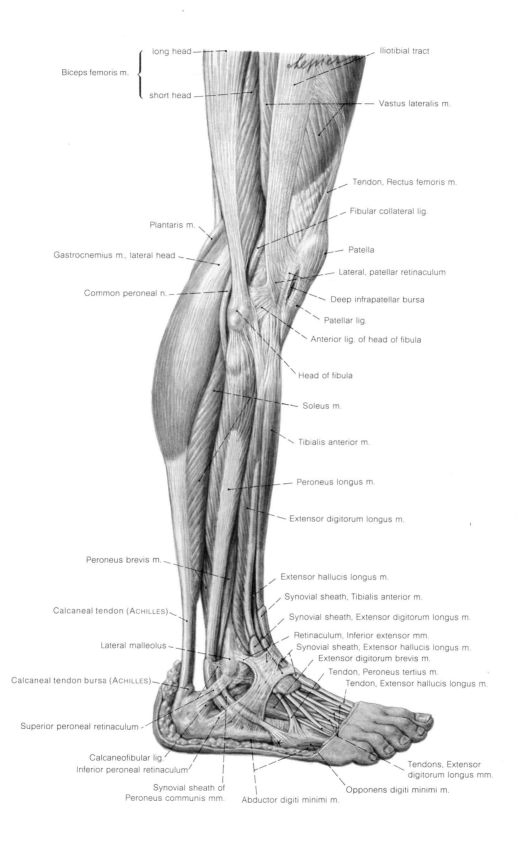

Biceps femoris m. { long head
short head

long head — Iliotibial tract

Vastus lateralis m.

Tendon, Rectus femoris m.

Fibular collateral lig.

Plantaris m.

Gastrocnemius m., lateral head

Patella

Lateral, patellar retinaculum

Common peroneal n.

Deep infrapatellar bursa

Patellar lig.

Anterior lig. of head of fibula

Head of fibula

Soleus m.

Tibialis anterior m.

Peroneus longus m.

Extensor digitorum longus m.

Peroneus brevis m.

Extensor hallucis longus m.

Synovial sheath, Tibialis anterior m.

Synovial sheath, Extensor digitorum longus m.

Calcaneal tendon (ACHILLES)

Retinaculum, Inferior extensor mm.

Synovial sheath, Extensor hallucis longus m.

Lateral malleolus

Extensor digitorum brevis m.

Tendon, Peroneus tertius m.

Calcaneal tendon bursa (ACHILLES)

Tendon, Extensor hallucis longus m.

Superior peroneal retinaculum

Calcaneofibular lig.

Inferior peroneal retinaculum

Synovial sheath of
Peroneus communis mm.

Abductor digiti minimi m.

Tendons, Extensor
digitorum longus mm.

Opponens digiti minimi m.

Fig. 465. The superficial layer of muscles of the right leg. Lateral view. The synovial sheaths (vaginae synoviales) are colored blue.
* = tuberositas of metatarsal bone.

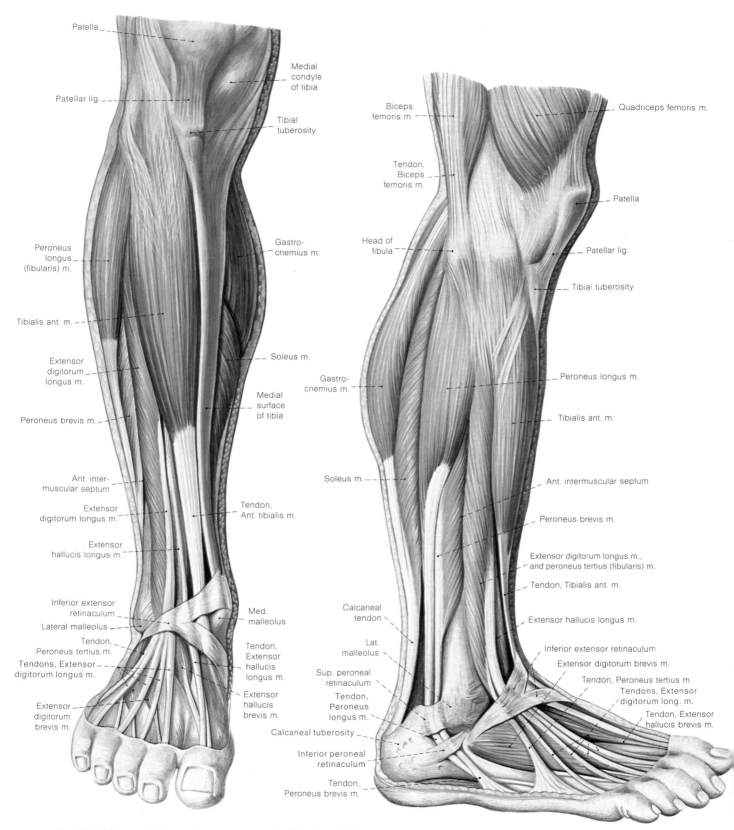

Fig. 466. Muscles of the anterior compartments of the leg and the dorsum of the foot. The superior extensor retinaculum was removed; the inferior extensor retinaculum was retained.

Fig. 467. Muscles of the leg and dorsum of the foot, seen from the lateral side. The fascia was removed as far as the retinacula.

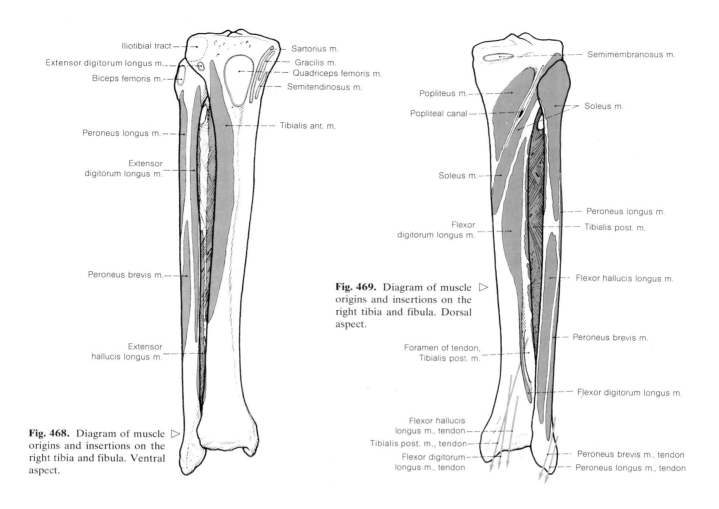

Fig. 468. Diagram of muscle ▷ origins and insertions on the right tibia and fibula. Ventral aspect.

Fig. 469. Diagram of muscle ▷ origins and insertions on the right tibia and fibula. Dorsal aspect.

Muscles of the Anterior Compartment of the Leg (Figs. 466, 467)

Name	Origin	Insertion
1. Tibialis anterior muscle With long tendon running under the retinaculum of the superior and inferior extensor muscles	Lateral condyle; upper half of lateral surface of tibia; interosseous membrane; crural fascia	Base of 1st metatarsal (medial edge); medial cuneiform (I) (plantar surface)
Nerve: Branch of deep peroneal (fibularis) nerve (L 4, 5; S 1)		
Function: Dorsally flexes and supinates (adducts and inverts) the foot		
2. Extensor hallucis longus muscle	Middle half of fibular and interosseous membrane; crural fascia	Base of distal phalanx of great toe
3. Extensor digitorum longus muscle Tendon fixed by the retinacula of the superior and inferior	Lateral condyle of tibia; proximal ¾ of fibula; interosseous membrane; crural fascia, anterior intermuscular septum of leg	Tendons to 2nd and terminal phalanges of 4 lateral toes
4. Peroneus (fibularis) tertius muscle	Distal third of shaft of fibula; interosseous membrane	Dorsal surface, fifth metatarsal bone (flat tendon)
Nerve: Deep peroneal (fibular) nerve (L 4, 5; S 1)		
Function: Extends toes; dorsiflexes ankle joint at the same time the Extensor digitorum longus muscle pronates and abducts the foot; also the Extensor hallucis longus muscle supinates the foot		

319

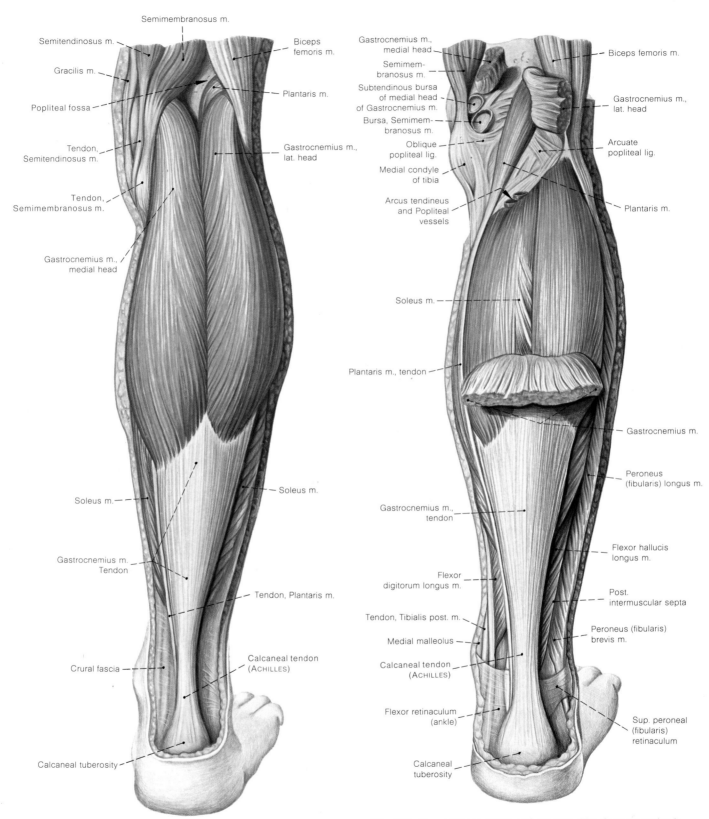

Semimembranosus m.

Semitendinosus m.

Gracilis m.

Popliteal fossa

Tendon, Semitendinosus m.

Tendon, Semimembranosus m.

Gastrocnemius m., medial head

Soleus m.

Gastrocnemius m. Tendon

Crural fascia

Calcaneal tuberosity

Biceps femoris m.

Plantaris m.

Gastrocnemius m., lat. head

Soleus m.

Tendon, Plantaris m.

Calcaneal tendon (ACHILLES)

Fig. 470. Superficial view of the muscular components of the calf.

Gastrocnemius m., medial head

Semimembranosus m.

Subtendinous bursa of medial head of Gastrocnemius m.

Bursa, Semimembranosus m.

Oblique popliteal lig.

Medial condyle of tibia

Arcus tendineus and Popliteal vessels

Soleus m.

Plantaris m., tendon

Gastrocnemius m., tendon

Flexor digitorum longus m.

Tendon, Tibialis post. m.

Medial malleolus

Calcaneal tendon (ACHILLES)

Flexor retinaculum (ankle)

Calcaneal tuberosity

Biceps femoris m.

Gastrocnemius m., lat. head

Arcuate popliteal lig.

Plantaris m.

Gastrocnemius m.

Peroneus (fibularis) longus m.

Flexor hallucis longus m.

Post. intermuscular septa

Peroneus (fibularis) brevis m.

Sup. peroneal (fibularis) retinaculum

Fig. 471. Second layer of the calf muscles. The Gastrocnemius is cut and reflected; the deeper layer of crural fascia was removed up to the retinacula.

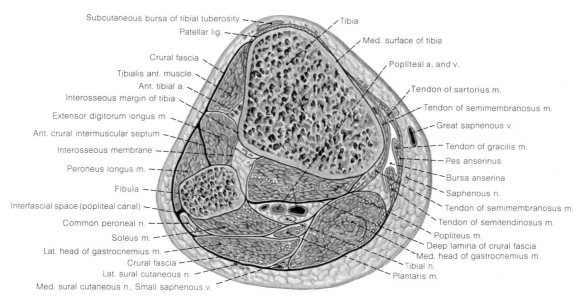

Fig. 472. Cross section through proximal third of right leg. Sectioned surface seen from distal.

Subcutaneous bursa of tibial tuberosity
Patellar lig.
Crural fascia
Tibialis ant. muscle
Ant. tibial a.
Interosseous margin of tibia
Extensor digitorum longus m.
Ant. crural intermuscular septum
Interosseous membrane
Peroneus longus m.
Fibula
Interfascial space (popliteal canal)
Common peroneal n.
Soleus m.
Lat. head of gastrocnemius m.
Crural fascia
Lat. sural cutaneous n.
Med. sural cutaneous n., Small saphenous v.

Tibia
Med. surface of tibia
Popliteal a. and v.
Tendon of sartorius m.
Tendon of semimembranosus m.
Great saphenous v.
Tendon of gracilis m.
Pes anserinus
Bursa anserina
Saphenous n.
Tendon of semimembranosus m.
Tendon of semitendinosus m.
Popliteus m.
Deep lamina of crural fascia
Med. head of gastrocnemius m.
Tibial n.
Plantaris m.

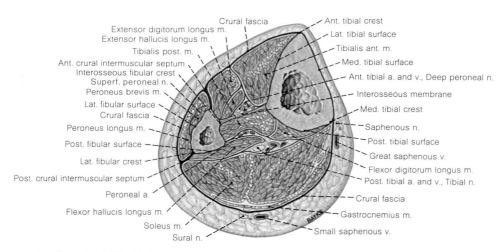

Fig. 473. Cross section through middle third of right leg. Sectioned surface seen from distal.

Crural fascia
Extensor digitorum longus m.
Extensor hallucis longus m.
Tibialis post. m.
Ant. crural intermuscular septum
Interosseous fibular crest
Superf. peroneal n.
Peroneus brevis m.
Lat. fibular surface
Crural fascia
Peroneus longus m.
Post. fibular surface
Lat. fibular crest
Post. crural intermuscular septum
Peroneal a.
Flexor hallucis longus m.
Soleus m.
Sural n.

Ant. tibial crest
Lat. tibial surface
Tibialis ant. m.
Med. tibial surface
Ant. tibial a. and v., Deep peroneal n.
Interosseous membrane
Med. tibial crest
Saphenous n.
Post. tibial surface
Great saphenous v.
Flexor digitorum longus m.
Post. tibial a. and v., Tibial n.
Crural fascia
Gastrocnemius m.
Small saphenous v.

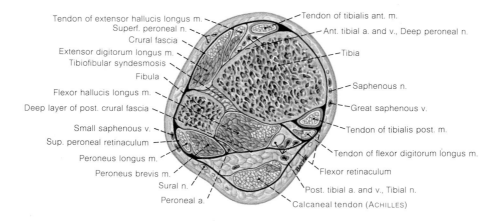

Fig. 474. Cross section through the right leg above the malleoli. Sectioned surface seen from distal.

Tendon of extensor hallucis longus m.
Superf. peroneal n.
Crural fascia
Extensor digitorum longus m.
Tibiofibular syndesmosis
Fibula
Flexor hallucis longus m.
Deep layer of post. crural fascia
Small saphenous v.
Sup. peroneal retinaculum
Peroneus longus m.
Peroneus brevis m.
Sural n.
Peroneal a.

Tendon of tibialis ant. m.
Ant. tibial a. and v., Deep peroneal n.
Tibia
Saphenous n.
Great saphenous v.
Tendon of tibialis post. m.
Tendon of flexor digitorum longus m.
Flexor retinaculum
Post. tibial a. and v., Tibial n.
Calcaneal tendon (ACHILLES)

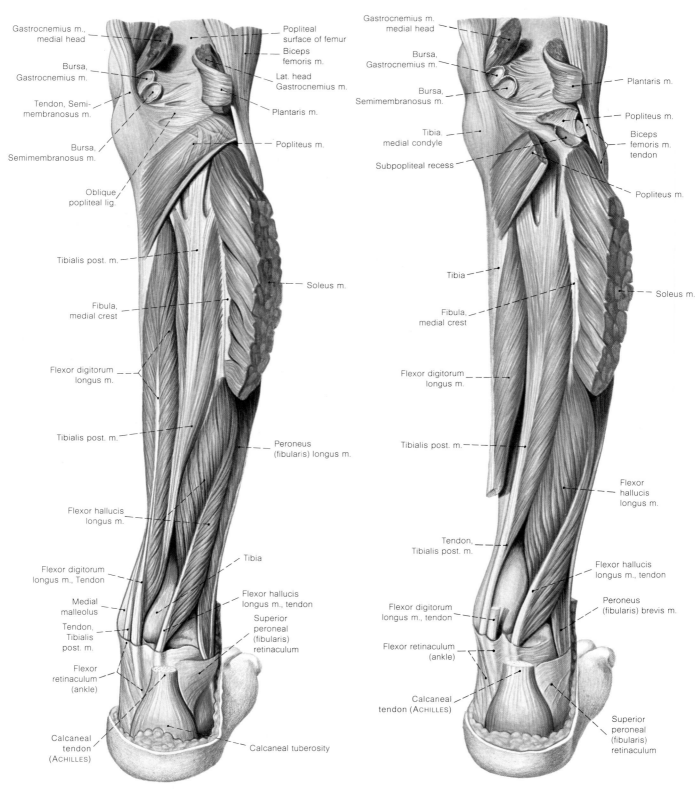

Gastrocnemius m., medial head

Bursa, Gastrocnemius m.

Tendon, Semimembranosus m.

Bursa, Semimembranosus m.

Oblique popliteal lig.

Tibialis post. m.

Fibula, medial crest

Flexor digitorum longus m.

Tibialis post. m.

Flexor hallucis longus m.

Flexor digitorum longus m., Tendon

Medial malleolus

Tendon, Tibialis post. m.

Flexor retinaculum (ankle)

Calcaneal tendon (ACHILLES)

Popliteal surface of femur

Biceps femoris m.

Lat. head Gastrocnemius m.

Plantaris m.

Popliteus m.

Soleus m.

Peroneus (fibularis) longus m.

Tibia

Flexor hallucis longus m., tendon

Superior peroneal (fibularis) retinaculum

Calcaneal tuberosity

Fig. 475. Deeper muscles of the posterior compartment of the leg. The Gastrocnemius, the Soleus, and the Plantaris muscles were removed or reflected.

Gastrocnemius m. medial head

Bursa, Gastrocnemius m.

Bursa, Semimembranosus m.

Tibia, medial condyle

Subpopliteal recess

Tibia

Fibula, medial crest

Flexor digitorum longus m.

Tibialis post. m.

Tendon, Tibialis post. m.

Flexor digitorum longus m., tendon

Flexor retinaculum (ankle)

Calcaneal tendon (ACHILLES)

Plantaris m.

Popliteus m.

Biceps femoris m. tendon

Popliteus m.

Soleus m.

Flexor hallucis longus m.

Flexor hallucis longus m., tendon

Peroneus (fibularis) brevis m.

Superior peroneal (fibularis) retinaculum

Fig. 476. Deepest layer of the muscular compartment of the calf. The Popliteus and Flexor digitorum longus muscles were transected.

Muscles of the Posterior Compartment of the Leg (Deep Layers) (Figs. 475, 476)

Name	Origin	Insertion
1. Tibialis posterior muscle	Posterior surface of the tibia (proximal part), interosseous membrane of the leg, medial surface of the fibula	Tuberosity of navicular bone; plantar surface of the 3 cuneiforms, sustentaculum tali of the calcaneus, bases of metatarsals 2 to 4

Function: Plantar flexes the foot, supinates (adducts and inverts)

2. Flexor digitorum longus muscle	Posterior surface and interosseus margin of the tibia, distal to soleal line with a tendinous arch from distal third of the fibula	By 4 tendons into bases of distal phalanges of toes 2 to 5

Function: Flexes terminal phalanges of toes 2–5, assists in plantar flexion, supination and adduction of the foot

3. Flexor hallucis longus muscle	Distal $^2/_3$ of posterior surface and margin of fibula, interosseus membrane of the leg, posterior intermuscular septum	Base of terminal phalanx of big toe

Nerve: Tibial nerve for all three muscles

Function: Flexes big toe, plantar flexion, supination, and adduction of foot

---

NOTE: The medial malleolar region contains from front to back: The tendons for the Tibialis posterior and Flexor digitorum longus muscles; the posterior tibial vessels, the tibial nerve and, deep dorsally, the tendon of the Flexor hallucis longus. A short tunnel is fashioned through the retinaculum, through which the structures of the deep calf region go to the sole of the foot (Fig. 505).

The lateral malleolar region contains the tendons of the Peroneus longus and Peroneus brevis muscles, which are fixed by a superior and inferior retinaculum (Fig. 504).

Muscles of the Lateral Compartment of the Leg (Figs. 467, 504)

Name	Origin	Insertion
1. Peroneus (fibularis) longus muscle The tendon is a cartilaginous thickening at the tuberosity of the cuboid bone	Head and upper $^2/_3$ of lateral surface and posterior margin of fibula; intermuscular septa	Long tendon ends on lateral side of the base of the 1st metatarsal bone and the lateral side of the medial cuneiform (Fig. 499)
2. Peroneus brevis muscle	Distal $^2/_3$ of the lateral surface and anterior margin of the fibula, intermuscular septa	Tuberosity at the base of the 5th metatarsal, tendon strip to little toe (Fig. 504)

Nerve: Superficial peroneal (fibularis) nerve

Function: Pronates (everts and abducts) and plantar flexes the foot

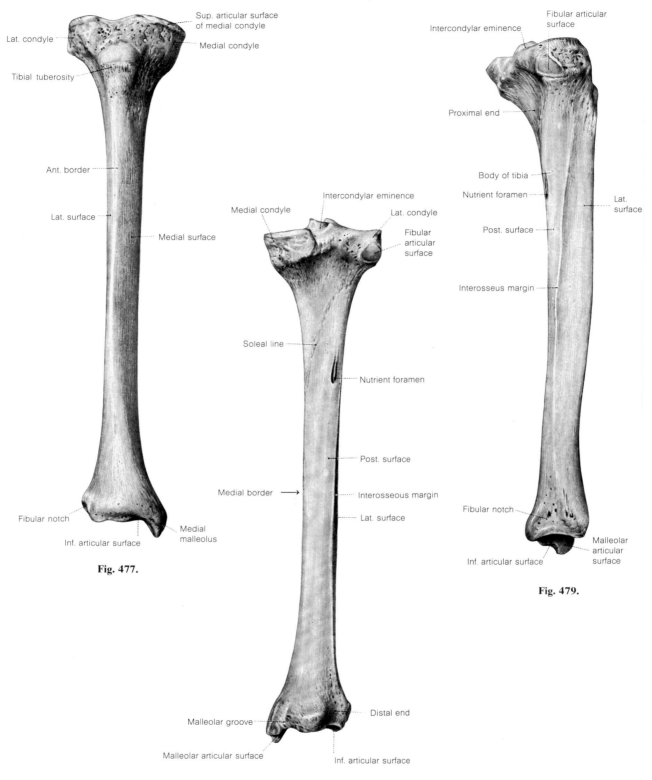

Fig. 477.

Sup. articular surface of medial condyle
Lat. condyle
Medial condyle
Tibial tuberosity
Ant. border
Lat. surface
Medial surface
Fibular notch
Inf. articular surface
Medial malleolus

Fig. 478.

Medial condyle
Intercondylar eminence
Lat. condyle
Fibular articular surface
Soleal line
Nutrient foramen
Post. surface
Medial border →
Interosseous margin
Lat. surface
Malleolar groove
Malleolar articular surface
Inf. articular surface
Distal end

Fig. 479.

Intercondylar eminence
Fibular articular surface
Proximal end
Body of tibia
Nutrient foramen
Post. surface
Lat. surface
Interosseus margin
Fibular notch
Inf. articular surface
Malleolar articular surface

Figs. 477–479. Right tibia. Fig. 477 Ventral view. Fig. 478 Dorsal view. Fig. 479 Lateral view.

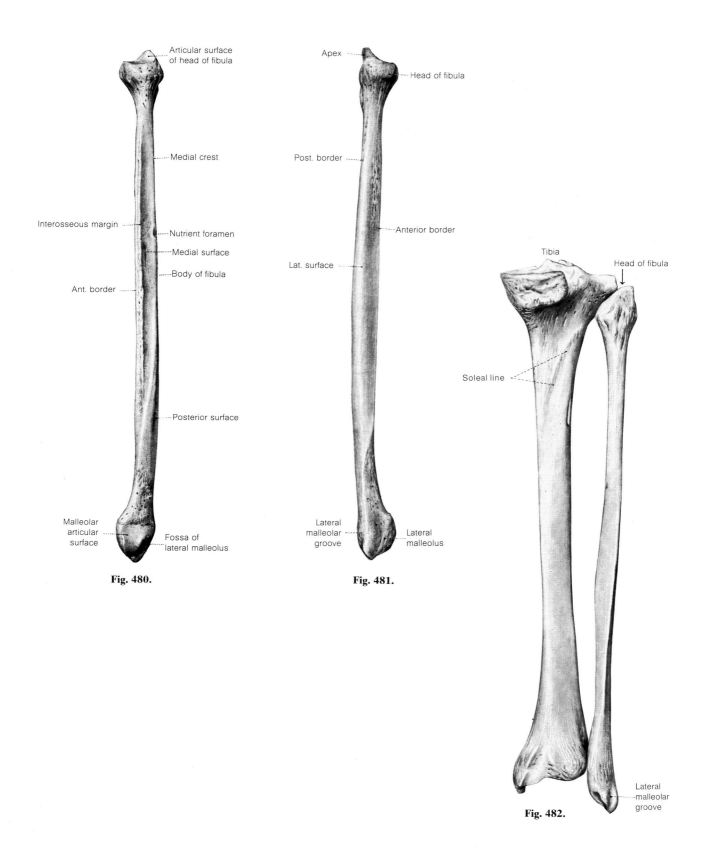

Fig. 480.

Fig. 481.

Fig. 482.

Figs. 480–482. Right fibula. Fig. 480. Medial view. Fig. 481. Lateral view. Fig. 482. Right tibia and fibula, dorsal view.

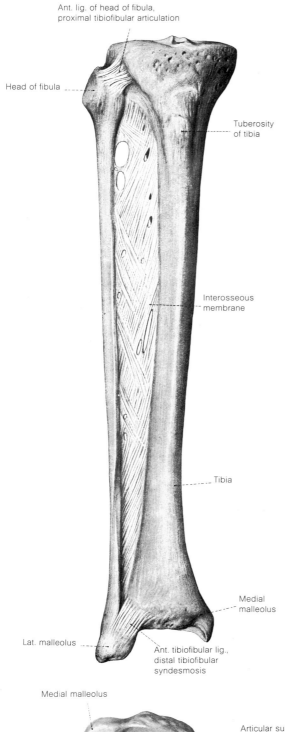

Ant. lig. of head of fibula, proximal tibiofibular articulation

Head of fibula

Tuberosity of tibia

Interosseous membrane

Tibia

Medial malleolus

Lat. malleolus

Ant. tibiofibular lig., distal tibiofibular syndesmosis

Medial malleolus

Articular surface, malleolus

Lat. malleolus

Medial malleolar articular surface

Inf. articular surface

◁ **Fig. 483.** The right tibiofibular articulations with their ligaments. Anterior view.

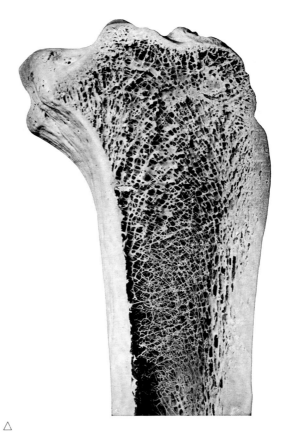

△ **Fig. 484.** Sagittal longitudinal section through the proximal end of the tibia.

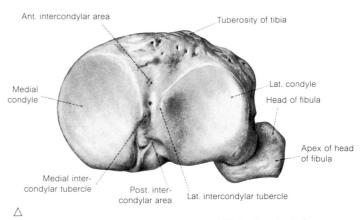

Ant. intercondylar area

Tuberosity of tibia

Medial condyle

Lat. condyle

Head of fibula

Apex of head of fibula

Medial intercondylar tubercle

Post. intercondylar area

Lat. intercondylar tubercle

△ **Fig. 485.** Proximal ends of the right tibia and fibula. Proximal view.

◁ **Fig. 486.** Distal ends of right tibia and fibula. Distal view.

Foot

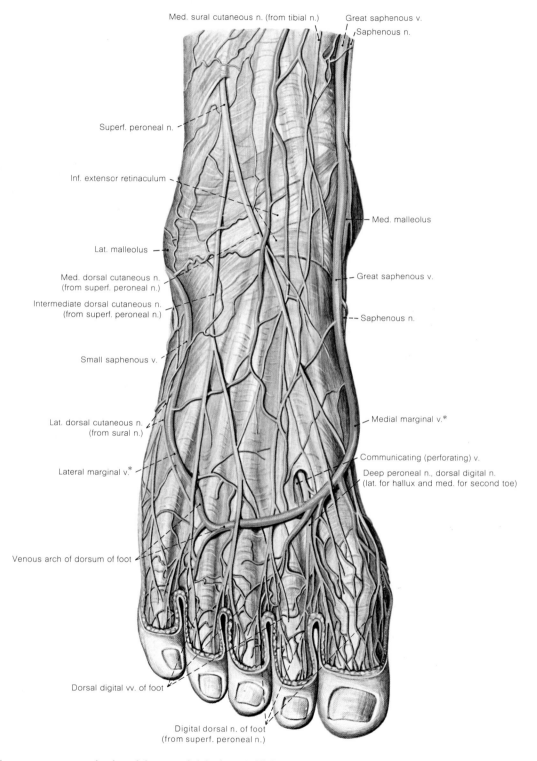

Med. sural cutaneous n. (from tibial n.)

Great saphenous v.

Saphenous n.

Superf. peroneal n.

Inf. extensor retinaculum

Med. malleolus

Lat. malleolus

Med. dorsal cutaneous n.
(from superf. peroneal n.)

Great saphenous v.

Intermediate dorsal cutaneous n.
(from superf. peroneal n.)

Saphenous n.

Small saphenous v.

Lat. dorsal cutaneous n.
(from sural n.)

Medial marginal v.*

Communicating (perforating) v.

Lateral marginal v.*

Deep peroneal n., dorsal digital n.
(lat. for hallux and med. for second toe)

Venous arch of dorsum of foot

Dorsal digital vv. of foot

Digital dorsal n. of foot
(from superf. peroneal n.)

Fig. 487. Cutaneous nerves and veins of dorsum of right foot. * Clinically important.

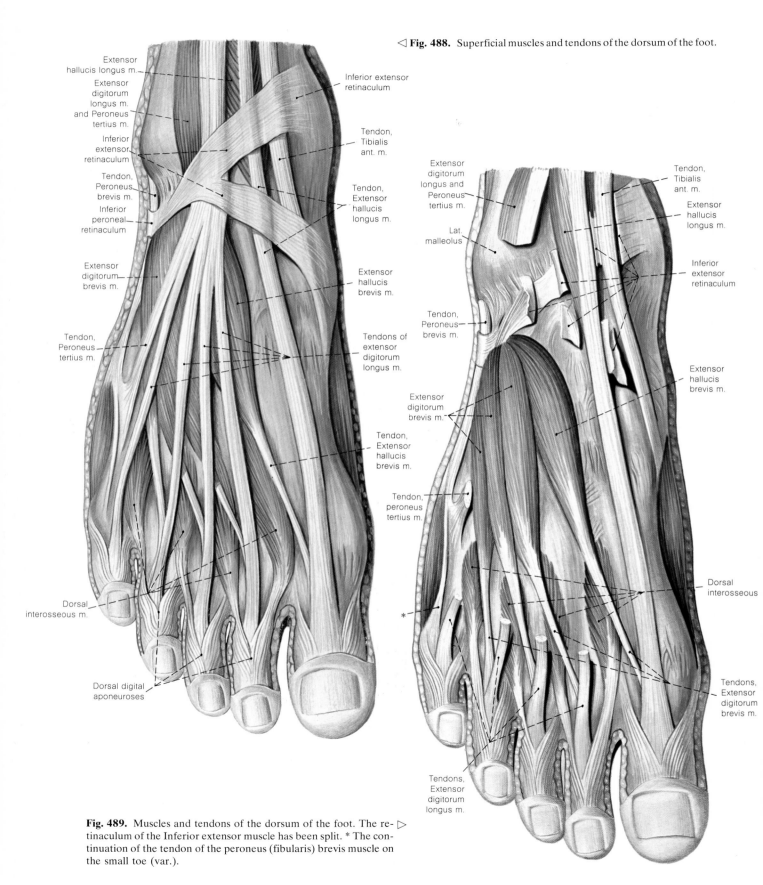

◁ **Fig. 488.** Superficial muscles and tendons of the dorsum of the foot.

Extensor hallucis longus m.

Extensor digitorum longus m. and Peroneus tertius m.

Inferior extensor retinaculum

Tendon, Peroneus brevis m.

Inferior peroneal retinaculum

Extensor digitorum brevis m.

Tendon, Peroneus tertius m.

Dorsal interosseous m.

Dorsal digital aponeuroses

Inferior extensor retinaculum

Tendon, Tibialis ant. m.

Tendon, Extensor hallucis longus m.

Extensor hallucis brevis m.

Tendons of extensor digitorum longus m.

Tendon, Extensor hallucis brevis m.

Extensor digitorum longus and Peroneus tertius m.

Lat. malleolus

Tendon, Peroneus brevis m.

Extensor digitorum brevis m.

Tendon, peroneus tertius m.

*

Tendon, Tibialis ant. m.

Extensor hallucis longus m.

Inferior extensor retinaculum

Extensor hallucis brevis m.

Dorsal interosseous

Tendons, Extensor digitorum brevis m.

Tendons, Extensor digitorum longus m.

Fig. 489. Muscles and tendons of the dorsum of the foot. The re- ▷ tinaculum of the Inferior extensor muscle has been split. * The continuation of the tendon of the peroneus (fibularis) brevis muscle on the small toe (var.).

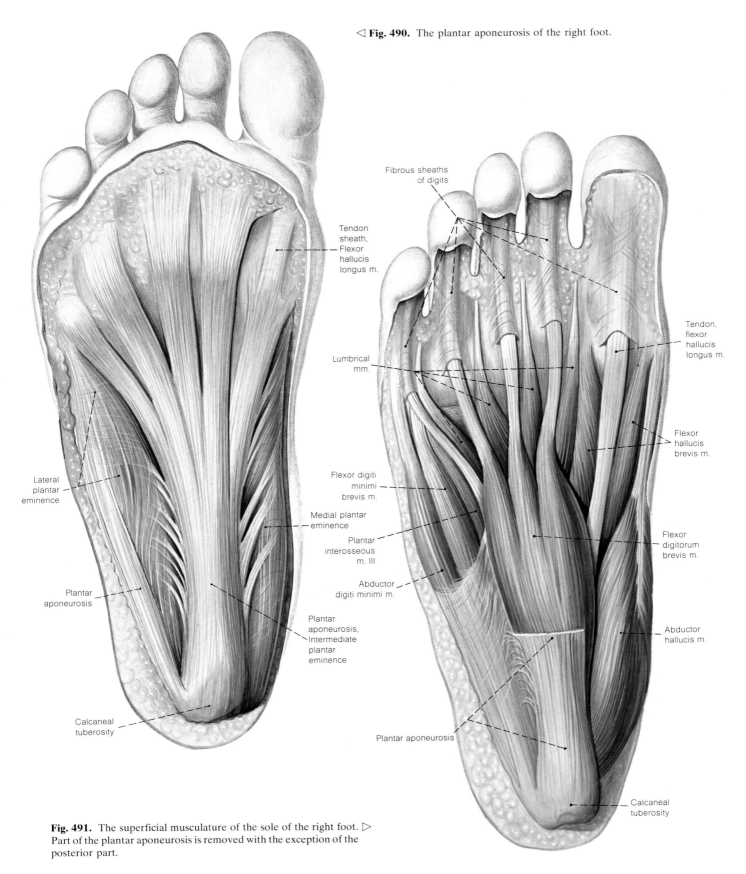

◁ **Fig. 490.** The plantar aponeurosis of the right foot.

Fibrous sheaths of digits

Tendon sheath, Flexor hallucis longus m.

Tendon, flexor hallucis longus m.

Lumbrical mm.

Flexor hallucis brevis m.

Lateral plantar eminence

Flexor digiti minimi brevis m.

Medial plantar eminence

Plantar interosseous m. III

Flexor digitorum brevis m.

Plantar aponeurosis

Abductor digiti minimi m.

Plantar aponeurosis, Intermediate plantar eminence

Abductor hallucis m.

Calcaneal tuberosity

Plantar aponeurosis

Calcaneal tuberosity

Fig. 491. The superficial musculature of the sole of the right foot. ▷ Part of the plantar aponeurosis is removed with the exception of the posterior part.

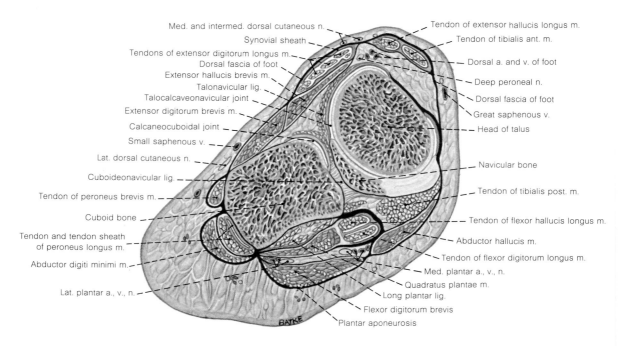

Med. and intermed. dorsal cutaneous n.
Synovial sheath
Tendons of extensor digitorum longus m.
Dorsal fascia of foot
Extensor hallucis brevis m.
Talonavicular lig.
Talocalcaveonavicular joint
Extensor digitorum brevis m.
Calcaneocuboidal joint
Small saphenous v.
Lat. dorsal cutaneous n.
Cuboideonavicular lig.
Tendon of peroneus brevis m.
Cuboid bone
Tendon and tendon sheath
of peroneus longus m.
Abductor digiti minimi m.
Lat. plantar a., v., n.

Tendon of extensor hallucis longus m.
Tendon of tibialis ant. m.
Dorsal a. and v. of foot
Deep peroneal n.
Dorsal fascia of foot
Great saphenous v.
Head of talus
Navicular bone
Tendon of tibialis post. m.
Tendon of flexor hallucis longus m.
Abductor hallucis m.
Tendon of flexor digitorum longus m.
Med. plantar a., v., n.
Quadratus plantae m.
Long plantar lig.
Flexor digitorum brevis
Plantar aponeurosis

Fig. 492. Cross section through the right tarsus in the area of the talus head. Sectioned surface seen from distal. Tendon sheaths and synovial membrane of joint capsules are shown in light blue.

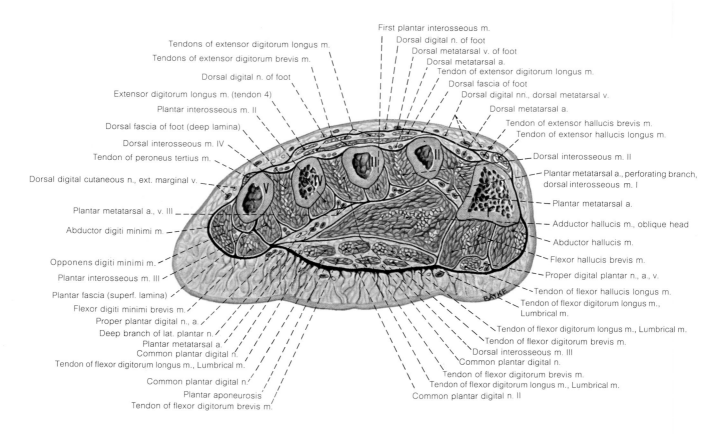

First plantar interosseous m.
Dorsal digital n. of foot
Dorsal metatarsal v. of foot
Dorsal metatarsal a.
Tendon of extensor digitorum longus m.
Dorsal fascia of foot
Dorsal digital nn., dorsal metatarsal v.
Dorsal metatarsal a.
Tendon of extensor hallucis brevis m.
Tendon of extensor hallucis longus m.
Dorsal interosseous m. II
Plantar metatarsal a., perforating branch,
dorsal interosseous m. I
Plantar metatarsal a.
Adductor hallucis m., oblique head
Abductor hallucis m.
Flexor hallucis brevis m.
Proper digital plantar n., a., v.
Tendon of flexor hallucis longus m.
Tendon of flexor digitorum longus m.,
Lumbrical m.
Tendon of flexor digitorum longus m., Lumbrical m.
Tendon of flexor digitorum brevis m.
Dorsal interosseous m. III
Common plantar digital n.
Tendon of flexor digitorum brevis m.
Tendon of flexor digitorum longus m., Lumbrical m.
Common plantar digital n. II

Tendons of extensor digitorum longus m.
Tendons of extensor digitorum brevis m.
Dorsal digital n. of foot
Extensor digitorum longus m. (tendon 4)
Plantar interosseous m. II
Dorsal fascia of foot (deep lamina)
Dorsal interosseous m. IV
Tendon of peroneus tertius m.
Dorsal digital cutaneous n., ext. marginal v.
Plantar metatarsal a., v. III
Abductor digiti minimi m.
Opponens digiti minimi m.
Plantar interosseous m. III
Plantar fascia (superf. lamina)
Flexor digiti minimi brevis m.
Proper plantar digital n., a.
Deep branch of lat. plantar n.
Plantar metatarsal a.
Common plantar digital n.
Tendon of flexor digitorum longus m., Lumbrical m.
Common plantar digital n.
Plantar aponeurosis
Tendon of flexor digitorum brevis m.

Fig. 493. Cross section through the right metatarsus. Sectioned surface seen from distal. I–V = first to fifth metacarpal bones.

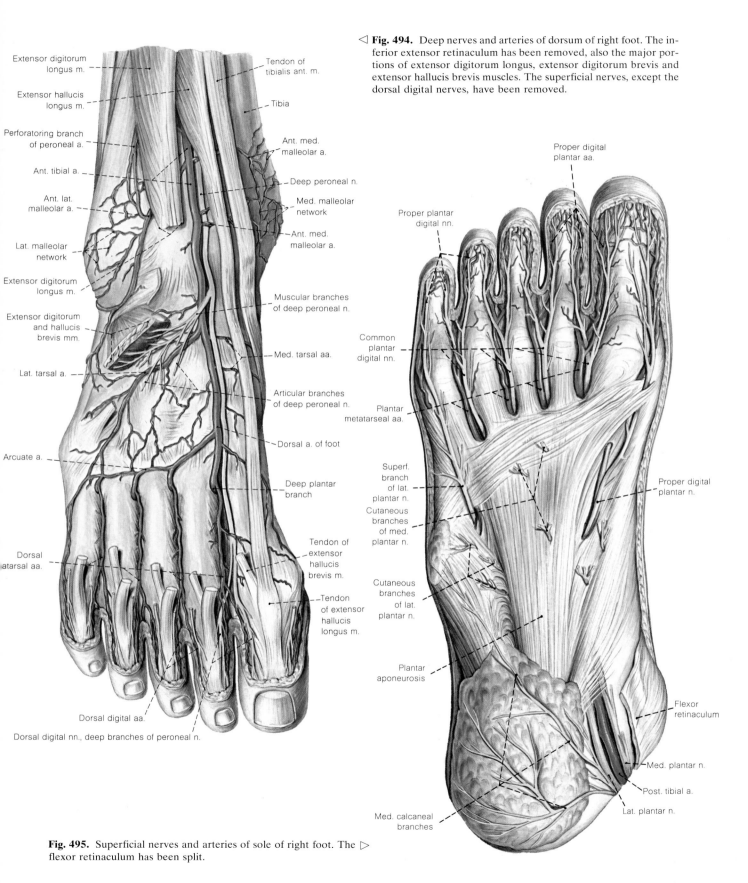

Extensor digitorum longus m.

Extensor hallucis longus m.

Perforatoring branch of peroneal a.

Ant. tibial a.

Ant. lat. malleolar a.

Lat. malleolar network

Extensor digitorum longus m.

Extensor digitorum and hallucis brevis mm.

Lat. tarsal a.

Arcuate a.

Dorsal atarsal aa.

Dorsal digital aa.

Dorsal digital nn., deep branches of peroneal n.

Tendon of tibialis ant. m.

Tibia

Ant. med. malleolar a.

Deep peroneal n.

Med. malleolar network

Ant. med. malleolar a.

Muscular branches of deep peroneal n.

Med. tarsal aa.

Articular branches of deep peroneal n.

Dorsal a. of foot

Deep plantar branch

Tendon of extensor hallucis brevis m.

Tendon of extensor hallucis longus m.

Fig. 494. Deep nerves and arteries of dorsum of right foot. The inferior extensor retinaculum has been removed, also the major portions of extensor digitorum longus, extensor digitorum brevis and extensor hallucis brevis muscles. The superficial nerves, except the dorsal digital nerves, have been removed.

Proper digital plantar aa.

Proper plantar digital nn.

Common plantar digital nn.

Plantar metatarseal aa.

Superf. branch of lat. plantar n.

Cutaneous branches of med. plantar n.

Cutaneous branches of lat. plantar n.

Plantar aponeurosis

Med. calcaneal branches

Proper digital plantar n.

Flexor retinaculum

Med. plantar n.

Post. tibial a.

Lat. plantar n.

Fig. 495. Superficial nerves and arteries of sole of right foot. The ▷ flexor retinaculum has been split.

331

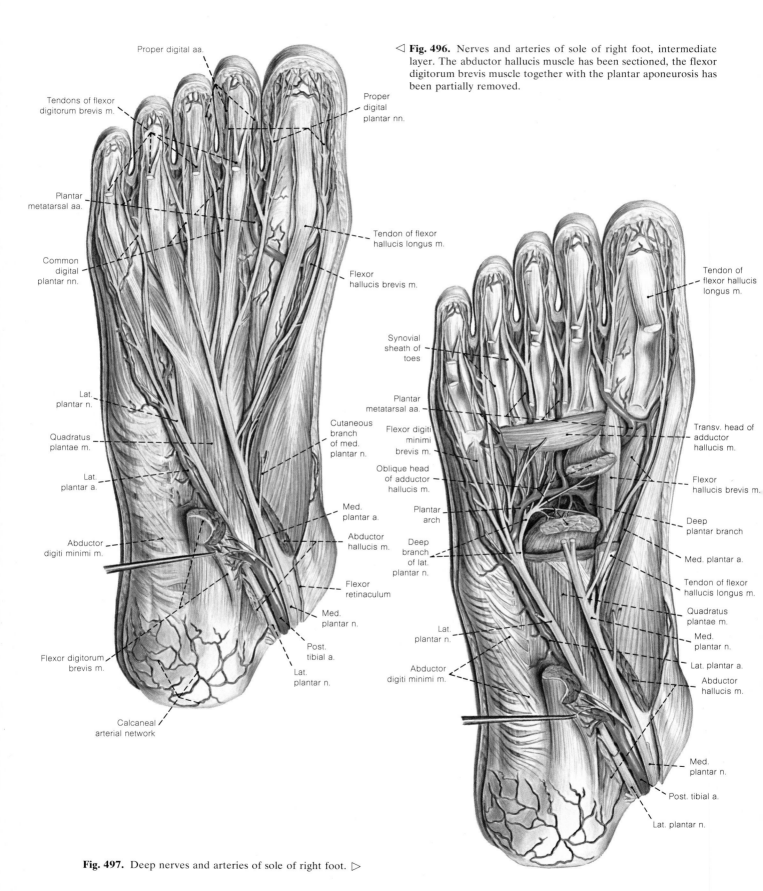

Proper digital aa.

Tendons of flexor
digitorum brevis m.

Plantar
metatarsal aa.

Common
digital
plantar nn.

Lat.
plantar n.

Quadratus
plantae m.

Lat.
plantar a.

Abductor
digiti minimi m.

Flexor digitorum
brevis m.

Calcaneal
arterial network

Proper
digital
plantar nn.

Tendon of flexor
hallucis longus m.

Flexor
hallucis brevis m.

Cutaneous
branch
of med.
plantar n.

Med.
plantar a.

Abductor
hallucis m.

Flexor
retinaculum

Med.
plantar n.

Post.
tibial a.

Lat.
plantar n.

◁ **Fig. 496.** Nerves and arteries of sole of right foot, intermediate
layer. The abductor hallucis muscle has been sectioned, the flexor
digitorum brevis muscle together with the plantar aponeurosis has
been partially removed.

Tendon of
flexor hallucis
longus m.

Synovial
sheath of
toes

Plantar
metatarsal aa.

Flexor digiti
minimi
brevis m.

Oblique head
of adductor
hallucis m.

Plantar
arch

Deep
branch
of lat.
plantar n.

Lat.
plantar n.

Abductor
digiti minimi m.

Transv. head of
adductor
hallucis m.

Flexor
hallucis brevis m.

Deep
plantar branch

Med. plantar a.

Tendon of flexor
hallucis longus m.

Quadratus
plantae m.

Med.
plantar n.

Lat. plantar a.

Abductor
hallucis m.

Med.
plantar n.

Post. tibial a.

Lat. plantar n.

Fig. 497. Deep nerves and arteries of sole of right foot. ▷

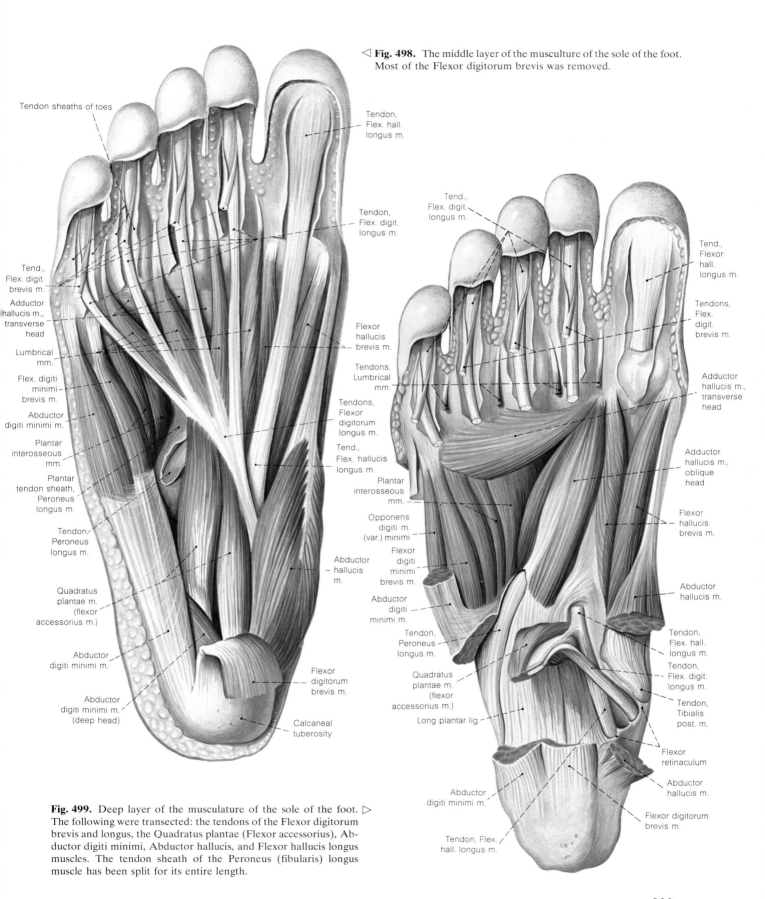

Tendon sheaths of toes

Tend., Flex. digit. brevis m.

Adductor hallucis m., transverse head

Lumbrical mm.

Flex. digiti minimi brevis m.

Abductor digiti minimi m.

Plantar interosseous mm.

Plantar tendon sheath, Peroneus longus m.

Tendon, Peroneus longus m.

Quadratus plantae m. (flexor accessorius m.)

Abductor digiti minimi m.

Abductor digiti minimi m. (deep head)

Tendon, Flex. hall. longus m.

Tendon, Flex. digit. longus m.

Flexor hallucis brevis m.

Tendons, Flexor digitorum longus m.

Tend., Flex. hallucis longus m.

Plantar interosseous mm.

Opponens digiti m. (var.) minimi

Flexor digiti minimi brevis m.

Abductor digiti minimi m.

Tendon, Peroneus longus m.

Quadratus plantae m. (flexor accessorius m.)

Long plantar lig.

Flexor digitorum brevis m.

Calcaneal tuberosity

Fig. 498. The middle layer of the musculture of the sole of the foot. Most of the Flexor digitorum brevis was removed.

Tend., Flex. digit. longus m.

Tend., Flexor hall. longus m.

Tendons, Flex. digit. brevis m.

Adductor hallucis m., transverse head

Adductor hallucis m., oblique head

Flexor hallucis brevis m.

Abductor hallucis m.

Tendons, Lumbrical mm.

Tendon, Flex. hall. longus m.

Tendon, Flex. digit. longus m.

Tendon, Tibialis post. m.

Flexor retinaculum

Abductor hallucis m.

Flexor digitorum brevis m.

Abductor digiti minimi m.

Tendon, Flex. hall. longus m.

Fig. 499. Deep layer of the musculature of the sole of the foot. ▷
The following were transected: the tendons of the Flexor digitorum brevis and longus, the Quadratus plantae (Flexor accessorius), Abductor digiti minimi, Abductor hallucis, and Flexor hallucis longus muscles. The tendon sheath of the Peroneus (fibularis) longus muscle has been split for its entire length.

Muscles of the Sole of the Foot *(planta pedis)* **(Figs. 491, 496–498)**

Name	Origin	Insertion
Flexor digitorum brevis muscle Plantar muscle forms the intermediate plantar eminence	Medial process, tuberosity of calcaneus; medial part of plantar aponeurosis	By 4 thin tendons (perforated by tendons of the Flexor digitorum longus muscle) on the middle phalanges of the 4 lateral toes

Nerve: Medial plantar nerve (L 4, 5)

Function: Flexes middle phalanges of the toes

Name	Origin	Insertion
Quadratus plantae muscle *(Flexor accessorius muscle)*	Two heads from plantar surface of calcaneus; long plantar ligament	Lateral margin of tendon of Flexor digitorum longus muscle

Nerve: Lateral plantar nerve (S 1, 2)

Function: Supports action of the Flexor digitorum longus muscle and corrects oblique direction of pull of its tendons

---

NOTE:

The muscle pattern on the sole of the foot is formed by 3 muscular eminences: Lateral, intermediate, and medial. In between are 2 longitudinal grooves: The medial and lateral plantar sulci which contain the lateral and medial plantar vessels and nerves having the same name (Figs. 496, 497). There is an abductor and flexor for the toe in its corresponding compartment.

The medial plantar eminence (compartment for the big toe) contains the belly of the Abductor hallucis muscle and the Flexor hallucis longus and brevis muscles.

The intermediate plantar eminence (central compartment for the sole of the foot) is the thickest and contains the belly of the Flexor digitorum brevis, which is covered by the plantar aponeurosis.

The lateral plantar eminence (compartment for the small toe) contains the Abductor digiti minimi and Flexor digiti minimi brevis muscles.

Muscles of the Great Toe (Figs. 491, 497, 499)

Name	Origin	Insertion
1. Abductor hallucis muscle Plantar muscle united to the medial plantar eminence	Medial process of tuberosity of calcaneus and plantar aponeurosis	Base of proximal phalanx of great toe
2. Flexor hallucis brevis muscle	Plantar surface of cuboid and lateral cuneiform bones; tendon of Tibialis posterior m.	Two heads on medial and lateral sides of proximal phalanx of big toe; sesamoid bones

3. Adductor hallucis muscle

Oblique head	Bases of metatarsal bones 2 to 4; sheath of tendon of Peroneus longus muscle	Lateral side of base of proximal phalanx of great toe; sesamoid bones
Transverse head	Metatarsophalangeal ligaments of the 3 lateral toes; deep transverse metatarsal ligament	

Nerve: For No. 1 and No. 2, the medial plantar nerve; No. 3 (and sometimes No. 2) lateral plantar nerve (S 1, 2)

Function: As the name implies: abducts, flexes, adducts big toe: above all, however, gives effective transverse and longitudinal tension to the plantar arch

Muscles of the Small Toe (Figs. 491, 497–499)

Name	Origin	Insertion
1. Abductor digiti minimi muscle (Plantar muscle united with lateral plantar eminence)	Medial and lateral process of tuberosity of calcaneus; plantar aponeurosis	Lateral side of proximal phalanx of small toe (and often into tuberosity of the 5th metatarsal bone)
2. Flexor digiti minimi brevis muscle	Base of 5th metatarsal bone; sheath of Peroneus longus tendon	Proximal phalanx of small toe
3. Opponens digiti minimi muscle (inconstant) (omitted by NA)		Lateral margin of 5th metatarsal

Nerve: Lateral plantar nerve

Function: As the name implies: abducts, flexes and opponed the small toe; above all, however, effective tension to the plantar arch

The **Lumbrical muscles** of the foot arise from the tendons of the Flexor digitorum longus. The first one by a single head from the medial ridge of the first tendon (2nd toe) and the other three by two heads. They join the dorsal aponeurosi of the toes in the region of the metatarsophalangeal joints from the medial side. Most small bursa of the lumbricals are found at their insertion. The medial plantar nerve (L 4, 5) supplies the first lumbrical and the other three lumbricals are supplied by the lateral plantar nerve (S 1, 2).
Function: Flex proximal phalanges, as in the hand.

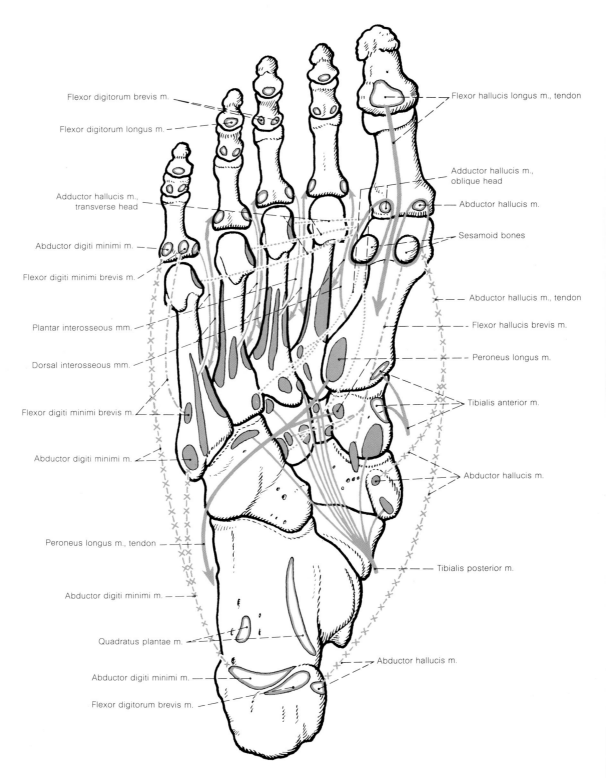

Flexor digitorum brevis m.

Flexor digitorum longus m.

Adductor hallucis m., transverse head

Abductor digiti minimi m.

Flexor digiti minimi brevis m.

Plantar interosseous mm.

Dorsal interosseous mm.

Flexor digiti minimi brevis m.

Abductor digiti minimi m.

Peroneus longus m., tendon

Abductor digiti minimi m.

Quadratus plantae m.

Abductor digiti minimi m.

Flexor digitorum brevis m.

Flexor hallucis longus m., tendon

Adductor hallucis m., oblique head

Abductor hallucis m.

Sesamoid bones

Abductor hallucis m., tendon

Flexor hallucis brevis m.

Peroneus longus m.

Tibialis anterior m.

Abductor hallucis m.

Tibialis posterior m.

Abductor hallucis m.

Fig. 500. Muscle origins and insertions mapped out on the sole of the right foot.

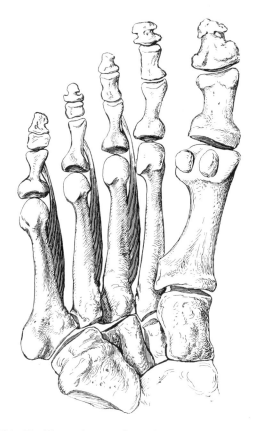

Fig. 501. The Plantar interossei muscles.

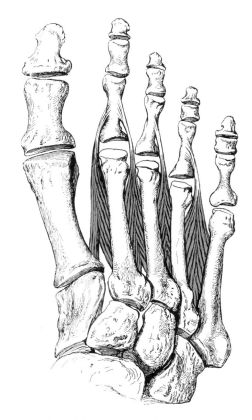

Fig. 502. The Dorsal interossei muscles.

The **Interosseus muscles** of the foot are arranged somewhat like those of the hand: There are four dorsal and three plantar muscles. The latter are relatively strong (stronger than the dorsal muscles of the foot) in contrast to those of the hand. All three Plantar muscles act in the same direction and arise from the medial border of the metatarsals III, IV, V, and all three are inserted in the dorsal aponeuroses of the toes of the same side. The relatively weak dorsal interosseus muscles arise by two heads as in the hand. The tendons (as in the hand) do not go in the same direction: I and II go to the second toe.

Nerve: The lateral plantar nerve.
Function: Similar to the muscles of the hand: Abduction, or else adduction and flexion.

Muscles of the Dorsum of the Foot (Figs. 488, 489)

Name	Origin	Insertion
Extensor digitorum brevis muscle	Lateral and dorsal surface of the calcaneus	Dorsal aponeurosis of 3 middle toes (3 thin tendons)
Extensor hallucis brevis muscle	Dorsal surface of calcaneus	Base of 1st phalanx of big toe
Nerve:	Deep peroneal (fibularis) nerve (L 5; S 1)	
Function:	Extension of the toes (dorsiflexion)	

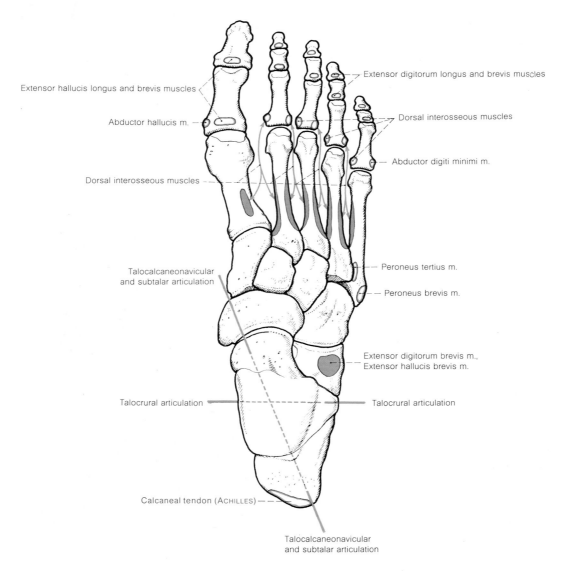

Fig. 503. Diagram of muscle origins and insetions on the dorsum of the right foot. Axes of the upper and lower ankle joint.

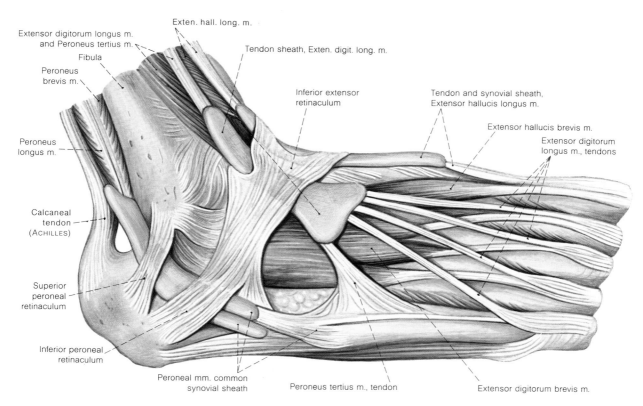

Fig. 504. The tendon sheaths of the ankle region and the dorsum of the foot. Lateral view. The tendon sheaths (vaginae synoviales) were filled in the living with a clear, colorless synovial fluid. The blue color is to differentiate the tendons and ligaments.

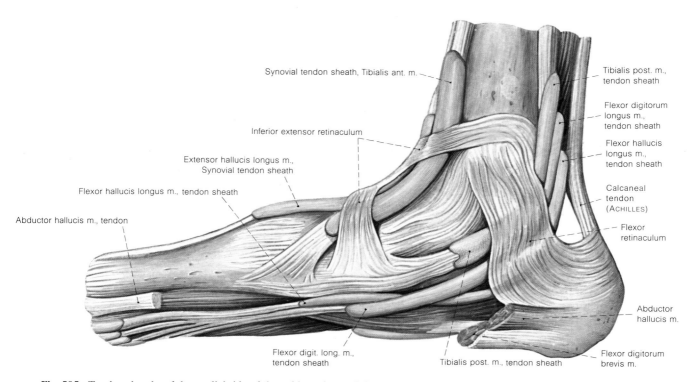

Fig. 505. Tendon sheaths of the medial side of the ankle region and the sole and dorsum of the foot. Partially schematic. The Abductor hallucis and the Flexor digitorum brevis muscles were partly removed.

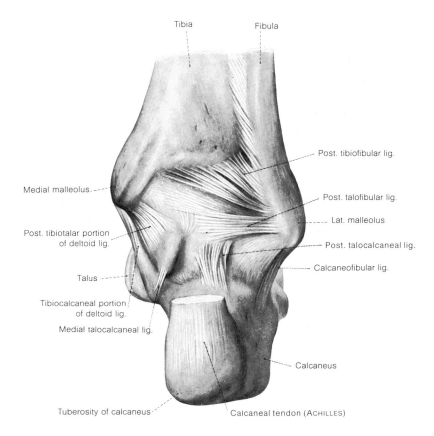

Tibia

Fibula

Post. tibiofibular lig.

Medial malleolus

Post. talofibular lig.

Lat. malleolus

Post. tibiotalar portion
of deltoid lig.

Post. talocalcaneal lig.

Calcaneofibular lig.

Talus

Tibiocalcaneal portion
of deltoid lig.

Medial talocalcaneal lig.

Calcaneus

Tuberosity of calcaneus

Calcaneal tendon (ACHILLES)

Fig. 506. The distal tibiofibular syndesmosis and ankle joint (articulatio talocruralis). Only a stump of the calcaneal tendon remains. Dorsal view.

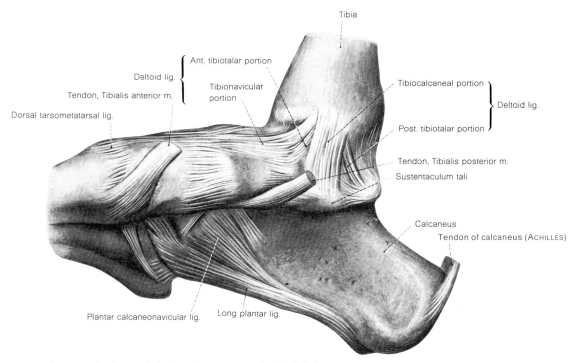

Tibia

Ant. tibiotalar portion

Deltoid lig.

Tibionavicular
portion

Tibiocalcaneal portion

Deltoid lig.

Tendon, Tibialis anterior m.

Post. tibiotalar portion

Dorsal tarsometatarsal lig.

Tendon, Tibialis posterior m.

Sustentaculum tali

Calcaneus

Tendon of calcaneus (ACHILLES)

Plantar calcaneonavicular lig.

Long plantar lig.

Fig. 507. Ligaments between the foot and the leg (ligamenta tarsi). Medial view.

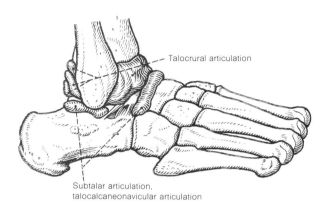

Fig. 508. Joint effusion of the upper and lower ankle joints of the right foot (articulatio talocruralis, articulatio subtalaris, articulatio talocalcaneonavicularis). Lateral view. (After BENNINGHOFF/GOERTTLER: Lehrbuch der Anatomie des Menschen, Vol. 1, 13th ed. [Eds. H. FERNER and J. STAUBESAND]. Urban & Schwarzenberg, Munich-Vienna–Baltimore 1980.)

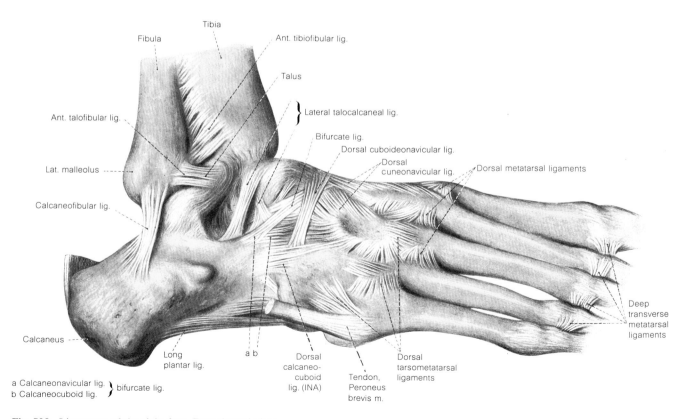

a Calcaneonavicular lig. } bifurcate lig.
b Calcaneocuboid lig.

Fig. 509. Ligaments of the right foot. Dorsolateral view.

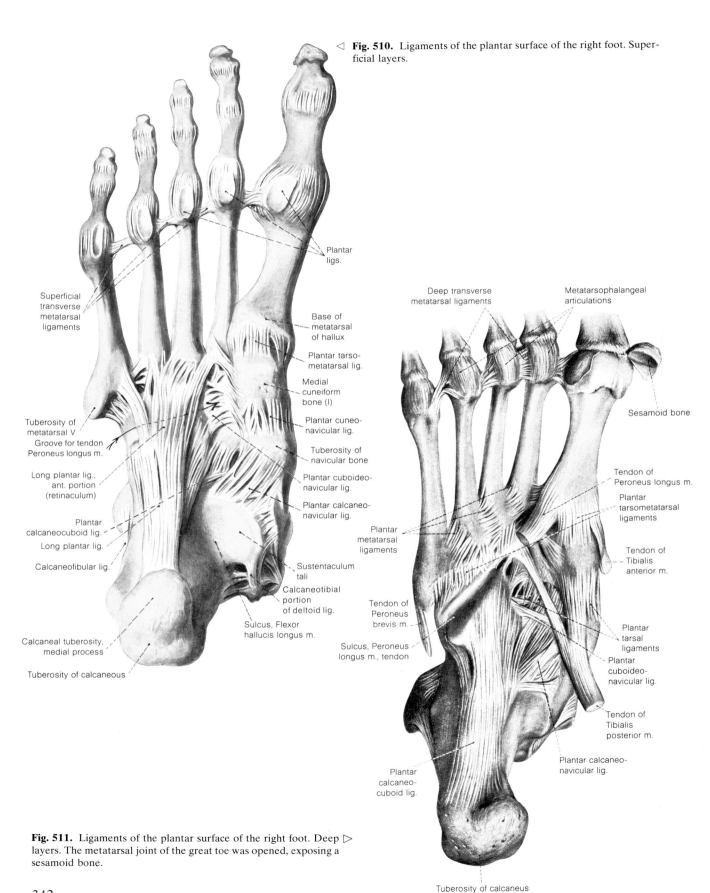

◁ **Fig. 510.** Ligaments of the plantar surface of the right foot. Superficial layers.

Plantar ligs.

Superficial transverse metatarsal ligaments

Base of metatarsal of hallux

Plantar tarso-metatarsal lig.

Medial cuneiform bone (I)

Plantar cuneo-navicular lig.

Tuberosity of navicular bone

Plantar cuboideo-navicular lig.

Plantar calcaneo-navicular lig.

Tuberosity of metatarsal V

Groove for tendon Peroneus longus m.

Long plantar lig., ant. portion (retinaculum)

Plantar calcaneocuboid lig.

Long plantar lig.

Calcaneofibular lig.

Sustentaculum tali

Calcaneotibial portion of deltoid lig.

Sulcus, Flexor hallucis longus m.

Calcaneal tuberosity, medial process

Tuberosity of calcaneous

Deep transverse metatarsal ligaments

Metatarsophalangeal articulations

Sesamoid bone

Tendon of Peroneus longus m.

Plantar tarsometatarsal ligaments

Tendon of Tibialis anterior m.

Plantar metatarsal ligaments

Plantar tarsal ligaments

Plantar cuboideo-navicular lig.

Tendon of Peroneus brevis m.

Sulcus, Peroneus longus m., tendon

Tendon of Tibialis posterior m.

Plantar calcaneo-navicular lig.

Plantar calcaneo-cuboid lig.

Tuberosity of calcaneus

Fig. 511. Ligaments of the plantar surface of the right foot. Deep ▷ layers. The metatarsal joint of the great toe was opened, exposing a sesamoid bone.

342

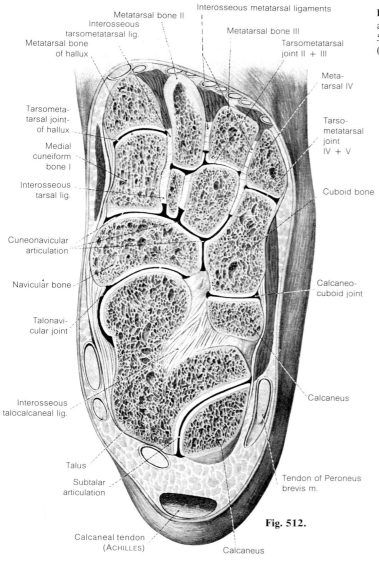

Metatarsal bone II

Interosseous tarsometatarsal lig.

Metatarsal bone of hallux

Tarsometatarsal joint of hallux

Medial cuneiform bone I

Interosseous tarsal lig.

Cuneonavicular articulation

Navicular bone

Talonavicular joint

Interosseous talocalcaneal lig.

Talus

Subtalar articulation

Calcaneal tendon (ACHILLES)

Interosseous metatarsal ligaments

Metatarsal bone III

Tarsometatarsal joint II + III

Metatarsal IV

Tarsometatarsal joint IV + V

Cuboid bone

Calcaneocuboid joint

Calcaneus

Tendon of Peroneus brevis m.

Calcaneus

Fig. 512.

Figs. 512 and 514. Horizontal sections through the joints of the ankle and foot (articulationes tarsi). Fig. 514. Bones and joints. Fig. 512. The cut is at a higher level so the calcaneus is cut in two places. (Fig. 514 depicted on next page.)

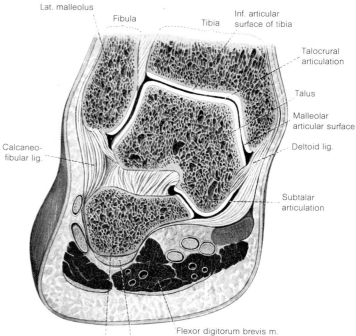

Lat. malleolus

Fibula

Tibia

Inf. articular surface of tibia

Talocrural articulation

Talus

Malleolar articular surface

Deltoid lig.

Subtalar articulation

Calcaneofibular lig.

Calcaneus

Long plantar lig.

Flexor digitorum brevis m.

Fig. 513. Frontal section through talocrural joint and the dorsal ▷ compartment of the subtalar joint.

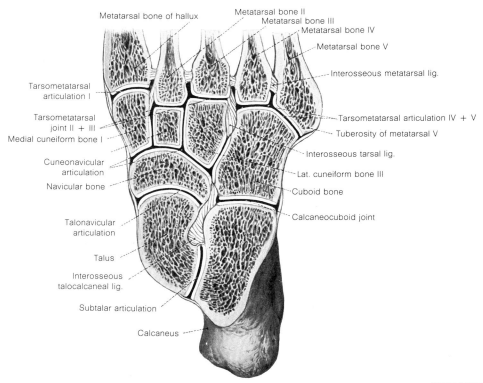

Metatarsal bone of hallux

Metatarsal bone II
Metatarsal bone III
Metatarsal bone IV
Metatarsal bone V

Interosseous metatarsal lig.

Tarsometatarsal articulation I

Tarsometatarsal joint II + III

Medial cuneiform bone I

Cuneonavicular articulation

Navicular bone

Talonavicular articulation

Talus

Interosseous talocalcaneal lig.

Subtalar articulation

Calcaneus

Tarsometatarsal articulation IV + V

Tuberosity of metatarsal V

Interosseous tarsal lig.

Lat. cuneiform bone III

Cuboid bone

Calcaneocuboid joint

Fig. 514. Caption see Fig. 512 (p. 343).

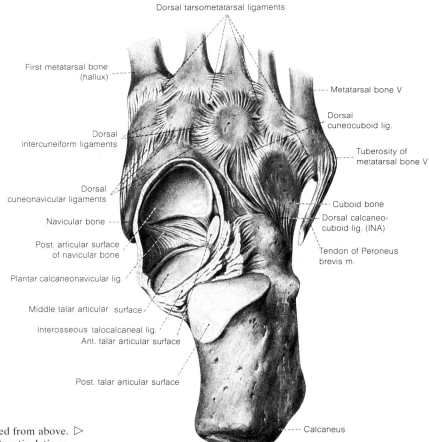

Dorsal tarsometatarsal ligaments

First metatarsal bone (hallux)

Dorsal intercuneiform ligaments

Dorsal cuneonavicular ligaments

Navicular bone

Post. articular surface of navicular bone

Plantar calcaneonavicular lig.

Middle talar articular surface

Interosseous talocalcaneal lig.
Ant. talar articular surface

Post. talar articular surface

Metatarsal bone V

Dorsal cuneocuboid lig.

Tuberosity of metatarsal bone V

Cuboid bone

Dorsal calcaneo-cuboid lig. (INA)

Tendon of Peroneus brevis m.

Calcaneus

Tuberosity of calcaneus

Fig. 515. Talocalcaneonavicular articulation. Viewed from above. ▷
The talus was disarticulated and removed to display its articulations,
especially the navicular socket for its head.

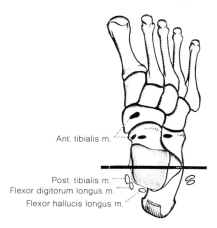

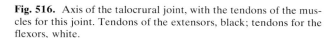

Ant. tibialis m.

Post. tibialis m.
Flexor digitorum longus m.
Flexor hallucis longus m.

Fig. 516. Axis of the talocrural joint, with the tendons of the muscles for this joint. Tendons of the extensors, black; tendons for the flexors, white.

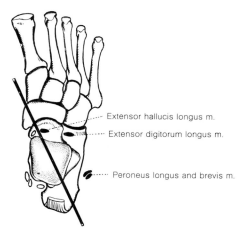

Extensor hallucis longus m.

Extensor digitorum longus m.

Peroneus longus and brevis m.

Fig. 517. Axis of the talocalcaneonavicular and subtalar articulations, with the tendons of the muscles for these joints. Tendons of the pronators, black; tendons of the supinators, white. (After S. MOLLIER from BENNINGHOFF/GOERTTLER: Lehrbuch der Anatomie des Menschen, Vol. 1, 13th ed. [Eds. H. FERNER and J. STAUBESAND]. Urban & Schwarzenberg, Munich–Vienna–Baltimore 1980.)

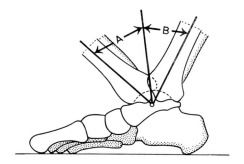

Fig. 518. Flexion and extension in the upper ankle joint, the talo- ▷ crural articulation, when the foot is solidly planted and the leg below the knee is moved back and forth. (After S. MOLLIER: Plastische Anatomie, 2nd ed. Bergmann, Munich 1938.)

The ankle joint (talocrural articulation) connects the two bones of the leg with the talus. In contrast to the relations in the upper extremity, only one bone of the foot, the tarsus, with its trochlea participates in this joint. The articular surface for the trochlea of the tarsus is formed by both crural bones: the tibia contributes with its inferior articular surface and the adjacent malleolar articular surface, the fibula contributes its malleolar articular surface. The joint capsule encloses the cartilaginous surfaces of the three bones and is thin. In some areas, especially in front, it is provided with synovial fat pads.

The ankle joint is always used during walking. The transverse axis of the hinge joint (Fig. 516) goes through both malleoli. From the normal position in which the foot forms a right angle with the leg, active elevation (= dorsal extension) of about 20° and plantar flexion of about 30° are possible.

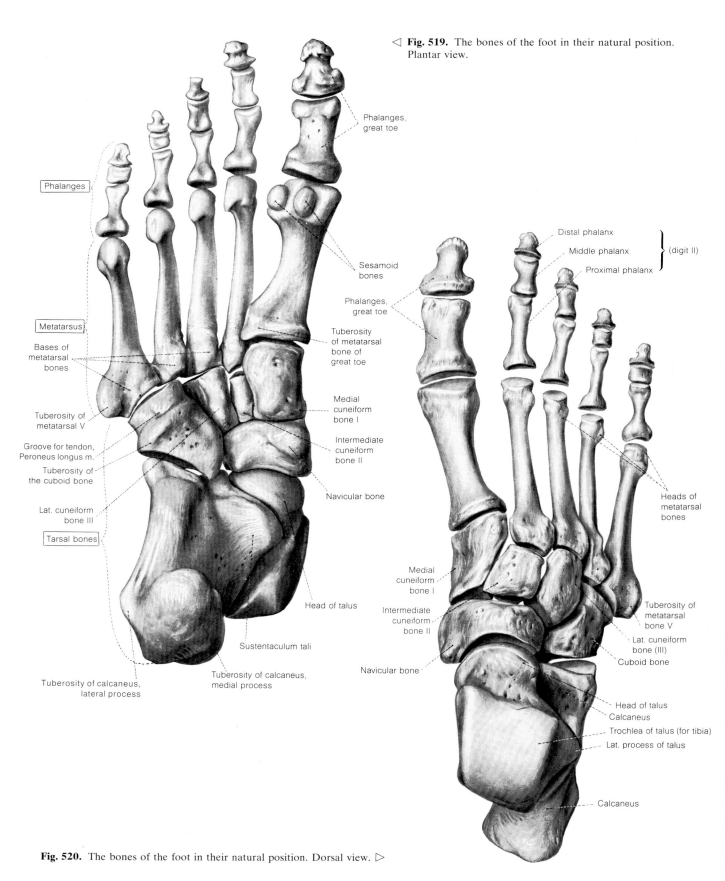

◁ **Fig. 519.** The bones of the foot in their natural position. Plantar view.

Phalanges, great toe

Phalanges

Sesamoid bones

Distal phalanx

Middle phalanx

(digit II)

Proximal phalanx

Phalanges, great toe

Metatarsus

Bases of metatarsal bones

Tuberosity of metatarsal bone of great toe

Tuberosity of metatarsal V

Medial cuneiform bone I

Groove for tendon, Peroneus longus m.

Intermediate cuneiform bone II

Tuberosity of the cuboid bone

Navicular bone

Lat. cuneiform bone III

Heads of metatarsal bones

Tarsal bones

Medial cuneiform bone I

Intermediate cuneiform bone II

Tuberosity of metatarsal bone V

Head of talus

Lat. cuneiform bone (III)

Navicular bone

Cuboid bone

Sustentaculum tali

Head of talus

Calcaneus

Trochlea of talus (for tibia)

Tuberosity of calcaneus, lateral process

Tuberosity of calcaneus, medial process

Lat. process of talus

Calcaneus

Fig. 520. The bones of the foot in their natural position. Dorsal view. ▷

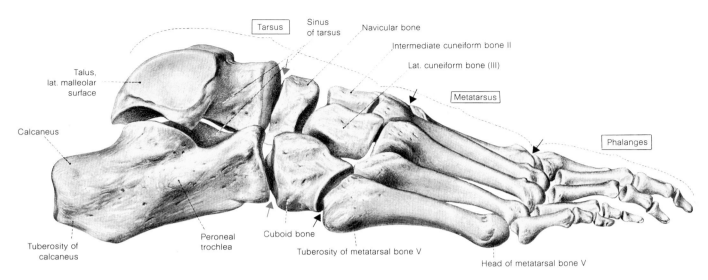

Fig. 521. Skeleton of the right foot. Lateral view. Chopart's amputation line = transverse tarsal articulation = cleft between talus and calcaneus on one side, cuboid and navicular bones on the other (marked by *red* arrows!). Lisfranc's amputation line corresponds to the tarsometatarsal articulation (marked by *black* arrows!).

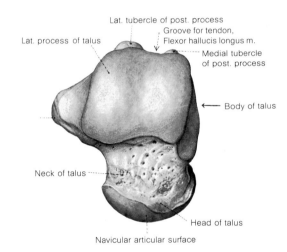

Fig. 522. The right talus. Proximal or dorsal view.

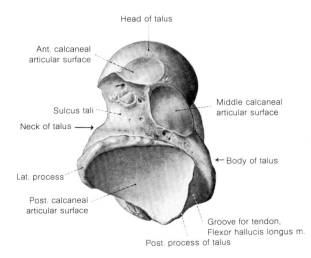

◁ **Fig. 523.** The right talus. Plantar view.

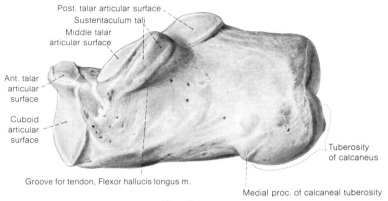

Post. talar articular surface
Sustentaculum tali
Middle talar articular surface
Ant. talar articular surface
Cuboid articular surface
Groove for tendon, Flexor hallucis longus m.
Tuberosity of calcaneus
Medial proc. of calcaneal tuberosity

Fig. 524.

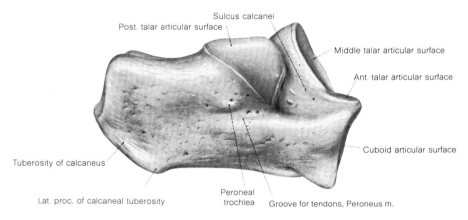

Sulcus calcanei
Post. talar articular surface
Middle talar articular surface
Ant. talar articular surface
Cuboid articular surface
Tuberosity of calcaneus
Lat. proc. of calcaneal tuberosity
Peroneal trochlea
Groove for tendons, Peroneus m.

Fig. 525.

Figs. 524 and 525. Right calcaneus. Fig. 524 Medial view. Fig. 525 Lateral view.

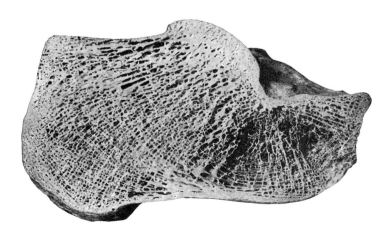

Fig. 526. Sagittal longitudinal section of the calcaneus. The trabeculae of the spongy bone are arranged along the lines of stress.

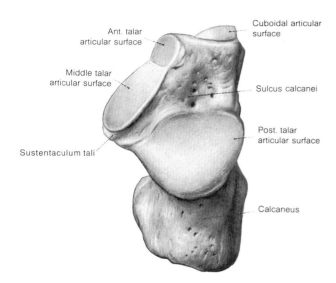

Ant. talar articular surface

Cuboidal articular surface

Middle talar articular surface

Sulcus calcanei

Post. talar articular surface

Sustentaculum tali

Calcaneus

Fig. 527. Right calcaneus. Dorsal view.

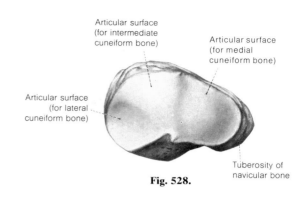

Articular surface (for intermediate cuneiform bone)

Articular surface (for medial cuneiform bone)

Articular surface (for lateral cuneiform bone)

Tuberosity of navicular bone

Fig. 528.

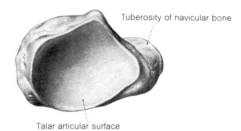

Tuberosity of navicular bone

Talar articular surface

Fig. 529.

Figs. 528 and 529. Right navicular bone.
Fig. 528: Distal view. Fig. 529: Proximal view.

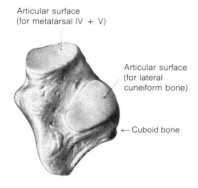

Articular surface (for metatarsal IV + V)

Articular surface (for lateral cuneiform bone)

← Cuboid bone

Fig. 530. Right cuboid. Medial view. (See also Fig. 521.)

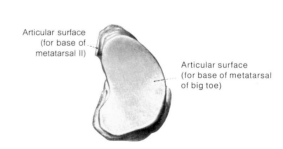

Articular surface (for base of metatarsal II)

Articular surface (for base of metatarsal of big toe)

Fig. 531.

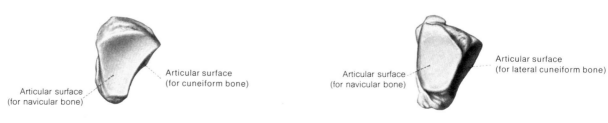

Articular surface (for cuneiform bone)

Articular surface (for navicular bone)

Fig. 532.

Articular surface (for lateral cuneiform bone)

Articular surface (for navicular bone)

Fig. 533.

Figs. 531–533. Right cuneiform bones. Fig. 531: Medial cuneiform, distal aspect. Fig. 532: Intermediate cuneiform, proximal aspect. Fig. 533: Lateral cuneiform, proximal aspect.

Skin

Figs. 534–536. Basic forms of papillary ridge patterns. ▷
Fig. 534: Arch, no delta. Fig. 535: Loop, one delta. Fig. 536:
Whorl, two deltas.

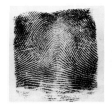

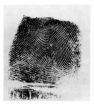

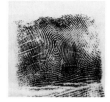

Fig. 534.   **Fig. 535.**   **Fig. 536.**

Fig. 537. Print of a right hand.

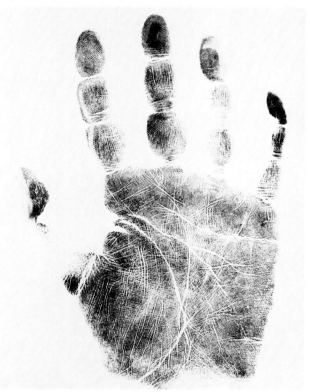

Fig. 537.

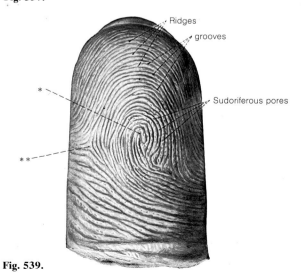

Fig. 539.

Fig. 538. Diagram of the skin ridge patterns, of the divisions of the
palm (thenar, hypothenar, interdigital spaces I–IV), of the carpal
deltas (a–d) and the axial delta (t).
Material for Figs. 534–543 and text in box on p. 351: Dr. T. GRIMM,
Institute for Human Genetics, University of Göttingen.

◁ **Fig. 539.** Grooves and ridges on palmar surface of finger tip. Papillary grooves and ridges on the palmar surfaces of fingers and toes are
arranged in patterns that are determined by the numbers of deltas
and the number of the papillary ridges between core and delta.
* core; ** delta

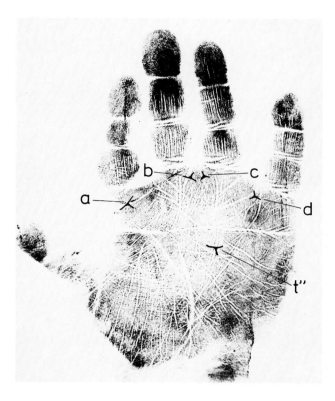

Fig. 540. Right palmar print with Simian line (four finger crease) in a female patient with Down's syndrome (Karyotype: 47, XX, + 21). Distally displaced t-Triradiation (t'').

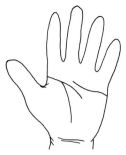

Fig. 541. Normal palmar grooves.

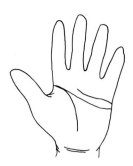

Fig. 542. SYDNEY line.

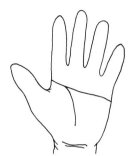

Fig. 543. Four-finger-sulcus. ▷

Frequency of Simian crease and SYDNEY crease:

	DOWN's Syndrome	Control
Simian crease	58.8%	5.5%
SYDNEY crease	21.9%	8.1%

The skin of the palmar surface of hand and fingers and of the plantar surface of foot and toes differs from the rest of the skin primarily in that it possess no sebaceous glands and no hairs, but shows a pattern of ridges and grooves. On top of the papillary ridges there are numerous openings of sweat glands (Fig. 539). The ridges originate from the touch pads during the third month of gestation. The patterns (Figs. 534–536) as well as the number of ridges remain constant for life. Because of the multiplicity of the combinations possible it is very improbable that two humans have the same conditon (identification of persons in police work). On the tips of fingers and toes, three main types of patterns may be distinguished: arches, loops and whorls (Figs. 534–536), whereby the number of ridges between core and delta determines the quantitative value of the pattern (Fig. 539). The sum of the quantitative values of all ten fingers forms the total ridge number of one person. Beyond the papillary ridges there is also a system of sulci on the palm and sole (Figs. 540–543). In chromosomal aberrations (e.g. Down's syndrome: 47, XY, + 21 or 47, XX, + 21, or Turner's syndrome: 45, XY) one finds typical changes in the distribution frequency of patterns (Fig. 540). There are interrelations between the total number of ridges (Total Finger Ridge Count = TFRC) of a person and the number of the X and Y chromosomes (TFRC = $187 - 30\,X - 12\,Y$; Penrose, L. S., Fingerprint patterns and the sex chromosomes, Lancet, I, 298, 1967). (Additional literature: B. Schaumann, M. Alter: Dermatoglyphics in Medical Disorders. Springer, New York–Heidelberg–Berlin 1976.)

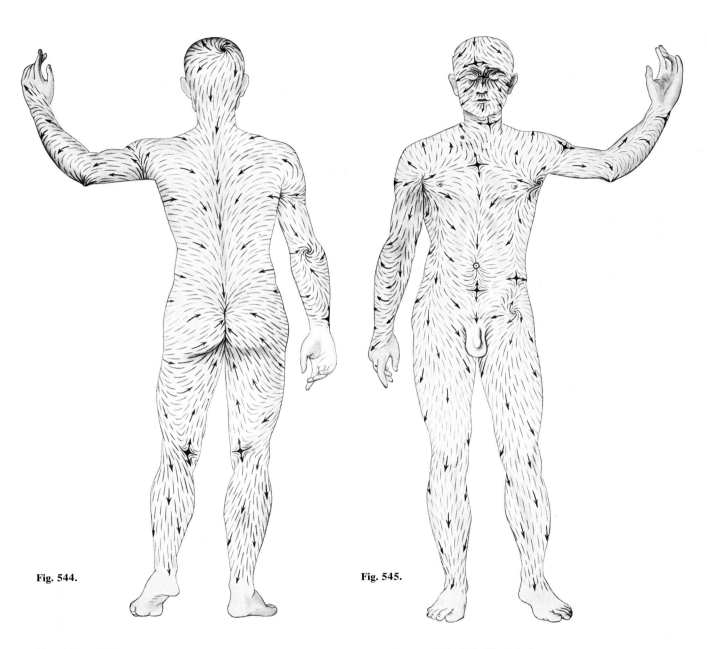

Figs. 544 and 545. Diagrams of hair streams and whorls. Fig. 544: Dorsal view, and Fig. 545: Ventral view.

Arterial Supply Areas

Arranged by Dr. Fr. PLATZ, Direktor, Anatomical Institute, University of Freiburg.

Curved brackets ( ) indicate anatomical variations, important alternative names and additions that are frequently omitted in the general use of certain anatomical names. Square brackets [ ] indicate synonyms or alternative names.

Arteries	Supply Areas
PULMONARY TRUNK	– Arterial trunk for right and left lungs
sinus of pulmonary trunk	– three sinuses on the wall of the pulmonary trunk above the attachments of the valve flaps
bifurcation of the pulmonary trunk	– division of the pulmonary trunk into right and left pulmonary artery
RIGHT PULMONARY ARTERY	– deoxygenated blood for right lung
apical branch	– apical segments
post. descending branch	– lower part of post. segment
ant. descending branch	– lower part of ant. segment
ant. ascending branch	– upper part of ant. segment
post. ascending branch	– upper part of post. segment
branch for middle lobe	– main branch for middle lobe
lat. branch	– lat. segment
med. branch	– med. segment
apical branch (superior) of inf. lobe	– apical segment of right inf. lobe
basal part	– basal segments of right inf. lobe
med. basal branch [cardiac]	– med. basal segment
ant. basal branch	– ant. basal segment
lat. basal branch	– lat. basal segment
post. basal branch	– post. basal segment
LEFT PULMONARY ARTERY	– deoxygenated blood for left lung
apical branch	– upper part of apicopost. segment
ant. descending branch	– lower part of ant. segment
post. branch	– lower part of apicopost. segment
ant. ascending branch	– upper part of ant. segment
lingular branch	– both lingular segments
sup. lingular branch	– sup. lingular segment
inf. lingular branch	– inf. lingular segment
apical [superior] branch of inf. lobe	– apical segment of left inf. lobe
basal part	– basal segments of right inf. lobe
med. basal [cardiac] branch	– med. basal segment
ant. basal branch	– ant. basal segment
lat. basal branch	– lat. basal segment
post. basal branch	– post. basal segment
(ductus arteriosus)	– fetal shunt between pulmonary trunk and arch of aorta
ligamentum arteriosum	– fibrous remnant of ductus arteriosus
AORTA	– main arterial trunk from the left ventricle
ASCENDING AORTA	– ascending portion of aorta within the pericardial sac
aortic bulb	– bulb-like enlargement of the aortic root above the aortic valve. Site of origin of right and left coronary arteries
aortic sinuses	– three enlargements of the aortic root above each aortic valve leaflet. Site of origin of right and left coronary arteries

Arteries	Supply Areas
right coronary a.[1]	– originates from the right aortic sinus; supplies right atrium, right ventricle, original parts of pulmonary trunk and ascending aorta, parts of the left atrium and the left ventricle as well as the conduction system
branch for conus arteriosus	– anteriorly running branch for conus arteriosus and base of the pulmonary trunk
branch for sinuatrial node	– sinuatrial node, right atrium, parts of left atrium
right marginal branch	– right cardiac margin, anterior wall of right ventricle
intermediate atrial branch	– right atrium, right auricle
post. interventricular branch	– branch in post. interventricular sulcus for post. wall of right and left ventricles and dorsal part of interventricular septum
interventricular septal branches	– interventricular septum
atrioventricular nodal branch	– atrioventricular node
(right posterolateral branch)	– right post. wall of left ventricle
left coronary a.	– originating from left aortic sinus, short stem; its ramifications supply parts of the left and right ventricle as well as areas of the interventricular system and left atrium
ant. interventricular branch	– main branch in ant. interventricular sulcus for ant. wall of right and left ventricles and ventral part of interventricular septum
branch for conus arteriosus	– conus arteriosus and base of pulmonary trunk
lat. branch	– lat. area of the ant. wall of the left ventricle
interventricular septal branches	– perforating branches for the ventral part of the interventricular septum
circumflex branch	– continuation of the left coronary a. in the left coronary sulcus for the post. wall of the left ventricle
anastomosing atrial branch	– anastomosis with branches from the left coronary a. for the left atrium
left marginal branch	– left cardiac margin and post. wall of left ventricle
intermediate atrial branch	– left atrium
(post. left ventricular branch)	– variable branch for post. wall of left ventricle
(sinuatrial nodal branch)	– irregular branch for the inflow area of the sup. vena cava
(atrioventricular nodal branch)	– occasional branch extending to the base of the heart and the lower part of the septum interatriale
AORTIC ARCH	– curved portion between ascending and descending aorta
aortic isthmus	– narrowing of the aortic arch between the left subclavian a. and the ligamentum arteriosum
para-aortic bodies	– irregularly distributed portions of chromaffine tissue next to the aorta

[1] The supply areas of the coronary arteries differ according to the type of their distribution. This tabulation is based on the "balanced distribution type" (see page 36). The clinically used coronarographic nomenclature is more extensive than the official anatomical nomenclature and deviates in part from the latter.

Arteries	Supply Areas
BRACHIOCEPHALIC TRUNK	– common trunk from the aortic arch for right common carotid a. and right subclavian a.
(lowest thyroid artery)	– variably (8–10%) occurring unpaired artery for thyroid gland
COMMON CAROTID ARTERY	– common trunk for external and internal carotid arteries
glomus caroticum	– chemoreceptor in the carotid fork
carotid sinus	– slight dilatation of the common carotid a., contains pressoreceptors
EXTERNAL CAROTID ARTERY	– ascending in the lateral cervical region for supply of neck and head
sup. thyroid a.	– first ant. branch of ext. carotid a. for thyroid gland and larynx
infrahyoid branch	– hyoid bone, insertions of intrahyal muscles
sternocleidomastoid branch	– sternocleidomastoid m.
sup. laryngeal a.	– upper interior larynx
cricothyroid branch	– cricothyroid m., interior larynx
ant. branch	– ant. part of thyroid gland
post. branch	– sup. and post. area of thyroid gland
ascending pharyngeal a.	– first dorsal a. from the ext. carotid a. for pharynx with additional branchlets for the dura mater in a small dorso-medial area of the middle cranial fossa
post. meningeal a.	– through the jugular foramen for dura mater of post. cranial fossa
pharyngeal branches	– wall of pharynx, longus capitis m.
inf. tympanic a.	– tympanic cavity
lingual a.	– second ant. branch of ext. carotid a. for tongue
suprahyoid branch	– hyoid bone, vascular network on the thyroid cartilage
sublingual a.	– sublingual gland and muscles in its vicinity, mucous membrane on the lower side of the tongue and the floor of the mouth, gingiva of the mandible
dorsal lingual branches	– lingual musculature and dorsum of tongue, epiglottis
deep lingual a.	– musculature and mucous membrane of tongue, especially of tip of tongue
facial a.	– third ant. branch of ext. carotid a., artery of the face
ascending palatine a.	– palatine arches, frequently also tonsils, ant. sup. pharyngeal wall below tuba auditiva
tonsillar branch	– tonsilla palatina
submental a.	– mylohyoid m., submandibular gland
glandular branches	– submandibular gland
inf. labial a.	– musculature, skin and mucous membrane of lower lip
sup. labial a.	– musculature, skin and mucous membrane of upper lip, lower ant. septum nasale
angular a.	– terminal branch of facial a.; medial angle of eye, parts of the root of the nose and cranial portion of the wings of the nose, anastomosis with ophthalmic a.
(linguofacial trunk)	– occasional common trunk for lingual a. and facial a. from the ext. carotid a.
occipital a.	– second dorsal branch from the ext. carotid a. for occiput and parietal area
mastoid branch	– diploe and mastoid air cells, through mastoid foramen to dura mater
auricular branch	– post. surface of external ear
sternocleidomastoid branches	– sternocleidomastoid m.
(meningeal branch)	– occasional branch through parietal foramen for dura mater of calvaria
occipital branches	– post. part of galea aponeurotica
descending branch	– upper nuchal musculature

Arteries	Supply Areas
post. auricular a.	– third dorsal a. from the ext. carotid a.: supplies the area of the ear
stylomastoid a.	– through stylomastoid foramen into canal: supplies middle and, partially, internal ear
post. tympanic a.	– through canaliculus of chorda tympani for mucous membrane of tympanic cavity and tympanic membrane
mastoid branches	– mastoid air cells
(stapedial branch)	– stapedius m.
auricular branch	– post. and, partially, ant. side of pinna, small muscles of ear
occipital branch	– occiput and parietal area
superficial temporal a.	– a terminal branch of the ext. carotid a.
parotideal branches	– parotid gland
transv. facial a.	– skin of the cheek and above the zygomatic arch, parotid gland
ant. auricular branches	– pinna, ext. auditory meatus, temporomandibular joint
zygomatico-orbital a.	– lat. margin of orbit and lat. area of eye-lids
med. temporal a.	– temporalis m., periosteum of the temporal squama
frontal branch	– Forehead, anastomoses with the supraorbital and supratrochlear aa. from the int. carotid a.
parietal branch	– parietal area
maxillary a.	– larger terminal branch of the ext. carotid a.
deep auricular a.	– temporomandibular joint, ext. auditory meatus, tympanic membrane
ant. tympanic a.	– through petrotympanic fissure for tympanic cavity
inf. alveolar a.	– bone and gingiva of lower jaw
dental branches	– teeth, periodontal tissue, gingiva and bone of lower jaw
mylohyoid branch	– origin of the mylohyoid m.
mental a.	– area of the chin
middle meningeal a.	– through foramen spinosum for dura mater and parts of the falx cerebri
(accessory meningeal branch)	– auditory tube; through foramen ovale for dura mater up to trigeminal ganglion
petrous branch	– through hiatus of facial canal for tympanic cavity, tensor tympani m., trigeminal ganglion
sup. tympanic a.	– together with lesser petrosal n. to tympanic cavity and mastoid antrum
frontal branch	– dura mater of middle and ant. cranial fossa
parietal branch	– dura mater of post. half of cranium
orbital branch	– connecting branch between frontal branch of middle meningeal a. and lacrimal a.
anastomosing branch (with lacrimal a.)	– through the sup. orbital fissure or a separate opening into the orbit where it anastomoses with the lacrimal a.
masseteric a.	– masseter m.
deep temporal aa.	– temporalis m., lat. wall of orbit
pterygoid branches	– med. and lat. pterygoid mm.
buccal a.	– cheek, gingiva, mucous membrane of lateral oral cavity
post. sup. alveolar a.	– molar teeth, gingiva and periosteum of maxilla, mucous membrane of maxillary sinus
dental branches	– upper molar teeth
infraorbital a.	– facial muscles and skin below the eye, floor or orbit
ant. sup. alveolar aa.	– ant. teeth of maxilla
dental branches	– branches into the teeth
a. of pterygoid canal	– through the pterygoid canal posteriorly to auditory tube and its surroundings

Arteries	Supply Areas	Arteries	Supply Areas
descending palatine a.	– through greater palatine canal to palate	supratrochlear a.	– forehead
greater palatine a.	– gingiva and mucous membrane in the area of the hard palate, palatine tonsil	dorsal nasal a. [ext. nasal a.]	– dorsum of nose; anastomosis via the angular a. with the facial a.
lesser palatine aa.	– soft palate and palatine tonsil	*ant. choroidal a.*	– originates in most cases from the int.
sphenopalatine a.	– through sphenopalatine foramen to nasal cavity		carotid a. proximally to the origin of the ant. cerebral a. (less frequently
lat. post. nasal and septal aa.	– lateral walls of nasal cavity, paranasal sinuses, nasal septum, anastomoses through incisive canal with greater palatine a.		from the middle cerebral a.): supplies the choroid plexus of the lat. ventricle and, partially, of the third ventricle, internal capsule and neighboring areas. Also parts of hippocampus, optic tract and optic radiation
INTERNAL CAROTID ARTERY	– brain and parts of dura mater, also orbit with contents, forehead and area of paranasal sinuses	lat. ventricular choroidal branches	– choroid plexuses of lat. ventricles
cervical portion	– from the bifurcation of the common carotid a. to the entry into the carotid canal	third ventricular choroidal branches	– choroid plexus of third ventricle
carotid sinus	– site of pressoreceptors	branches for ant. perforate substance	– thin branches entering the brain through the ant. perforate substance
petrous portion	– within the carotid canal of the petrous bone	optic tract branches	– optic tract
caroticotympanic aa.	– co-supply of tympanic cavity	branches for lat. geniculate body	– lat. geniculate body
artery of pterytoid canal	– through pterygoid canal for auditory tube and surroundings	internal capsular branches	– predominantly to post. limb of internal capsule
cavernous portion	– within the cavernous sinus	branches for globus pallidus	– dorsal area of globus pallidus
basal tentorial branch	– tentorium cerebelli	branches for tail of caudate nucleus	– tail of caudate nucleus
marginal tentorial branch	– margin of tentorium cerebelli		
meningeal branch	– dura mater of tentorium cerebelli	branches for tuber cinereum	– tuber cinereum
trigeminal ganglionic branch	– trigeminal ganglion	branches for hypothalamic nuclei	– branches to the hypothalamus that also supply parts of the thalamus
trochlear and trigeminal branches	– roof of trigeminal nerve and dura mater in its vicinity, trochlear n.	branches for substantia nigra	– substantia nigra
cavernous sinus branch	– perivascular tissue around the int. carotid a. within the cavernous sinus	branches for nucleus ruber	– red nucleus
		amygdaloid branches	– amygdala, pes hippocampi
inf. hypopohyseal a.	– basal portion of posterior lobe, periosteum and bone of the hypophyseal fossa, dorsum sellae	*ant. cerebral a.*	– at first rostrally directed and then above the corpus callosum dorsally running terminal branch of the int. carotid a.; supplies the medial
cerebral portion	– from exit out of cavernous sinus to the division into ant. and med. cerebral aa.		surface of the frontal and parietal lobes and, extending over the pallial crest, the adjacent areas of the
sup. hypophyseal a.	– hypophysis, diaphragma sellae; forms arterial ring around the hypophyseal stalk; supplies parts of the hypothalamus in the area of the infundibulum as well as optic n. and optic chiasm		convexity of the hemisphere. Major portion of the corpus callosum. Co-supply of caudate nucleus, thalamus, hypothalamus, optic chiasm and optic tract
clivus branch	– dura mater of cranial clivus (may also arise from the inf. hypophyseal a.)	precommunical portion	– that portion from the origin of the artery from the int. carotid a. to the origin of the ant. communicating a.
ophthalmic a.	– from the intracranial part of the int. carotid a., runs with the optic nerve through the optic canal into the orbit	antero-medial central aa. [antero-medial thalamo-striate aa.]	– branches originating from the middle area of the precommunical portion and entering the brain through the ant. perforate substance
central retinal a.	– optic n. and retina	short central a.	– medial part of the ant. perforate substance, optic chiasm
lacrimal a.	– lacrimal gland and neighboring musculature of the orbit, conjunctiva, lat. angle of eye	long central a. [recurrent a.]	– originates from the ant. cerebral a. in the area of the origin of the ant. communicating a.; supplies medial,
anastomosing branch	– anastomosis with the frontal branch of the middle meningeal a.		and in part also lateral areas of the ant. perforate substances as well as ant.
lat. palpebral aa.	– eyelids and conjunctiva		and med. parts of the lentiform
short post. ciliary aa.	– choroid coat		nucleus, ant. crus of internal capsule,
long post. ciliary aa.	– ciliary body and iris		hypothalamus, head of caudate
muscular aa.	– sup. and lat. rectus mm., levator palpebrae sup. m.		nucleus
ant. ciliary aa.	– sclera, choroid coat, ciliary body	ant. communicating a.	– unpaired connection between right and left ant. cerebral a.
ant. conjunctival aa.	– conjunctiva	antero-medial central branches	– ant. perforate substance, olfactory trigone, basal parts of caudate nucleus
post. conjunctival aa.	– conjunctiva	postcommunical portion [pericallosal a.]	– portion of the ant. cerebral a. after the origin of the ant. communicating a.
episcleral aa.	– sclera	med. frontobasal a. [med. orbitofrontal branch]	– originates from the ant. cerebral a. at the level of the subcallosal area;
supraorbital a.	– upper orbit and forehead		supplies medial areas of the orbital
post. ethmoidal a.	– post. ethmoidal air cells, post. part of nasal cavity		gyri and olfactory tract
ant. ethmoidal a.	– lat. wall and septum of nasal cavity; frontal sinus		
(ant. meningeal a.)	– dura mater of ant. cranical fossa		
med. palpebral aa.	– med. portion of upper and lower lid		
sup. palpebral arch	– connection between med. and lat. palpebral aa. in the upper eyelid		
inf. palpebral arch	– connection between med. and lat. palpebral aa. in the lower eyelid		

Arterial Supply Areas

Arteries	Supply Areas
callosa-marginal a.	– pallial crest, superolateral surface of cerebrum, frequently also paracentral lobulus
antero-medial frontal branch	– branch originating in the subcallosal area and running to the medial area and the superolateral area of the pallial crest in the region of the frontal lobe
intermedio-medial frontal branch	– originates at the level of the genu of the corpus callosum and runs to the medial side of the frontal lobe and the superolateral surface of the cerebrum
postero-medial frontal branch	– originates at the posterior portion of the genu of the corpus callosum and runs to the medial portion side of the frontal lobe
cingular branch	– to cingulate sulcus and neighboring areas
paracentral artery	– from the postcommunical part of the ant. cerebral a., frequently also from the cingular branch, to the area of the cingulate gyrus, paracentral lobule, and upper portions of the precentral and postcentral gyri
precuneal artery	– mostly originating as a doublet from the posterior third of the pericallosal a.; supplies parts of the cingulate gyrus and the precuneus
parieto-occipital artery	– parieto-occipital sulcus
middle cerebral artery	– lateral larger end branch of the int. carotid a. running over the insula to the lateral cerebral fissure. Supplies the superolateral surface of the cerebrum with the exception of the pallial crest and the occipital lobe as well as a small strip at the lower margin of the temporal lobe. Supplies also the anterior areas of the basal ganglia and the internal capsule
sphenoidal part	– approximal horizontally running portion from the origin of the ant. cerebral a. to the limen insulae
anterolateral central aa. [anterolateral-thalamo-striate aa.]	– branches entering the brain through the ant. perforate substance and supplying the basal ganglia and internal capsule
medial branches	– medial group of the anterolateral central aa.
lateral branches	– lateral group of the anterolateral central aa.
insular part	– that portion of the middle cerebral a. on the surface of the insula
insular aa.	– branches running dorsally and upward on the surface of the insula
lateral frontobasal a. [lat. orbitofrontal branch]	– through the lateral fissure to inf. frontal gyrus and orbital gyri
ant. temporal a.	– sup., med., and inf. temporal gyri
intermediate temporal a.	– middle and ant. parts of sup. and med. temporal gyri, middle part of the inf. temporal gyrus
a. temporalis posterior	– runs over sup. and med. temporal gyri downward and backward to the middle and post. parts of the sup. and med. temporal gyri
terminal part [cortical part]	– part of the middle cerebral a. ramifying on the cerebral surface
artery of central sulcus	– artery in the central sulcus to the precentral and postcentral gyri as well as bordering areas of the frontal and parietal lobes
artery of precentral sulcus	– originating in the anterior part of the lateral fissure and supplying the post.

Arteries	Supply Areas
	areas of the middle frontal gyrus and the basal half of the precentral gyrus
artery of postcentral sulcus	– postcentral gyrus and neighboring areas of the parietal lobe
ant. and post. parietal aa.	– ant. and post. parts of the parietal lobe, upper half of the postcentral gyrus, inf. parietal lobule
artery of angular gyrus	– runs in the lateral fissure obliquely backward and upward to the angular gyrus and gives off a lower branch for the upper half of the occipitotemporal gyri
SUBCLAVIAN ARTERY	– originates on the right side from the brachiocephalic trunk and on the left side from the aortic arch and runs to the lateral margin of the first rib; co-supply of thorax, neck and brain; supplies shoulder girdle and upper extremity
vertebral a.	– from the subclavian a. running through the transverse foramina of the sixth to the first cervical vertebrae, perforates the post. atlanto-occipital membrane and reaches the neurocranium
prevertebral part	– portion between origin from the subclavian a. and entry into the transverse foramen of the sixth cervical vertebra
transverse [cervical] part	– that portion running through the transverse foramina
spinal [radicular] branches	– branches running through the intervertebral foramina into the vertebral canal to supply spinal cord and its meninges as well as epidural space and periosteum of vertebral bodies
muscular branches	– deep regional muscles of the neck
atlantic part	– that portion from the exit from the transverse foramen of the atlas to the entry into the post. atlanto-occipital membrane
intracranial part	– that portion running within the subarachnoid space
ant. meningeal branch	– an anterior branch originating at the level of the foramen magnum and supplying the dura mater of the post. cranial fossa
post. meningeal branch	– post. branch for dura mater of post. cranial fossa and falx cerebri
ant. spinal a.	– forming through the union of paired branches of the vertebral a., mostly at the level of C_2; runs in the ant. median fissure and supplies ant. and lat. areas of the spinal cord
post. inf. cerebellar a.	– lower surface of the cerebellar hemispheres, medulla oblongata
choroidal branch of fourth ventricle	– choroid plexus of fourth ventricle
cerebellar tonsillar branch	– cerebellar tonsil
med. and lat. medullary branches [branches for medulla oblongata]	– med. and lat. parts of medulla oblongata
(post. spinal a.)	– artery coming off the post. inf. cerebellar a. or the vertebral a. and supplying the gracilis and cuneate fascicles as well as the corpus restiforme
basilar artery	– forming through the union of right and left vertebral a. for the supply of rhombencephalon, midbrain and internal ear

Arteries	Supply Areas
ant. inf. cerebellar a.	– lower, lat. and ant. parts of the cerebellum, floccule, pons, upper medulla oblongata, cerebello-pontine angle, choroid plexus of fourth ventricle, internal ear, facial and vestibulo-cochlear nn.
labyrinthine a. [branch of internal acoustic meatus]	– internal ear with branchlets for dura mater and petrous bone
pontine aa.	– branches for pons and midbrain
mesencephalic aa.	– cerebral peduncles and midbrain
sup. cerebellar a.	– upper surface of cerebellum, parts of the cerebellar vermis, cerebellar nuclei, cerebellar peduncles, sup. medullary velum, branches to pineal body and choroid tela of fourth ventricle
post. cerebral a.	– resulting from the bifurcation of the basilar a., supplying occipital lobe, two-thirds of the temporal lobe, midbrain, post. perforate substance, parts of the cerebral peduncles and of the thalamus
precommunical part	– portion between the origin of the artery and its union with the post. communicating a.
posteromedial central aa.	– in the interpeduncular fossa originating branches with twigs for oculomotor and trochlear nn. as well as mammillary bodies; through the post. perforate substance to the diencephalon with parts of the thalamus and to the midbrain (red nucleus, substantia nigra, tectal lamina)
postcommunical part	– portion after the union with the post. communicating a.
posterolateral central aa.	– cerebral peduncles, med. and, in part, lat. geniculate bodies. Co-supply of thalamus, dentate gyrus, parahippo-campal gyrus as well as hippocampus
thalamic branches	– central thalamic nuclei as well as parts of the medial and ventrolateral nuclei
med. post. choroidal branches	– choroid plexus of third and lateral ventricles, epiphysis, superior collicles
lat. post. choroidal branches	– choroid plexus of lateral ventricles, branchlets to thalamus and fornix
peduncular branches	– cerebral peduncles
terminal [cortical] part	– that portion of the post. cerebral a. beginning at the division into lat. and med. occipital aa.
lat. occipital a.	– lat. main branch for lower surface of temporal and occipital lobes
ant. temporal branches	– ant. and lat. underside of the temporal lobe and uncus
intermediate medial temporal branches	– middle and post. underside of the temporal lobe, occipital lobe
post. temporal branches	– underside of the occipital lobe
med. occipital a.	– med. main branch for parts of the corpus callosum, calcarine sulcus and occipital pole
dorsal corpus callosal branch	– isthmus of cingulate gyrus, splenium and middle and post. part of the body of corpus callosum, cortical region of precuneus and lingual gyrus
parietal branch	– post. areas of the precuneus
parieto-occipital branch	– neighboring superficial and deep cerebral structures in the area of the parieto-occipital sulcus, lateral side of the occipital lobe, cuneus, occipital pole
calcarine branch	– calcarine sulcus, occipital pole as well as lateral surface of the occipital lobe
occipitotemporal branch	– med. occipitotemporal gyrus

Arteries	Supply Areas
circulus arteriosus of brain (Willis)	– arterial circle at the base of the brain, consisting of the connection of both int. carotid aa. with the addition of the vertebral aa. via the basilar a. and the post. cerebral aa.
int. carotid a.	– it contributes, with a part of its intra-cranial portion, to the formation of the circle of WILLIS
ant. cerebral a.	– ant. terminal branch of the int. carotid a.
ant. communicating a.	– unpaired shunt between right and left ant. cerebral a.
anteromedial central aa.	– originating near the ant. communi-cating a. and entering into the lamina terminalis
middle cerebral a.	– lat. terminal branch of the int. carotid a. continuing in the direction of the main vessel
post. communicating a.	– paired arterial channel connecting on each side the post. cerebral a. with the int. carotid a. or the middle cerebral a.
chiasmatic branch	– optic chiasm and optic tract
branch for oculomotor nerve	– oculomotor n.
thalamic branch	– co-supply of the thalamus
hypothalamic branch	– hypothalamus with mammillary bodies and tuber cinereum
branch for tail of caudate nucleus	– tail of caudate nucleus
post. cerebral a.	– paired terminal branch of the basilar a., connected to the post. communi-cating a.
int. thoracic a.	– from subclavian a. descending to the inner ant. thoracic wall
mediastinal branches	– mediastinum, mediastinal pleura
thymic branches	– thymus
bronchial branches	– root of the lung, hilar lymph nodes, bronchi
pericardiophrenic a.	– pericardium, ant. part of diaphragm, mediastinal pleura
sternal branches	– arterial network on sternum
perforating branches	– skin in the medial chest area, pectoralis major m.
mammary branches	– mammary gland
(lat. costal branch)	– lat. upper inner chest wall
ant. intercostal branches	– ant. intercostal spaces
musculophrenic a.	– 7th to 10th intercostal spaces, diaphragm, cranial areas of the abdominal muscles
sup. epigastric a.	– rectus abdominis m., rectus sheath
thyrocervical trunk	– common trunk for inf. thyroid a., transverse cervical a. and supra-scapular a.
inf. thyroid a.	– thyroid gland, larynx, pharynx, esophagus
inf. laryngeal a.	– pharyngeal surface, post. musculature and mucous membrane of larynx, hypopharynx
glandular branches	– lower and dorsal surface of thyroid gland and parathyroid glands
pharyngeal branches	– parts of the pharyngeal wall
esophageal branches	– upper esophagus
tracheal branches	– upper area of trachea
ascending cervical a.	– scalenus, longus colli and neighboring mm.
spinal branches	– vertebral canal and spinal cord in the area of the lower cervical vertebral column
transverse cervical a.	– from the subclavian a. or the thyro-cervical trunk for the cervical and shoulder regions
superficial branch [superf. cervical a.]	– trapezius and neighboring mm.

Arterial Supply Areas

Arteries	Supply Areas
dorsal scapular a.	– originating frequently (67%) from the subclavian a. or from the transverse cervical a. for the rhomboid and neighboring mm.
suprascapular a.	– supraspinatus and infraspinatus mm., acromion
acrominal branch	– acromion
costocervical trunk	– dorsally directed trunk for the deep cervical a. and supreme intercostal a.
deep cervical a.	– semispinalis capitis m. and deep nuchal musculature
supreme intercostal a.	– common trunk for the first and second post. intercostal aa.
first post. intercostal a.	– first intercostal space
second post. intercostal a.	– second intercostal space
dorsal branches	– dorsal skin, deep cervical and dorsal musculature
spinal branches	– vertebral canal and spinal cord
AXILLARY ARTERY	– continuation of the subclavian a. from first rib to lower margin of pectoralis major m.
subscapular branches	– supscapularis m.
sup. thoracic a.	– variable branch for subclavius m., muscles of the first and second intercostal spaces, serratus ant. m., pectoralis major m.
thoracoacrominal a.	– chest and shoulder area
acrominal branch	– through the deltoid m. to acromion, deltoid m., shoulder joint and parts of pectoralis major and minor mm.
acrominal arterial net	– arterial network on the acromion
clavicular branch	– clavicle and subclavius m.
deltoid branch	– deltoid and pectoralis major mm.
pectoral branches	– serratus ant. m., pectoral mm.
lat. thoracic a.	– pectoral mm., serratus ant. m.
lat. mammary branches	– mammary gland
subscapular a.	– latissimus dorsi, teres minor and serratus ant. mm.
thoracodorsal a.	– subscapularis, latissimus dorsi, teres major, serratus ant. mm.
scapular circumflex a.	– infraspinatus, supraspinatus mm., shoulder joint and capsule
ant. circumflex humeral a.	– coracobrachialis, biceps brachii, deltoid mm., shoulder joint
post. circumflex humeral a.	– shoulder joint, deltoid m., long and lat. head of triceps brachii m.
brachial a.	– continuation of the axillary a. beginning at the lower margin of the pectoralis major m.
(superficial brachial a.)	– variation in which the brachial a. lies on top instead of under the median n.
deep brachial a.	– deltoid and triceps brachii m., humerus
humeral nutrient aa.	– humerus
deep branch	– lower part of deltoid m.
med. collateral a.	– distal segment of triceps brachii m., humeral parts of the extensor musculature of the forearm, cubital arterial network
radial collateral a.	– distal brachial and proximal antebrachial extensor muscles, cubital arterial network
sup. ulnar collateral a.	– brachialis m., med. head of triceps m., cubital arterial network
inf. ulnar collateral a.	– brachialis and neighboring mm., cubital arterial network
radial a.	– predominantly antebrachial flexor musculature, hand
radial recurrent a.	– brachioradialis m., brachialis m., proximal parts of forearm extensors, cubital arterial network
carpal palmar branch	– pronator quadratus m., palmar carpal arterial network

Arteries	Supply Areas
superficial palmar branch	– thenar, superficial palmar arch
dorsal carpal branch	– dorsal carpal arterial network
dorsal carpal rete	– arterial network on the dorsal surface of carpus
dorsal metacarpal aa.	– second to fourth interosseous space, dorsal interosseous mm.
dorsal digital aa.	– back of the fingers up to middle phalanx
pollicis princeps a.	– originating from the radial a. and supplying the palmar side of the thumb and radial margin of the index finger
radial a. of index	– radial side of index finger
deep palmar arch	– deep arterial arch of palmar
palmar metacarpal a.	– interosseous and lumbrical mm.
palmar perforating branches	– branches to the dorsal metacarpal aa.
ulnar a.	– extensor and flexor muscles of forearm
ulnar recurrent a.	– flexor carpi ulnaris m., articular cubital network
ant. branch	– brachialis m., cubital articular network
post. branch	– cubital articular network
cubital articular network	– predominantly dorsal arterial net around elbow joint
post. interosseous a.	– short stem for the post. and ant. interosseous aa.
	– extensor muscles of forearm, dorsal carpal network
recurrent interosseous a.	– anconeus m., proximal parts of forearm extensor mm., cubital articular network
ant. interosseous a.	– pronator quadratus m., dorsal carpal network
comitant a. of median n.	– thin twig for median n.
palmar carpal branch	– palmar side of carpus
dorsal carpal branch	– dorsal carpal network
deep palmar branch	– branch for deep palmar arch
superficial palmar arch	– superficial arterial arch of palm
common palmar digital aa.	– from the superficial palmar arch to the palmar digital aa.
proper palmar digital aa.	– palmar side of fingers, dorsal side of middle and end phalanges
DESCENDING AORTA	– continuation of the aortic arch and descending to the aortic bifurcation in front of the 4th lumbar vertebra
THORACIC AORTA	– from aortic arch to aortic hiatus of diaphragm
bronchial branches	– root of lung, bronchi, pulmonary tissue, visceral pleura
esophageal branches	– esophagus
pericardiac branches	– post. wall of pericardial sac
mediastinal branches	– lymph nodes and connective tissue of posterior mediastinum, pericardial sac
sup. phrenic aa.	– dorsal part of diaphragm
post. intercostal aa.	– posterior contributions for 3rd to 11th intercostal spaces
dorsal branch	– musculature and skin of back
spinal branch	– spinal cord and meninges
med. cutaneous branch	– skin near spinous processes
lat. cutaneous branch	– skin for the lateral to spinous processes
collateral branch	– branch originating near the costal angle and running to the upper margin of the next deeper rib
lat. cutaneous branch	– skin of lateral chest wall
mammary branches	– branches of the lat. cutaneous branches for mammary gland
subcostal a.	– branch below the 12th rib
dorsal branch	– musculature and skin of back
spinal branch	– through 12th thoracic intervertebral foramen to spinal cord and meninges

Arteries	Supply Areas
ABDOMINAL AORTA	– from the aortic hiatus of diaphragm to division into the common iliac aa.
inf. phrenic aa.	– underside of the lumbar part of the diaphragm, abdominal portion of esophagus
sup. suprarenal aa.	– suprarenal glands, on the right side also to pancreas, on the left side also to abdominal portion of esophagus
lumbar aa.	– four arteries corresponding to intercostal aa. for iliopsoas and quadratus lumborum mm. as well as to flat abdominal mm.
dorsal branch	– medial musculature and skin of the back
spinal branch	– vertebral canal, spinal cord and meninges
median sacral a.	– thin median continuation of the abdominal aorta down to the coccygeal body
lowest lumbar a.	– a vessel corresponding to a fifth lumbar artery with anastomoses with lat. sacral a.
corpus coccygeum	– a nodule of anastomosing vessels and epitheloid cells at the tip of the coccyx
celiac trunk	– common trunk from the abdominal aorta for the common hepatic, splenic and left gastric aa.
left gastric a.	– cardiac portion and lesser curvature of stomach, lesser omentum
esophageal branches	– portion of esophagus above cardia
common hepatic a.	– branch of the celiac trunk for liver as well as parts of duodenum, stomach and pancreas
proper hepatic a.	– liver, gall bladder, stomach
right gastric a.	– pylorus, lesser gastric curvature; anastomosis with left gastric a.
right branch	– right hepatic lobe and gall bladder
cystic a.	– gall bladder
a. of caudate lobe	– caudate lobe of liver
ant. segmental a.	– ventral hepatic segment
post. segmental a.	– dorsal hepatic segment
left branch	– left hepatic lobe
a. of caudate lobe	– caudate lobe of liver
a. of caudate lobe	– med. hepatic segment
lat. segmental a.	– lat. hepatic segment
gastroduodenal a.	– parts of stomach, duodenum and pancreas
(supraduodenal a.)	– upper portion of duodenum, often also pyloric part of stomach
post. sup. pancreaticoduodenal a.	– head of pancreas, duodenum, common bile duct
pancreatic branches	– head of pancreas, duodenum especially descending portion
duodenal branches	– dorsal side of upper and descending parts of duodenum
retroduodenal aa.	– dorsal side of head of pancreas and duodenum, common bile duct
right gastroepiploic a.	– greater curvature of stomach, greater omentum
gastric branches	– greater curvature of stomach, pyloric portion, pyloric antrum
epiploic branches	– long branches for greater omentum
ant. sup. pancreaticoduodenal a.	– superior, descending and beginning horizontal parts of duodenum, ventral side head of pancreas and right area of body of pancreas
pancreatic branches	– extending from ventral into pancreas
duodenal branches	– especially medial and ventral parts of the horizontal portion of duodenum
splenic a.	– spleen, stomach, pancreas
pancreatic branches	– numerous branches to body of pancreas
dorsal pancreatic a.	– body of pancreas
inf. pancreatic a.	– dorsal underside of body of pancreas
great pancreatic a.	– body of pancreas, especially dorsal surface
caudal pancreatic a.	– tail of pancreas
left gastroepiploic a.	– greater curvature of stomach and greater omentum
gastric branches	– greater curvature of stomach in the area of the body of stomach
epiploic branches	– long branches for greater omentum
short gastric aa.	– cardia and fundus of stomach
splenic branches	– spleen
sup. mesenteric a.	– gut down to the area of the left flexure of the colon
inf. pancreaticoduodenal aa.	– head of pancreas, duodenum
jejunal aa.	– jejunum
ileal aa.	– ileum
ileocolic a.	– terminal part of ileum, cecum, beginning of ascending colon
ascending a.	– ascending colon
ant. cecal a.	– ant. surface of cecum
post. cecal a.	– dorsal surface of cecum
appendicular a.	– appendix vermiformis
right colic a.	– ascending colon
med. colic a.	– transverse colon
inf. mesenteric a.	– supplies the gut from the left colon flexure to the rectum
left colic a.	– left one-third of the transverse colon, descending colon
sigmoidal aa.	– sigmoid colon
sup. rectal a.	– rectum down to internal anal sphincter
med. suprarenal a.	– suprarenal gland
renal a.	– kidney, adipose capsule, suprarenal gland
inf. suprarenal a.	– suprarenal gland
ant. branch	– upper, ant. and lower renal segment
a. of sup. segment	– upper renal segment
a. of sup. ant. segment	– ant. upper renal segment
a. of inf. ant. segment	– ant. lower renal segment
a. of inf. segment	– lower renal segment
post. branch	– dorsal renal segment
a. of post. segment	– dorsal renal segment
ureteric branches	– initial portion of ureter
testicular a.	– testic and epididymis
ureteric branches	– ureter
ovarian a.	– ovary, ampulla of uterinic tube
ureteric branches	– ureter
BIFURCATION OF AORTA	– division of the abdominal aorta into right and left common iliac aa.
COMMON ILIAC ARTERY	– common a. for pelvis and lower extremity
INTERNAL ILIAC ARTERY	– pelvic viscera, muscle of the pelvic girdle, genitalia, musculature of the thigh
iliolumbar a.	– musculature of post. abdominal wall iliopsoas m., branch to vertebral canal
lumbar branch	– psoas major and minor mm., quadratus lumborum m.
spinal branch	– between sacral bone and 5th lumbar vertebra to vertebral canal
iliac branch	– iliopsoas m., peritoneum, bones of the pelvic girdle
lat. sacral aa.	– pelvic musculature on the surface of the sacral bone, pelvic bones and nerves
spinal branches	– through the pelvic sacral foramina into the sacral canal and from here after ramification in the bone through the dorsal foramina to the musculature of the back

Arterial Supply Areas

Arteries	Supply Areas
obturator a.	– psoas and obturator int. mm., after passage through obturator canal branches to hip joint, proximal areas of adductor and neighboring mm.
pubic branch	– anastomosis with inf. epigastric a.
acetabular branch	– lig. capitis femoris, hip joint
ant. branch	– symphysis, adductor brevis m., proximal areas of remaining adductors
post. branch	– below the adductor brevis m. to the deep muscles of the hip
sup. gluteal a.	– through the suprapiriform foramen to the gluteal region
superficial branch	– gluteus maximus and medius mm.
deep branch	– gluteus medius and minimus mm., piriformis m., hip joint
sup. branch	– gluteus minimus and tensor fasciae latae mm.
inf. branch	– gluteus medius and piriformis mm., hip joint, area of the greater trochanter
inf. gluteal a.	– exiting through the infrapiriform foramen and supplying lower part of gluteus maximus m., sup. and inf. gemelli mm., obturator inf. m., and skin of buttocks
comitant a. of sciatic n.	– sciatic n.
umbilical a.	– placenta; postnatally obliterated distal to the origin of the sup. vesical a.
a. of ductus deferens	– ductus deferens, seminal vesicles
ureteric branches	– ureter
sup. vesical aa.	– upper and middle region of urinary bladder
med. umbilical lig.	– fibrous remnant of the umbilical artery
inf. vesical a.	– fundus of urinary bladder, in the male prostate gland and seminal vesicle; in the female branch to vagina
uterine a.	– from the int. iliac a. to uterus, cervix, uterine tube, ovary and vagina
(vaginal a.)	– upper part of vagina
ovarian branch	– ovary; anastomosis with ovarian a.
tubar branch	– uterine tube, mesosalpinx
vaginal a.	– upper part of vagina, frequently originating immediately from the int. iliac a.
middle rectal a.	– middle and lower area of rectum, rectal ampulla, branches to levator ani m., post. side of urinary bladder, in the male to prostate and seminal vesicle, in the female to lower part of vagina
int. pudendal a.	– exiting through the infrapiriform foramen and running in the pudendal canal (ALCOCK) along the lateral wall of the ischiorectal fossa
inf. rectal a.	– anal skin, and canal, int. and ext. sphincter ani mm.
perineal a.	– skin and musculature of perineum, urogenital diaphragm, bulbospongiosus and ischiocavernosus mm.
post. scrotal branches	– post. surface of scrotum
post. labial branches	– labia majora
urethral a.	– corpus spongiosum of penis to glans
penile bulbar a.	– bulb of penis, transversus perinei profundus m., bulbourethral glands
vestibular bulbar a.	– bulb of vestibule
deep a. of penis	– corpora cavernosa of penis
dorsal a. of penis	– beneath deep penile fascia to glands penis
deep clitoral a.	– corpora cavernosa of clitoris
dorsal clitoral a.	– back of clitoris and corpora cavernosa
EXTERNAL ILIAC ARTERY	– ant. and lat. abdominal wall, ext. genitalia, lower extremity
inf. epigastric a.	– rectus abdominis m., rectus sheath, inside of abdominal wall

Arteries	Supply Areas
pubic branch	– branch to symphysis
obturator branch	– anastomosing with pubic branch
[accessory obturator a.]	– occasionally originating from inf. epigastric a.
cremasteric a.	– cremaster m. and testicular sheaths
a. of round lig.	– connective tissue and smooth musculature of lig. teres
deep circumflex iliac a.	– along the inguinal ligament and iliac crest with branches to the neighboring muscles and to transversalis fascia
ascending branch	– ant. abdominal wall, int. oblique and transverse abdominal mm.
FEMORAL ARTERY	– continuation of the ext. iliac a. after leaving the lacuna vasorum
superficial epigastric a.	– Skin of ant. abdominal wall
superficial circumflex iliac a.	– skin along the inguinal ligament to the ant. sup. iliac spine, iliac lymph nodes
ext. pudendal aa.	– abdominal wall above symphysis, external genitalia
ant. scrotal branches	– skin of scrotum
ant. labial branches	– labia majora
inguinal branches	– inguinal region and inguinal lymph nodes
PROFUNDA FEMORIS ARTERY	– deep femoral structures
med. circumflex femoral a.	– proximal area of femur and adductor mm., capsule of hip joint
deep branch	– quadratus femoris and adductor magnus mm., ischiocrural musculature
ascending branch	– adductor brevis and magnus mm., obturator ext. m.
transverse branch	– ischiocrural musculature
acetabular branch	– ligamentum capitis femoris
lat. circumflex femoral a.	– proximal area of femur and neighboring musculature
ascending branch	– sartorius, rectus femoris, tensor fasciae latae, gluteus med. mm., capsule of hip joint
descending branch	– quadriceps femoris m., skin of the thigh down to knee
transverse branch	– vastus lateralis m.
perforating aa.	– femoral adductor and flexor mm., dorsal skin of thigh, branches to femoral bone
descending a. of knee	– originating from the femoral a. within the adductor canal, perforating the vastoadductorial membrane and supplying the arterial network of the knee joint
saphenous branch	– comitant artery of saphenous n., distal musculature of thigh
articular branches	– arterial network of knee joint and neighboring musculature, especially vastus medialis m.
POPLITEAL ARTERY	– continuation of the femoral a. from the end of the adductor canal to the lower margin of the popliteus m.
lat. sup. a. of knee	– knee joint, arterial network of knee joint, distal parts of biceps femoris and vastus lateralis mm.
sup. med. a. of knee	– muscles originating from the med. epicondyle of tibia, knee joint, arterial network of knee joint
middle a. of knee	– capsule of knee joint, cruciate ligaments, fat body of knee and neighboring tissues, menisci, distal femur and proximal tibia
sural aa.	– sural skin and musculature, especially gastrocnemius m., tendon of biceps femoris m.

Arteries	Supply Areas	Arteries	Supply Areas
lat. inf. a. of knee	— knee joint, lat. meniscus, arterial network of knee joint, distal end of biceps femoris m., lat. head of gastrocnemius m., plantaris m.	circumflex fibular branch	— arterial network of knee
		med. malleolar branches	— post. area of med. malleolus, med. malleolar network
med. inf. a. of knee	— knee joint, arterial network of knee, muscles inserting on medial side of tibia	calcaneal branches	— med. surface of calcaneus and calcaneal network
		peroneal [fibular] a.	— branches for deep flexor musculature of leg, peroneus mm., soleus m., fibula, lat. side of calcaneus
arterial network of knee joint	— principally on the anterior side of the joint, joint capsule, menisci and collateral ligaments		
		perforating branch	— through the interosseous membrane to lat. malleolar network, lat. margin and dorsum of foot
patellar network	— arterial network on the patella; periosteum and patellar bone		
ant. tibial a.	— through interosseous membrane to extensor musculature and skin of leg	communicating branch	— connecting branch to post. tibial a.
		lat. malleolar branches	— lat. malleolus, Achilles tendon, fat body in front of Achilles tendon
(post. tibial recurrent a.)	— post. surface of knee joint, capitulum of fibula		
ant. tibial recurrent a.	— ant. area of the arterial network of knee joint, proximal parts of the extensor musculature and skin of leg	calcaneal branches	— principally lat. side of calcaneus
		calcaneal network	— arterial network on post. side of calcaneus
ant. malleolar a.	— arterial network on the lateral malleolus, talotibial joint	*med. plantar a.*	— bones and ligaments of med. margin of foot as well as med. plantar musculature
med. ant. malleolar a.	— arterial network on the med. malleolus, talotibial joint		
		deep branch	— deep plantar muscles, flexor hallucis m., connects with plantar arch and sends branch around first metatarsal bone to dorsum of foot
med. malleolar network	— arterial network on the med. malleolus		
lat. malleolar network	— arterial network on the lat. malleolus		
dorsal artery of foot	— continuation of the ant. tibial a. beneath the extensor retinaculum to dorsum of foot	superficial branch	— skin of med. plantar margin of foot, abductor hallucis m., med. area of big toe
lat. tarsal. a.	— lat. dorsum of foot, extensor digitorum and hallucis brevis mm.	*lat. plantar a.*	— med. and lat. plantar musculature
		plantar arch	— arterial arch formed by lat. plantar a. and deep branch of med. plantar a., supplies oblique head of adductor hallucis m., plantar interosseous mm. and neighboring muscles as well as bones and joints of metatarsus
med. tarsal aa.	— med. margin of foot, bones and ligaments of the tarsus, branches to abductor hallucis m.		
arcuate a.	— dorsum of foot, extensor digitorum brevis m., metatarso-phalangeal joints		
dorsal metatarsal aa.	— metatarsal dorsal area of foot, dorsal interosseous mm.	plantar metatarsal aa.	— plantar interosseous mm., adductor hallucis m. and distal parts of flexor hallucis m.
dorsal digital aa.	— dorsal margins of toes		
deep plantar branch	— large perforating branch to plantar arch	perforating branches	— mostly paired connecting vessels, between the metatarsal bones, with arteries on dorsum of foot
post. tibial a.	— beneath the tendinous arch of the soleus m. to med. malleolus with branches for deep, and partially also superficial, flexor musculature, tibia and skin on the medial side of the leg	common plantar digital aa.	— connecting the plantar metatarsal aa. to the proper plantar digital aa.
		proper plantar digital aa.	— running along the med. and lat. sides of the toes and supplying them

Index

All numbers refer to the numbers of figures